Psychotherapy and the Social Clinic in the United States

William M. Epstein

Psychotherapy and the Social Clinic in the United States

Soothing Fictions

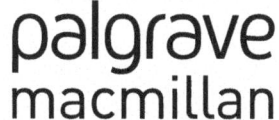

William M. Epstein
University of Nevada, Las Vegas
Las Vegas, NV, USA

ISBN 978-3-030-32749-1   ISBN 978-3-030-32750-7   (eBook)
https://doi.org/10.1007/978-3-030-32750-7

Cover illustration: Pobytov/gettyimages

This Palgrave Macmillan imprint is published by the registered company Springer Nature Switzerland AG
The registered company address is: Gewerbestrasse 11, 6330 Cham, Switzerland

What rough beast, its hour come round at last, slouches toward Bethlehem to be born?
W. B. Yeats *The Second Coming*

Liz
My love

Preface

American institutions and the national ethos are basically romantic rather than pragmatic. Extreme individualism—the classic myth of self-reliance—maintains that people essentially invent themselves and are thus proportionately responsible for where they end up in the American stratification. The nation sees itself as exceptional and chosen by both God and Darwin; its people the best of the species; its society and government the latest blessed evolutions of human organization; and its destiny to lead the world assured as a covenant with the Fates in recognition of its many good works. All this is known through romantic processes that elevate emotion over reason: the lived experience, insight, intuition, revelation, epiphany, clairvoyance, and the spiritual, but still a physical inheritance of knowledge common to all mankind. The exceptionalism of the American people, just like space and time, is certain, synthetic a priori knowledge that constitutes a universal archetype of the collective unconscious. The United States has enshrined ideology as social theology. And as embedded belief, the social clinic emerges as a favored mission of American romanticism and social policy to address a variety of social problems.

The social clinic is a sanctioned agency of both public and private policies that offer services ostensibly to address a variety of personal and social problems. Clinical services are usually dominated by some form of talk therapy even when the agency offers other programs such as food banks, temporary housing, short term cash assistance and surveillance as in cases of probation and parole. The social clinic is also a general strategy of social welfare policy as well as an icon of social attitudes toward the problems and the people who suffer them. Even broader, as an institution of American society, it dramatizes the boundaries of individual and social responsibility that mark out long-standing American policy toward social and economic inequality.

The preference for talk therapy of one sort or another expresses the social clinic's broader commitment to the principle of social efficiency, the notion that services for people in need should be inexpensive, compatible with social values, and usually of temporary or short duration. Social efficiency does not imply effectiveness but only conformity with broadly popular social values.

Even without explicitly offering talk therapy, many social welfare agencies that provide material assistance still mimic the social clinic in their intentions to address recipients' attitudes. As examples, the eligibility limits and operating rules of Temporary Assistance for Needy Families and the Supplemental Nutrition Assistance Program (also known as food stamps), two prominent public sector welfare programs, both incorporate the logic of behavior change implicit in talk therapy and not least because recipients are put through a discretionary supervised process of case management. Similarly, when voluntary agencies—religious affiliates such as Catholic Charities or secular agencies like women's shelters—provide food, housing, or clothing as examples, the context of service often reinforces the rules of social stratification. The application of those rules often carries along the stigma attached to lower status—the sense of personal failure that attends handouts and consequently the deeper isolation of recipients from the American communion.

To the extent to which the social clinic is charity, it constrains the rights of citizenship and reiterates recipients' low social status. Yet social clinics are often dedicated to wealthier populations who pay for services through insurance or out of pocket. These clinics often provide psycho-therapy but also provide some form of life coaching, guided self-help, counseling, or theologically driven counseling. Yet even when address-ing wealthier citizens, the social clinic affirms America's romantic ethos by encouraging people to see themselves as self-inventive, self-reliant, and self-determinative. It seems to matter little that the self-positing ego is an illusion and that the social clinic customarily fails in its service mission. Social and personal problems persist with a ubiquitous tenacity that is oblivious to the distinction between the poor and the wealthy.

Shifting blame from society to the individual is not a frank narra-tive, an objective plan, or an annual collective policy that public and private bodies vote on or even frankly discuss. Rather, it is the cumu-lative result of a multitude of micro-decisions that citizens make daily. Those micro-decisions build to the long-term choices that define pref-erences. The preferences aggregate to social institutions, in this case, the programs and roles of social clinics.

A popular social institution is as difficult to modify as the embed-ded individual preferences that created it. Too many people are over-weight and sedentary; many smoke and take harmful, illicit drugs; and many drive too fast while impaired. Many others are undisciplined, inattentive, hedonistic, and selfish. Many children are born to inad-equate parents and live in inadequate communities. Many of the per-sonal problems associated with unfortunate behaviors have become widespread social problems of addiction, poverty, violence, crime, men-tal disease, and emotional dysfunctions that are threats to the safety, security, and basic functions of American society. Few of these people have been talked out of their problems. Just like common pleasures and customs, the momentum of the social clinic seems impervious to argu-ments about ineffectiveness and even harm.

America seems largely content with the social clinic and the way things are. Perhaps the complacency is inevitable and wise. Nonetheless, other societies, some wealthy and some not, seem to have done a bet-ter job of things: less violence and crime, a better-educated population, fewer family failures, fewer imprudent births, and even greater expressed pleasure in living. They also tend to take a systemic approach to their social problems.

Except in rare instances that are impossible to replicate, the social clinic does not help, cure, prevent, rehabilitate, or assist people to adjust, cope, or adapt. Nonetheless, the thoroughgoing failure of the social clinic has not impeded its popularity. Indeed, the social clinic reflects the determinative values of the American people that recast systemic imperfections as the obdurate character flaws of those with problems. More than any other modern industrial nation, the United States has long preferred to shift the onus of social problems from public policy to the individual and private charity. In this way, the minimalism of social clinic interventions—largely talk therapy of one sort or another—reflects popular tastes and diminishes the possibility of systemic reform while ratifying the great inequalities of American stratification. The important point is that the social clinic is not a stray enthusiasm of a social minority but a long-dominant expression of the defining preferences of American citizens. National convenience is often masked by noble ideals and soothing fictions such as the social clinic that remain unrealized and even disingenuous.

The social clinic appears to embrace the rational enterprise of clinical sciences such as medicine, dentistry, and physical therapy along with the logic of the social sciences. The rational enterprise of the clinical sciences requires the identification of the sustaining and initial causes of a social problem then the design of interventions to address them and finally but crucially the evaluation of outcomes, that is, whether the interventions succeed or not. In turn, scientific and thus credible evaluation of the clinic necessitates first and foremost the true application of randomized controlled trials, the apotheosis of rationality in the applied sciences. Randomization entails at best a random selection of research subjects that represent the problem population and then the random assignment of these subjects to comparison groups that are equivalent except for the receipt of the experimental condition and the types of controls (nontreatment and placebo). Together with randomization and controls, additional protections of neutral evaluation, reliable and valid test instruments, and others assure that any outcomes of the research can be attributed only to the experimental condition which in the case of the social clinic refers to its services. The replication of research is singularly important both periodically and for new interventions. As a result of numerous design requirements including replication, scientifically valuable research in human services generally is often impractical, expensive, illegal, unethical, and theoretically ambiguous.

While the scientific enterprise is unevenly realized throughout the social sciences (Armstrong and Green 2017), randomized procedures and good research are in fact frequently possible in clinical practice and notably because the value of its various interventions has not been established. Thus, withholding service from a control group, at least for a while, is ethically defensible. In fact, randomized procedures have become common in evaluation of the social clinic. Unfortunately, randomization even when appropriately implemented has not been sufficient to protect against a variety of invalidating problems—large attrition, biased measurement, demand characteristics, and others. Even experimental psychology with its exquisite sensitivity to research design has been able to replicate only a small percent of its core discoveries. The Open Science Collaboration was able to successfully replicate only 39% of 100 psychology studies with "high powered designs" (*Science* 2015 p. 1 http://science.sciencemag.org/content/349/6251/aac4716.full). Moreover, as the quality of research improves, the size of reported positive outcomes often shrinks.

Summaries of the primary research—meta-analyses and systematic reviews—in most of the disciplines of the social clinic often conclude that progress has been made and that patient outcomes are improving. Yet these reviews, even when they only include research that incorporates randomized controls, usually accept primary research with serious, invalidating flaws. The summaries tend to be bulletins of professional loyalty more than careful analyses. For these reasons, prudent analysis after inspection of the best of the primary research contradicts the summaries.

At best, the rational enterprise of the social clinic remains immature, tentative, and nascent, not least because rational tests of effectiveness often challenge professional and social orthodoxy. When all is said and done, there is little scientifically credible evidence that affirms the effectiveness of the social clinic. By the same token, there is little empirical data that sustain the prudence of alternatives, namely generous systemic reforms. Nevertheless, the burden to prove effectiveness and safety rests with the innovator, that is, with those who claim that a procedure or product confers a benefit. The burden is quite different for a social institution that is accepted by use and tradition. In this case, the task of proof becomes the responsibility of those who seek change. Thus, it is quite apparent that the social clinic testifies to the triumph of the political.

The analysis of the social clinic as an expression of social policy making is also limited by a variety of factors that reduce the issue of political choice to ideology. The social clinic is obviously the product of social policy but there are different theories of what determines social choice. These different theories defy rational testing, that is, the application of randomized controlled trials among other requirements of science. The nation cannot be divided into small samples that are randomly assigned to the different conditions of American policy making to find out which theory prevails. Even if this were possible, the trials would be prohibitively expensive and coercive and thus illegal and unethical. They would also be theoretically ambiguous since the conditions of the research will probably affect social perceptions and motives in unpredictable and material ways. Moreover, causes exist in causal chains and the decision to select one for testing is itself ideologically dependent.

The present analysis makes the assumption that social policy in the United States is largely a reflection of mass preference. There are obviously powerful people and groups that enjoy unequal influence. However, their position is granted not usurped. By and large Americans have consented to American stratification despite its many apparent problems. What is often seen as the propaganda of wealth and privilege is perhaps more accurately identified as the long-standing ethos of the nation itself. The content of the national ethos, more romantic than pragmatic, is not imposed by coercive elites. Rather, embedded social values in the United Sates continue the tradition of the nation's culture that apparently dominates the free expression of the population. The United States with near universal suffrage has developed and protects perhaps the most open society in the world. It is a daunting task to prove that the population has been compelled into obedience, let alone oppressed, and that power is usurped by conspiratorial elites that frustrate popular intents (discussed at some length in Epstein 2017).

The social clinic is thus more prudently derived from culture and society as a consensual institution than from the common romantic drama of heroic goodness or illegitimate power. The heroic narrative typically ignores programmatic effectiveness and seems content to lay the wreath of success on programs that are socially accepted—the reward for a noble quest. Yet social acceptance is not necessarily a sign of successful treatment. To the contrary, the programs of the social clinic are nearly always ineffective. The inability to address their defining problems underscores the plausibility of explanations for their acceptance that involve considerations other than the achievement of their service goals.

The ambiguities of information restrict any criticism of social policy to speculation. All that remains is the ability to limn out a point of view— an alternative series of values realized in a different range of social provisions but one, alas, that implies a different civic culture. The injunction to consider the possibility that the alternatives will improve society is very modest. Rationality contends weakly with the political and even the reasonable seems an episodic fashion in American decision making that concerns social welfare. The intellectual's bias for ideas and open narratives may be less determinative than expressive of ceremonial social preferences while innovation is usually accepted only when underlying conditions are ripe. Yet there is always hope that the American grip on the romantic can be loosened enough to consider the material needs of many fellow citizens and the possibility that greater equality will stimulate a more gracious, coherent, and kind society with fewer problems. Still and all, the solution probably does not lie with eloquence or grand proof since the former usually flatters social stability and the latter is quite unlikely.

Chapters

This work is an analytic monograph that is not intended to serve as a comprehensive textbook. Its discussion of a large and representative selection of prominent social clinic interventions relies on the most scientifically credible information.

The internal chapters that discuss the different incarnations of the social clinic follow a similar pattern and employ a common standard of scientific discovery. Each chapter begins by describing the context of practice usually in reference to continuing debates within each field and then goes on to handle the issue of effectiveness. Effectiveness is initially addressed first by reporting each area's sense of its value as stated in the best of the summaries—meta-analyses and systematic reviews—of the primary research that tests effectiveness. The value of these conclusions is then assessed on the basis of the scientific credibility of the very best of the research cited in the summaries. The research is held to the standards of randomized controlled trial. On the one hand, each area of social clinic practice has come ostensibly to value randomized controlled trials. On the other hand, the logic and protections of randomized controlled trials are routinely violated and often with the impudence that the social clinic deserves a special dispensation from the canons of science.

The absence of accurate assessments of outcomes provides no warrant to assert a needed role in cure, prevention, or rehabilitation. Indeed, in light of its characteristic biases, the poor research often leads to reasonable conclusions that services have failed and at times raise the specter of harm. In fact, the broad and long-standing acceptance of faulty research and groundless claims of effective service has become a profound statement of the social preferences that engender contemporary social policy.

The chapters are more easily separated than the actual practice of social clinics. They often employ a variety of professional disciplines and treat many different social conditions and patients. The same social clinic may handle patients who present themselves voluntarily and others who come under threat of incarceration or benefit losses; private pay patients, insured patients, and public welfare patients; patients with complex problems and those with simple ones. Yet in the end, the book offers a comprehensive view of the activities and social role of the social clinic.

Each chapter also discusses alternatives to clinical services—usually publicly provided surrogates for the protections and caring of absent or failed families and communities. These surrogates are implicit in the few personal services that have credibly achieved their goals. Unfortunately, the successes in their present forms cannot be easily replicated. They are usually very expensive and involve uniquely talented professionals.

More importantly, their success often depends on large voluntary efforts of family and community that are very expensive to replicate.

A curious conflict plays itself out in the evaluative research of social clinics. A clinical intervention bears the burden to prove its effectiveness and safety, and a scientist accepts the task of implementing investigative methods that protect scientific credibility. Thus, in the role of treatment, the obligation to prove effectiveness rests with the social clinic. However, the task of proving deficiency rests with the critic of a social institution. The chapters contrast the social clinic's inability to cure, to prevent, and to rehabilitate with the prominence of its ceremonial role in affirming social values. As an institution of social belief, the long existence of the social clinic is sufficient proof of acceptability. Existence is often its own justification and begins to suggest that social consent has provided the sanction that resolves the tension between the production function of the social clinic and its ceremonial role.

Chapters 2 through 5 address psychotherapy and clinical psychology. Three prominent areas of practice are examined: treatment for post-traumatic stress disorder, for depression, and for opioid addiction. In each area, they assess the best of the recent outcome research and consider the field's ceremonial role as an affirmation of embedded romantic values.

Chapters 6 through 8 concern clinical social work. Chapter 5 provides an evaluation of the principal social welfare programs that were precursors to clinical social work practice. The historical analysis demystifies the usual heroic treatment of the social worker fighting the forces of social evil. Chapters 6 through 8 evaluate clinical social work through an analysis of the outcome literature in a variety of the field's most important clinical manifestations. These include counseling in defined social clinics but also the use of clinical techniques in foster care, family reunification and preservation, and school social work. Clinical social work as a form of the social clinic is not independent of social preferences; both are social institutions of the culture. They express the society's deepest attitudes that ratify its economic and social stratification.

Chapter 9 handles community psychology and community psychiatry. While the fields imagine themselves to embrace a systematic, objective coherence, their practice is circumscribed by social preferences that express themselves in the limitations of public funding. They are largely replications of clinical social work while presiding over the problems of community care for the chronically mentally ill. The chapter also addresses psychotherapeutic approaches to corrections, that is, for delinquents and criminals. Chapter 10 evaluates examples of the more marginal interventions of the social clinic—spiritualism, mindfulness and meditation, guided self-help, past life regression therapy, hypnosis to treat the traumatic effects of alien abduction, and ho'oponopono among others. Some are standard practices in standard social clinics; others are strange practices in even unusual clinics that are often attached to gift shops. The distinction between clinical practice on the margins of respectability and mainline psychotherapeutic practice is one of style rather than substance—between laughably deficient tests of effectiveness and pretenses to science.

The concluding chapter, *Soothing Fictions*, provides a critical synthesis. Each of the chapters attempts to grab onto something substantial in clinical practice. The hand closes; the fingers meet but there is nothing between them. The insubstantiality of the social clinic mirrors the emptiness of the American soul, the nation's unconcern with the suffering of its own citizens and the pervasive will to ignore the problems it creates. The social clinic is itself a soothing fiction—a dream of order—that justifies the nation's failure to address its many problems, notably including the large material and social inequalities of its citizens.

Every grand national purpose that ends up violating human dignity comes along with demulsifying fictions. The white man's burden justified imperialism and colonialism in Africa while in the United States, white supremacy and states' rights justified slavery and apartheid, eugenics justified sterilization and worse, the free market justifies the class system, imperfect character justifies inadequate public support, economic growth justifies ignoring social need, diversity, multiculturalism, and "the language of race" justify sectarianism and bigotry at the expense of the freedoms and basic rights of a liberal democracy. Many other unfortunate myths cut against basic social decency and the goal of a sustaining civic culture.

Noble ideals are often masks for a predatory reality. Myth itself is a hypocrisy that allows the reconciliation of reality with aspiration or perhaps that simply ennobles a troublesome reality as transitory, developmental, deserved, or otherwise easily tolerated. Joseph Conrad's Kurtz in *The Heart of Darkness* may have been a Peace Corps volunteer gone rogue, an errant son, a straying lamb, or a recognition of deviance that preserved the comforting notion of Europe's moral duty to rule Africa.

The alternative to the social clinic lies in providing the material supports of greater equality. In fact, the few successful personal social services provide unacknowledged testimony to the necessity of material support—usually surrogates for the voluntary efforts of family and community—in achieving educational parity, community-based mental health services, successful emotional adaptation, and others. However, surrogate care in contrast with clinical services is extremely expensive and thus unlikely in the long-standing political climate of the United States. Yet slow realization of the need for greater equality may come along with recognition of shared national peril, perhaps in response to climate change but also in recognition that the American dream depends upon fulfilling the American promise to provide greater opportunity through greater social equality.

A predatory elite dominating social policy in defiance of national will does not exist in the United States. The impediment to change lies in the broadly cherished political romanticism of the American people—a civic fundamentalism—that undermines the promises of liberal democracy to protect political minorities and the role of government in economic redistribution—positive and negative liberty in Berlin's terms.[1]

Las Vegas, USA   William M. Epstein

---

[1]Political romanticism in American social welfare, society and politics was the core of *The Masses are the Ruling Classes* (2017), my previous book, and provides a framework for this one.

References

Armstron, J. S., & Green, K. C. (2017). *Guidelines for Science: Evidence and Checklists Scholarly Commons*. https://papers.ssrn.com/sol3/papers.cfm?abstract_id=3055874.

Epstein, W. M. (2017). *The Masses are the Ruling Classes: Policy Romanticism, Democratic Populism, and Social Welfare*. New York, NY: Oxford University Press.

Acknowledgements

The book is indebted to intelligent first readers for encouragement and wise suggestions: Anne-Marie Abruscato, Robert E. Becker, Ronald A. Farrell, Joel Fischer, Tomi Gomory, Stuart A, Kirk, Paul Moloney, and David Stoesz. My research assistants—Naomi Elliott and Patricia Scherer—were patient, astute, and industrious. Hokwon Cho, Seongmin Park, Sandra Catlin, and Carlton D. Craig provided gracious technical assistance, notably with the interpretation of statistics and quantitative models. A nod of gratitude for the flattering and helpful comments by anonymous reviewers and by Beth Farrow, my editor at Palgrave Macmillan. As ever, the energetic, hardworking, intelligent, and careful reference librarians at UNLV saved me enormous amounts of time and identified many works that I had missed. A special thanks to my wife, Elizabeth—a skilled journalist and rare social worker—for patience, copyediting, and love. Despite the bleakness of *Soothing Fictions*, there are some in the field who dare to walk their own way. May their journey continue. The errors in the book remain mine, all mine.

Contents

Abstracts

Preface

The social clinic is a sanctioned program strategy to handle social and personal problems. It is defined as programs that employ some form of talk therapy. Even without explicitly offering talk therapy, many social welfare agencies that provide material assistance still mimic the social clinic in their intentions to address recipients' attitudes through psychological interventions. The broad popularity of the treatment assumptions social clinic is coextensive with a national ethos of policy romanticism—extreme individualism, a sense of chosenness, and the primacy of emotion over objective coherence.

The book's analysis relies on the very best of the clinical outcome literature—randomized controlled trials and other criteria of credible scientific research—to evaluate the effectiveness of the social clinic in core areas of social concern.

Chapter 1 Introduction

The social clinic employs the disciplines of social work, counseling, clinical psychology, community psychology and community psychiatry, community nursing, and others. Its programs of psychotherapy and personal support usually attend to mental and emotional disorders but also adjustment problems, criminal rehabilitation, motivation, and to a much lesser degree social support. It typically functions as free-standing agencies and solo practices but also within prisons, reformatories, courts, mental hospitals, churches, universities, the military, police forces, public and private schools, community centers, and others. The social clinic has also seeped into unexpected areas of American life—organized religion, the workplace and even professional and amateur sports organizations that employ clinical techniques to motivate their athletes. Services are funded through a variety of public programs and private insurance as well as cash.

Chapter 2 Psychotherapy and the Social Clinic in the United States

The greatest fault of the field is the failure to develop and implement a credible science that monitors its effectiveness and guides its development. As a result, psychotherapy remains an alternative, even unorthodox medical practice in the manner of acupuncture, chiropractic, herbal cures, and others.

While research has become more sophisticated and objective over the decades, the field of psychotherapy remains complacent, even smug, in assurance of clinical effectiveness. This confidence, carried into the community of scholars responsible for the field's literature and research, overwhelms any systemic attempt at truly credible research. Nonetheless, as a black box of treatment, the ability of talk therapy to cure, prevent, or rehabilitate can be evaluated even when the precise therapeutic content of treatment can be neither specified nor tested.

Chapter 3 Psychotherapy and the Social Clinic in the United States

The best of the PTSD outcome research is deeply flawed—researcher and institutional biases, lack of blinding, large attrition, questionable patient self-report, and others. Analysts who are not committed to psychotherapy, that is, neutral critics, might interpret the same primary evidence as a profound challenge to the clinical claims that any form of psychotherapy provides effective treatment for PTSD. It is worth considering that the VA and NIMH, as agencies of government that presumably bear the obligation for objective and neutral assessment in protection of the health of the nation, are simply carrying forward the stakes of the treatment community and apparently the priorities of the society. The caring alternative to psychotherapy: expensive and largely unexplored.

Chapter 4 Psychotherapy for Depression and Addiction

Substantively as well as symbolically, psychotherapy for depression and addiction repeats the clinical record of post-traumatic stress disorder. The best of the best studies of psychotherapy for depression fails as science, lacking true tests of treatment while routinely exaggerating the effectiveness of psychotherapy. The research does not dispel the likelihood that psychotherapy for depression fails to improve on the processes that account for natural remission.

Psychotherapy offers no apparent cure for drug addiction. The variation in reported addiction rates from year to year, suspect in itself, may be due to generational learning and changing fashions in social attitudes to illicit drug use more than to any form of treatment. The small amount of remission and true long-term abstinence reported in psychotherapy trials are likely determined by rare patient motivation and their situations rather than treatment itself.

Chapter 5 Psychotherapy and the Social Clinic in the United States

The critical analysis of psychotherapy, the core intervention of the American social clinic, indicts each link in the chain of American social welfare policy making: the inability of the social clinic itself to achieve the remission or prevention of mental and emotional disorders; the community of scholars that fails to offer scientifically credible tests of its outcomes; and the American culture that endorses the affirming myths of the social clinic thus encouraging the distortions of its research community and the fecklessness of its interventions.

Psychotherapy rather than care and the failure of critical psychology: Mental and emotional problems remain embedded in society and not amenable to isolation for clinical treatment.

Chapter 6 Precursors to Modern Social Work

Histories of social work and the social clinic face a number of barriers to fulfill the most basic tasks of description. Little can be surmised about the extent of operations, the details of service, the number served and most important the effects of the services on recipients or more broadly on the culture itself. Even the more recent program evaluations, and notably those that attempted to address outcomes are themselves tortuously biased. Their methods, data, and conclusions can be untwisted to provide a general estimate of outcomes that usually reduce their modest claims to levels of ineffectiveness. All that is left is the field's beleaguered adherence to popular values—a pantomime of ineffective talking cures in denial of the material claims of those in need.

Chapter 7 Contemporary Social Work and the Social Clinic

Rather than the scientific practice of philanthropy, charity or caring, social work has institutionalized an obedience to policy minimalism by the choice of talk therapy of one sort or another as its base of practice knowledge. The very strongest evaluations of clinical social work published during the past twenty years in the most highly regarded research journals within social work are trivial both as practice and as theory. They are deficient as science. Despite a near-constant claim to credible knowledge, social work has never done so.

Chapter 8 Psychotherapy and the Social Clinic in the United States

The clinical social work outcomes in the traditional practice areas of foster children, schools, and family reunification are disappointing—a multitude of poorly conducted studies that fail to support the field's claims of effective practice but that perpetuate the soothing fictions of social welfare in America. There is little credible evidence that social work practice actually pursues let alone achieves any of its grand goals, notably including its clinical promises of successful treatment. In fact, American social welfare policy has rarely if ever endorsed the field's aspirations as a paladin of the poor and the oppressed in the actual job descriptions of social workers.

Chapter 9 Community Psychological Practice and a Note on Rehabilitation in Corrections

Community psychological practice fails but largely because funds are inadequate to sustain its programs, notably housing, and supportive care. The resistance to adequate funding has not been surmounted by strategies of political activism. The organization of vulnerable, needy, and poorer people for political power is very unlikely to succeed. The list of similar attempts contains a greater number of heroic tragedies and tyrannies than successes. There is no successful discipline of political, social, or psychological liberation.

Community psychological practice and rehabilitation in corrections have failed to achieve their goals for two principal reasons. The wrong interventions are pursued and the American public is unwilling to allocate appropriate resources. The provision of decent community care, notably for offenders as well as patients with chronic mental and emotional disorders is very expensive. The social clinic is much less expensive. Neglect is even cheaper.

Chapter 10 Psychotherapy and the Social Clinic in the United States

The mind and spirit interventions of the social clinic are a type of alternative, fringe, complementary, integrative, folk, adjunctive, unconventional, unorthodox, nonmainstream, or irregular procedure that promises to treat mental, emotional, or physical ailments. What isolates past life therapy, MariEl (sic) healing, Reiki healing, light and sound therapy, gestalt psychotherapy, therapy for post-alien abduction syndrome, ho'oponopono, spiritualism, mindfulness, and many others from the mainstream is not their strangeness but rather their use of alternative science to validate their outcomes. Yet many marginal interventions are traveling the same track on which psychoanalysis, psychotherapy, and social work moved from the odd to the commonplace and all without compelling scientific evidence of effectiveness. The achievement of clinical acceptance is a social phenomenon more often than a rational one—validation through faith and use often in defiance of clinical evidence.

Chapter 11 Psychotherapy and the Social Clinic in the United States

With broad consent, enduring and prevalent soothing fictions—white superiority, eugenics, states' rights, salvation, volunteerism, charity, social growth, progress, manifest destiny, diversity, multiculturalism, affirmative action, entrepreneurship, free markets, self-determination, self-reliance, self-help, self-invention, self-actualization, individual responsibility, extreme individualism, moral hazards, helping, social treatment, voluntary good works, and, repeatedly, some form of America First and increasingly in conformity with the tenets of "volksgemeinshaft"—express the cultural values embedded in the United States. The American dream of fair equality depends on the American promise of a decent civic culture: free speech, equal application of the law, respect for the individual, common decency, and most important the constant responsibility seated in government to monitor and reduce great social and economic inequalities. Engendered by persistent social fictions, the social clinic institutionalizes denial of the American promise.

Afterword

Social fictions obscure and minimize the existential threat of global warming.

1

Introduction

In its long and frequent expression in the United States, the social clinic has become a broadly sanctioned, well-funded, and often attended institution of society. It is a touchstone, a defining totem of American values that is carved into the goals and practices of the social services and social policy itself; it circumscribes many of the functions of charity and public social welfare. The social clinic is also a frequent instance of the sacred beliefs and tenets of American citizenship. Even more subtly, it defines the national psyche.

The social clinic manifests itself most obviously as programs of psychotherapy (including its behavioral adaptations), mentoring, and counseling to address a variety of mental, social, and personal problems such as substance abuse, trauma and depression, mental and psychiatric problems, weight problems, major and minor criminal transgressions, and many others. Less often, it also provides supportive services and other nonmedical interventions designed to change undesirable behavior. Indeed, the view has long persisted in American social welfare that poverty itself is principally a result of character flaws—laziness, promiscuity, and hedonism—that require clinical attention. In addition, an enormous group of people voluntarily seek care from the social clinic

© The Author(s) 2019
W. M. Epstein, *Psychotherapy and the Social Clinic in the United States*,
https://doi.org/10.1007/978-3-030-32750-7_1

to better their lives, to find greater psychic comfort, to improve performance at work, to sharpen social skills, and to enrich family life. Without any appreciation for irony, the social clinic frequently offers professional counseling to improve self-help.

The social clinic employs the disciplines of social work, counseling, clinical psychology, community psychology and community psychiatry, community nursing, and others. Its programs of psychotherapy and personal support usually attend to mental and emotional disorders but also adjustment problems, criminal rehabilitation, motivation, and to a much lesser degree social support among many others. It typically functions as free-standing agencies and solo practices but also within prisons, reformatories, courts, mental hospitals, churches, universities, the military, many police forces, public and private schools, community centers, and others. The social clinic has also seeped into unexpected areas of American life. It is present in organized religion as pastoral counseling and in the workplace often as employee assistance programs, industrial psychology, the disciplines of management such as organizational development programs that rely on worker counseling and motivation. Many professional and amateur sports organizations seek clinical assistance to motivate their athletes. It is paid for through a variety of public programs—e.g., Medicaid, Medicare and Title XX of the Social Security Act—as well as through private insurance, local and state subsidies, charitable contributions, and cash.

Even while the central talk therapies of the social clinic are creations of clinical psychology, the majority of professional talk therapy and perhaps administrative leadership is provided by social workers. Bledsoe and Grote (2006) report that social workers account for more than 60% of psychotherapists (p. 114). The interventions of the social clinic are largely based on one form of talk therapy or another since the social clinic rarely if ever dispenses material support and rarely provides supportive care. Indeed, clinical services are usually predicated on the assumption that attitude change, achieved through processes of "rational induction," that is, discussions and evaluations of the patient's behavior, precedes behavioral change. The corollary assumption prevails in the United States that material support and thus public welfare create a moral hazard that inhibits behavioral change while encouraging deviant behavior, particularly dependency on charity and public welfare.[1]

The history of social work mirrors the other occupations of the social clinic, contradicting an institutionalized role as the heroic advocate of systemic change. If anything, it consistently looked toward a revolution in human consciousness, if even that, rather than in politics. Social work and the other clinical disciplines have customarily been obedient to romantic social norms—notably the pursuit of human perfection through self-help and counseling based on the possibility of self-invention. The social clinic did not choose its goals, service groups, or types of intervention. It yielded to dominant social and cultural changes. Indeed, social work as one typical example continues to take refuge in established tolerances, promoting social causes such as diversity and empowerment when they are safely two generations old and have matured from pursuits of liberation to practices of restraint. Advocacy is rare; programmatic success is even rarer, idiosyncratic, and thus sterile.

The social clinic was easily realized. It was not a fiercely contended victory over the forces of rebarbative tradition by the professions of helping. There was little if any opposition to a practice of social reform that put the onus of change on the service recipient. Its popularity was presaged by established practices and assumptions of American religion. Even before the advent of modern psychotherapy, the tenets of the social clinic—notably a sense of personal responsibility for personal failure and need—customarily defined the center of social work. The field sought professional standing early on by adopting a psychological practice, initially Freudian therapy, and then others built on assumptions of individual agency rather than social causation. Social work found convenience in the romantic traditions of psychological practice—insight,

---

[1]Social work does have a presence outside of the clinic—in hospitals, schools, and some public legal practices as well in programs that provide supportive services such as in foster care and adoption, adult and child protection, and nonpsychotherapuetic programs in public schools. Note difficult of describing social work practice. Community work has become vestigial, and agency management is becoming so with deference to schools of management. However, even in these ostensibly nonclinical settings talk therapy is a frequent intervention. Even case management often drifts into clinical practice.

intuition, subjectivity, and self-evident truth—that rejected the substance of science but conveniently adopted its form.

Nonetheless, social welfare histories, when they touch on the social clinic or are addressed largely to it, pay little attention to the issue of service effectiveness. This is not surprising since program evaluation until fairly recently relied on intuitive assessments by practitioners and administrators as well as other nonsystematic and unreliable reviews. At best, partial descriptions of personal, recipients, and services were drawn from institutional accounts. Moreover, with few exceptions the histories fail to appreciate the obedience of the social clinic to the romantic tenets of American society and its immense popularity. Instead, most impose a biblical narrative on the history of the social clinic in the United States, imagining a heroic struggle of virtuous social reform in overcoming rebarbative resistance. However, the journalism of David and Goliath is insufficient to address the actual role of the social clinic or to acknowledge that willingly, quietly, and knowingly it purveys inadequate services to needy populations. Paraphrasing the late president Lyndon Johnson, getting ahead depends on getting along and the social clinic was an obliging miracle of congeniality rather than effective opposition to racism, poverty, and social inequality.

At least superficially, the social clinic was modeled on the medical clinic and accepted its core assumption of practice that the presenting problem could be treated in isolation from its social context. That is, the individual's problems could be successfully and efficiently addressed without the immense expense of addressing either the initial or sustaining social causes. Yet the medical clinic is twinned with public health while the social clinic is devoid of scientific coherence.

Throughout their development, the medical clinic and the social clinic faced similar challenges but took different paths. Medical practice embraced science. Social treatment rejected it in reality, reducing science to a ritual of evidence-based practice and its even weaker form, evidence-informed practice. Through credible science, medicine achieved the ability to treat physical disease. In contrast, the social clinic has failed to develop scientifically credible evidence of success. Yet neither field chose freely. Each realized different prevailing social goals, expectations, and roles in becoming institutions of popular consent. In short, the practice of medicine is sustained by a pragmatic ability to treat physical disease. The social clinic performs a ceremonial role in affirming romantic social preferences.

Medicine has professionalized applied science. The social clinic, employing the techniques of belief and cultural loyalty rather than evidence of reason, has professionalized a form of religion but one in which theology is displaced by an ideology of dominant social values. The conclusion of ideological consistency would not be justified if the social clinic pursued vastly different goals that reflected different social assumptions and values. However, American social policy choices including the goals, assumptions, and interventions of the social clinic are dependably romantic. As a result of its loyalty to social values, the social clinic has achieved a sanctioned and licensed franchise to treat individual behavioral problems that imitates the near-monopoly granted to medicine and the allied health professions to treat physical disease.

As part of its ritual of science, the social clinic claims professional standing on the basis of specialized knowledge that is effective in treating personal and social problems. Yet deprived of credible science, its knowledge remains uncertain and contrived. Not surprisingly, the defining goals of the social clinic are not achieved. Nonetheless, the alleged specialized knowledge of the social clinic constitutes the core of professional training in a variety of university-based programs—prominently social work, child and family practice, clinical and counseling psychology—and contributes peripherally to others—public administration, management, public health, and even psychiatry and physical therapy.

Part of the reason for the social clinic's lack of good information lies with the corruption of its research, its failure to successfully apply randomized designs even when they are possible. The social clinic like the medical clinic seems ideal for the application of controlled research to test whether interventions are successful—whether recipients of social clinic services have recovered or improved. Both treat large numbers of individuals and both are testing interventions that are not proven to be effective. However, much of the social clinic's knowledge problem rests with intractable and near intractable issues of testing.

At its root, the social clinic emerged from the Enlightenment hope of realizing a science of the individual and society. Yet it is customarily impossible to apply credible science to discover the cause of most social problems and thus to eliminate the "germs" of social pathology. In contrast, medical science has progressed because of a theory of disease that led to the identification of its causes and then successful treatment and containment. Yet it is not possible to divide any society into testable groups over long periods of time—generations—to test the degree to which structural or personal conditions create problematic outcomes. Furthermore, much of the instrumentation of the social clinic—the tools to measure service effects—is impaired and inadequate. As a result, much of its outcome data, solicited without corroboration from service recipients, is presumably unreliable and subject to reporting and measurement biases. Even worse, replications are rare, uncertain, and uneven; protections against biases are weak; and research intended to test the state of the art is customarily conducted as optimal demonstrations that include rigorous accountability and that employ presumably gifted clinicians. Thus, these demonstrations fail to test the outcomes of the social clinic's interventions under the customary, suboptimal conditions of practice. Yet even taken at its word, the most credible of the research usually reports only small gains. It is difficult to ignore the conclusion that the social clinic is a cultural form without much of an ability to talk people out of their problems or to convince them to conform with approved social norms.

The social clinic makes a number of basic assumptions about the individual and society, in particular that many social problems if not most are caused by character deficits, rather than imperfections in the structure of society and its conspicuous economic and social stratification. Understandably, then if individuals have freely made bad choices then they are free to change their problem behavior. Furthermore, self-invention and personal agency imply that attitude change precedes behavioral change. Most tellingly, these assumptions build to the bedrock imperative of belief in the capacity of talk therapy to address individual problems and thus social problems. The success is measured as both remission and abatement of problems as well as prevention and rehabilitation. Yet even when patently not successful, for example in treating drug and alcohol addictions and sexually predatory behaviors, the social clinic is sustained as a beacon of moral truth and restraint, that is, a mission of the civic religion to the misbegotten, improvident, perverse, and others who need to see the light of virtue and come home to the communion of Americans. Much to the point, the assumptions of the social clinic have failed to inspire an effective practice.

These assumptions—flawed character, sufficient individual freedom and thus personal agency, the primacy and possibility of attitude change, and the efficacy of practice—are symmetrical with the broad American credo. The credo is romantic—a fact of tradition and belief—far more than committed to pragmatism based in objective coherent evidence. American policy romanticism has three tenets: extreme individualism that defines an extreme sense of personal responsibility, the dominance of gnostic insight, and the assurance of exceptionalism both in the celestial sense of God's chosen people but also as the nation's Darwinian superiority. Thus more than simply addressing unwanted and deviant individual behaviors, the social clinic is an inspiration of public and private policy that defines the nature of American citizenship. In this broad sense, the social clinic is a powerful metaphor of America that institutionalizes its romantic core of belief, its ethos. The assumptions of clinical practice are better understood as reflections of popular ideology that justifies complacency with the nation's enormous social and economic inequalities. Indeed, to the extent that social problems are engendered by flaws in the American system, the social clinic is a bulwark against pragmatic, reasoned social reform.

The history of the social clinic, commonly coextensive with social work and the variety of counseling and mental health professions, stands witness to public neglect since at least the early twentieth century but also before. All the American helping fields although certainly not all of their members have nourished their privileged professional standing on the principle of social efficiency. Indeed, despite breastplates of liberality, progressiveness, and concern for those in need, the social clinic and its professionals have endorsed institutionalized roles that realize a conservative agenda of neglect, low expense, and social compatibility. This is hardly surprising since the auspices of the social clinic reside in the dominant society that provides its mandates, franchises, and financial support. Indeed, the social clinic as a substitute for a material social welfare strategy as well as a metaphor of extreme personal responsibility persists because of its obedience to the national will. It is precisely these myths of effective care that constitute its soothing fictions, assurances that all is well with the nation's ethos. The social clinic does not invent itself and human beings do not either. Both the social clinic and the nation's romantic ethos are triumphs of cultural momentum and emotion over reason.

It is a puzzle that so many of the analyses of psychotherapy so very lightly pass over the issue of effectiveness or handle it without rigorous skepticism toward the body of clinical research. Because that body of research is thoroughly flawed and consistently biased, it stands as a rebuke to the claim that the field is effective. At best, the outcomes of psychotherapy are indeterminate. However, far more likely, it is ineffective and perhaps even routinely harmful. In short, there is no scientifically credible evidence that psychotherapeutic treatment is effective. The small critical tradition that looks at the field skeptically is routinely ignored, and the clinical role is accepted with a priori faith. The effectiveness of the social clinic is an incidental concern; its ceremonial role in sustaining the national ethos is primary and explains its persistence.

The same conclusion is strengthened after critical analyses of outcome research covering the different programs of the social clinic. People's nasty little ways are not changed. Depression, eating disorders, trauma, addictions, and others persist after treatment. Work performance, family functioning, and marriage do not improve. Abused and forlorn children are not comforted or made whole by treatment. Indeed, the outcome literature of the personal social services is biased and tendentious rather than a lofty example of scholarly disinterest, humane concern and neutral, independent evaluation.

Considerable and credible evidence testifies to the stubbornness of habit that diminishes the possibility of reasoned personal change. Embedded human behaviors that are problematic—crime and substance abuse as well as dysfunctional economic choices that promote global warming and the pollution of the environment—are persistent and often impervious to argument. Indeed, attitude change is perhaps more an adaptation to new situations than their cause.

Yet in fact alternatives to the social clinic are more likely to be effective against social and individual problems. They are suggested by the few social programs that have been successful but they have not been replicated. By and large, they provide greater comparability and access to standard cultural experience. Rather than the inexpensive and failed shortcuts of the social clinic, greater equality may be the tool to repair the problems caused by the long-standing deficits of the nation's society and economy. However, greater equality—caring and material supports in contrast with treatment—entails considerable expense and challenges long-standing priorities, attitudes, and customs. It is routinely denied by the American public.

Writing about colonialism, Joseph Conrad (1988) maintained that

> the conquest of the earth, which mostly means the taking it away from those who have a different complexion or slightly flatter noses than ourselves, is not a pretty thing when you look into it too much. *What redeems it is the idea only.* An idea at the back of it, not a sentimental pretense but an idea; and an unselfish belief in the idea—something you can set up, and bow down before, and offer a sacrifice to. (emphasis in original, ibid., p. 10)

Perhaps the "white man's burden" or the benevolence of spreading advanced civilization to presumed barbarians served as the ideas at the back of colonialism. Conrad's statement seems true whether he was an apologist for colonialism or a harsh critic. Yet national depravity customarily comes along with ennobling ideals—soothing fictions. The social clinic incorporates the demulsifying ideals of helping, social treatment, charity, benevolence, concern, and, always, individual agency, the autonomous will, and self-invention.

These myths perpetuate exaggerated, romantic belief in personal rather than collective responsibility—the determinative influence of the autonomous individual rather than the enveloping circumstances of socialization and the conditions of citizenship. Even when not hypocritical but merely oblivious, soothing fictions—the blandishments of the helping professions—ease the social conscience with virtuous intent and heroic overcoming that lubricate the frictions of American social and economic inequality. Rather than the fictions that mask neglect and unconcern as virtue, in the end it comes down to an issue of common decency.

References

Bledsoe, S. E., & Grote, N. K. (2006). Treating Depression During Pregnancy and the Postpartum: A Preliminary Meta-Analysis. *Research on Social Work Practice, 16,* 109–120. https://doi.org/10.1177/1049731505282202.

Conrad, J. (1988). *Heart of Darkness* (3rd ed.). London: W. W. Norton.

Part I

Psychotherapy

2

Psychotherapy and Tests of Effectiveness

A wise listening ear that soothes the heaving breast, comforts the troubled soul and redirects the wayward heart has always been a blessing of sociability. However, it is doubtful that the psychotherapy industry has professionalized the natural caring of a well-ordered society. Patients do not routinely profit from any of the various forms of psychotherapy; some patients apparently deteriorate during treatment. Yet the greatest fault of the field is the failure to develop and implement a credible science that monitors its effectiveness and leads its development. As a result, psychotherapy remains an alternative, even unorthodox medical practice in the manner of acupuncture, chiropractic, herbal cures, and others. Yet, despite its many failures, psychotherapy is immensely popular.

Psychotherapy, encompassing all the different forms of talk therapy, is the defining although not the sole intervention of the social clinic. According to the influential *History of Psychotherapy* (Norcross et al. 2011), "broadly defined, psychotherapy refers to the treatment of emotional or physical ills by psychological means, implying a belief in the influence of the mind on the mind and of the mind on the body" (p. 3). Wallerstein (1995) in his comprehensive analysis of psychoanalysis and

© The Author(s) 2019
W. M. Epstein, *Psychotherapy and the Social Clinic in the United States*,
https://doi.org/10.1007/978-3-030-32750-7_2

psychoanalytically inspired psychotherapies covers the different therapies in detail while assuming an implicit common definition expressed in the title of the book—*The Talking Cures*—that seems widely shared. In a generic sense, psychotherapy is speech between a patient and a trained therapist intended to resolve the patient's mental and emotional problems. It is a tribute to the institutional popularity of talk therapy that Wallerstein pays little attention to the question of effectiveness beyond his own research. He shows more respect for the insights of essentially qualitative studies of the therapeutic process—its evidence from the couch—than for rigorously controlled tests of effectiveness. On its part, the *History of Psychotherapy*, an 800-page tome published by the American Psychological Association, also devotes little space or attention to the issue of effectiveness, accepting with even less skepticism seriously impaired research. Yet while subsequent research has become more sophisticated and objective, the field of psychotherapy remains complacent, even smug, in assurance of clinical effectiveness. This confidence, carried into the community of scholars responsible for the field's literature and research, overwhelms any systemic attempt at truly credible research.

After all, people do get better during psychotherapy and many patients report satisfaction with treatment. However, there is little if any credible proof that improvement documented during treatment is due to the therapy itself. Other considerations rather than the therapy per se may account for the improvement: the seasonality of the psychological problem, the maturation and changing circumstances of the patient, bias in measuring symptoms, fortuitously small samples, demand characteristics of the research situation, placebo effects, unrepresentative samples, large attrition, the absence of appropriate controls for the intervention, demonstration effects, and others. Moreover, many of those diagnosed with problems may not in fact suffer from them since psychological diagnoses are often inappropriate or unreliable (Kirk and Kutchings 1992; Horwitz and Wakefield 2007). The field's clinical research has been unable to disprove these alternative explanations for measured improvement in outcomes by way of establishing with scientific credibility the effectiveness of psychotherapeutic treatment.

Nonetheless, as a black box of treatment, the ability of talk therapy to cure, prevent, or rehabilitate can still be evaluated even when the precise therapeutic content of treatment can be neither specified nor tested. With this in mind and in light of great budgetary pressure for inexpensive cures, attention to the effectiveness of psychotherapeutic treatment has increased greatly over the past decades. Still and all, the research remains porous and self-serving. While Wallerstein largely ignores the crucial role of rigorous research methods in establishing clinical authority, subsequent studies acknowledge the value of science but then suborn its requirements in the actual tests of practice. With rare skepticism, the psychotherapeutic community appears convinced that the talk therapies are valuable and that the job of the outcome research is to demonstrate rather than test their obvious virtues.

Addressing complementary and alternative medicine, Bausell (2007) emphasizes the necessity of randomized controlled trials and the crucial importance of appropriate controls, notably placebos, to separate false science from true science, effective clinical practice from bogus clinical practice. Yet placebos in psychotherapy's clinical research are rare and customarily inadequate since effectiveness is assumed and thus withholding treatment is considered to be unethical. The field prefers delayed treatment waitlist controls. These controls come along with several problems. First, they prevent follow-up but more importantly they are not placebos for treatment. Moreover, they cannot control for alternative sets of plausible biases that may falsely manufacture evidence of effectiveness by pulling in opposite directions. Those on the waitlist may exaggerate their symptoms to stay eligible for treatment while the treated group may exaggerate their reported gains in gratitude for free service, as a compliment to their engaging, supportive therapists, or even out of a sense of personal obligation to improve. Since the differences between the outcomes of waitlist subjects and treated patients measure success, their biases would falsely inflate reported treatment effectiveness. Yet, Mohr et al.'s (2014) meta-analysis argued for the propriety of waitlist controls on grounds that subjects on waitlists will not seek treatment from other sources. However, Mohr et al. do not sustain this assumption, not least because waitlist attrition is common and large, nor do they address the plausible skepticism attending inaccurate self-reports of those on waitlists.

Until the field matures past reliance on questionable, customarily uncorroborated, and patently subjective patient self-reports to measure most clinical effects of psychotherapy, it cannot mature as a science. The difficulty of developing reliable and valid measures of symptoms provides no warrant for the field to graduate weak evidence of effectiveness into definitive proofs. Moreover, publication bias—the suppression of reports and findings by researchers and journals that challenge psychotherapy's effectiveness—is a recurrent finding of studies throughout the field. Nonetheless, the obligation to demonstrate clinical effectiveness on credible scientific grounds rests with the clinician, not the skeptic. Without a community of scholars acculturated to skepticism, there is no science, clinical, or otherwise (Ravetz 1971). Indeed, without skepticism and freedom to question established truths, there is little chance of any progress, clinical, social, or otherwise.

Skepticism is more than the hallmark of a scientific community. It is the bedrock value of a modern democracy, realized in the First Amendment of the US Constitution, as a protection against self-serving power and the tyranny of incontestable truth. The scientific value of freedom of expression is symmetrical with its political and social value. Within a community of scholars, it is not merely the freedom to question authority but indeed the obligation to do so: to test truth. A creative and fruitful community of scholars thrives by challenging regnant orthodoxies. The psychotherapy community of scholars has failed in this regard. It protects its social authority through corrupt science that is little better in the end than the bogus "proofs" of alternative medicine. Yet it acts with a broad social consent to propagate soothing fictions that endorse the romantic values of American society.

The lack of a community of psychotherapy scholars committed to skepticism explains the absence of neutral tests of psychotherapy's effectiveness. This profound rejection of the most basic function of science—the pursuit of objective truth through credible challenges to the authority of established practice—erects an impregnable barrier to credible research. It is even more problematic than the absence of credible placebos and the other essentials of research. At the same time, the society's deep affection for the mythic role of psychotherapy removes the obligation for credible tests of its effectiveness from the social clinic and places it on the shoulders of the skeptic. Psychotherapy has become a social institution in the manner of religion, family, and baseball rather than a pragmatic tool of treatment with clinical meaning. Popularity, social utility, and satisfaction have displaced clinical effectiveness; soothing fictions are more important than effective cures.

Over the past few decades, the statistical sophistication of research that tests the effectiveness of the social clinic has continued to improve, usually in small elegant ways. However, the methods of investigation remain porous and reported results are customarily inflated estimates of actual success. Thus, attempts to summarize an immense body of outcome research, customarily through statistical meta-analyses, come along with serious analytic challenges (Nugent 2017).

There have in fact been compelling criticisms of psychotherapy although the few critics have been largely ignored both within the field and by a society that finds the message of ineffectiveness to be largely irrelevant if not actually disloyal to abiding social values. From its beginning in the late nineteenth century, psychoanalysis and then the many descendant forms of psychotherapy were not serious scientific endeavors although the practitioners were dead serious about promoting their craft of psychic healing. They pursued a social and clinical standing equivalent to their medical colleagues with all it entails for professional credibility and prestige. The psychotherapists promised what few medical practitioners could: relief of psychic pain and often the achievement of contentment if not happiness itself. Both the promises of the field and its failures to achieve them have remained constant over the many decades during which its popularity has grown along with that of many other alternative forms of medical practice. Complementary and alternative medicine remains widespread and lucrative despite its lack of credible clinical proofs of effectiveness (Eisenberg et al. 1993, 1998; Bausell 2007; Gardner 1998; Singh and Ernst 2008). Indeed, "alternative" refers less to the oddities of the intervention and more to the alternative-to-science methods employed to test its outcomes. With regard to the quality of research, psychotherapy is companionable with acupuncture, aromatherapy, and chiropracty more than with mainline medicine.

Freudian psychoanalysis has been largely debunked even while its offspring of psychodynamic psychotherapy remains popular. Eysenck and Rachman (1965) then Grunbaum (1984) and subsequently many others mounted the argument that Freudian theory was not adequately tested by reports of patients "from the couch" but required standard methods of clinical proof, namely randomized controlled trials along with other protections against bias. Moreover, Ernest Nagel (in Hook 1959) pointed out that Freudian theory defies empirical testing since many of Freud's basic constructs—e.g., the unconscious, repression, id and so forth—are often unspecified as material entities. In this way, much of psychoanalytic practice is devoid of clinical meaning if the standard is medical practice. Still and all, if treatment promises to change behavior and not simply provide personal insights, it is amenable to testing as a black box through randomized clinical trials. Indeed, this is the logic of most tests of clinical effectiveness: even while the precise elements of therapeutic effects are elusive, treatment approaches can be compared to controls that do not provide the black box of therapeutic techniques.

Two monumental works by Crews (1993, 2017) and another by Macmillan (1997) have largely put to rest any rational belief in the clinical value of psychoanalysis. Crews shows up Freud as a charlatan and quack, dishonest and self-serving, who through chicanery, intelligence, and charm succeeded in promoting what became an immensely profitable and popular clinical practice of little if any value. He took advantage of patients, colleagues, and a credulous public. Rather than a commitment to science, Freud expressed a "gradually emergent affinity for the paranormal:" the occult, "the symbolic presentiment of unknown realities," telepathy, the miraculous and others (pp. 632–633). Crews treats Freud and psychoanalysis as if it were a violation of social values, a consumer fraud perpetrated on a naïve population. Yet, despite the personal faults of the shaman Freud, psychotherapy and psychoanalysis expressed in its myths of deviance and treatment broadly popular notions of the individual and social roles. It demulsified the emergent individualism of modern society, and notably the appalling romantic assumption that people create themselves captured in Fichte's idea of the self-positing ego.

On his part, Macmillan (1997) provides a detailed critique of Freudian theory but a limited presentation of the empirical literature that tests outcomes. He empties Freudian theory of any value but like Crews he seems to suggest that its popularity is a meander in social and cultural choices. Macmillan does not address the fact that the absence of compelling empirical evidence of the field's clinical value has been largely ignored by the society. Crews, Macmillan and with a few notable exceptions, most other critics of psychotherapy largely fail to explore the underpinnings of the field's popularity instead discuss its advent as treatment. In contrast, the social tenets of psychotherapy—its mythology of individual prowess and self-determination—seem more important in explaining its prevalence than its clinical outcomes, especially since there is little if any credible scientific evidence to sustain its effectiveness.

Grunbaum (1984) specifically rejected Freud's insistence on testing the effectiveness of psychotherapy with the "consilience" of data obtained from patients during therapy. To the contrary, Grunbaum argued that consilience could be produced through the influence of the therapist. It is however worth pointing out that Grunbaum never succeeded in demonstrating even this since his observations were about the theories of psychoanalysis and psychotherapy more than the clinical reality of either. Most telling, to the extent to which the therapist mediates social norms, the process becomes one that realizes Rieff's (1966) criticism of individualism supplanting more noble communal ends. What began as a personal release from social strictures in the pursuit of creativity had become the practice of restraint, the "triumph of the therapeutic,...that a sense of well-being has become the end, rather than a by-product of striving after some superior communal end" (Rieff, p. 261). Rather than analyzing the potency of tools through which "character can be transformed" (p. 36)—its clinical meaning—Rieff actually defined the ascendant soothing fictions of the social clinic. He argued that those fictions of extreme individualism were displacing collective responsibility for the general welfare and perhaps even the most basic communitarian obligations of religious faith.

This transformation of emphasis from the social to the individual along with the rise of the psychotherapeutic clinic has not taken place through insidious influences imposed on an innocent population through evil conspiracies. Rather, the extreme individualism of American society in particular reflects the gradual, consensual, willing acculturation of the masses to innumerable economic and social circumstances. A more caring and sharing society has been repeatedly rejected through ballots and the choices of daily living that accumulate into social policy and social institutions (Epstein 2017).

Freudian psychoanalysis and the emergent popularity of psychotherapy were contemporaries of Madam Blavatsky's theosophy and Mary Baker Eddy's Christian Science each of which appealed to wealthy, influential classes. None of them led missions to the poor or sought social reform. Theosophy was practiced in séances to communicate with the spirits of the dead and Christian Science invoked radical reliance on God's will to cure physical disease. The field of psychotherapy prospered while Theosophy and Christian Science faded away after a few fashionable seasons but not due to any differences in material reality, objectivity, or successful achievement of avowed goals. All of them shared the subjectivities of faith healing and were constructed on metaphysical foundations.

Yet psychoanalysis and the social clinic better affirm popular values, in particular, extreme individualism but also intuitive, implicit sources of truth and a sense of chosenness both personally and as a society. Ironically, Crews' explanation of the ascendancy of psychoanalysis that relies on Freud's extraordinary personal skill as a huckster and shameless conniver—the irresistible momentum of the heroic will—the culture's romantic core of individualism and better accounts for Freud's popularity. Psychotherapy closely replicates the core mythic themes of the culture: self-reliance and thus personal responsibility. The séance was simply too fantastic and the spirits were often discovered behind the curtains as Madam Blavatsky's helpers. For its part, radical reliance was a foolish defiance of the successes of medicine that led at times to death. In contrast, the social clinic directs patients to look inside themselves for truth that with the help of the clinician reveals (or at least comes to an agreement about) their unrealized prowess. In the manner of the typical American religion, personal transformations become acts of individual insight, understanding, and, in the end, individual will. It is no accident that the enormous self-help industry in the United States often pairs its lessons and exhortations with psychotherapy that frequently invokes Jung's mystical constructs of a collective unconscious and the material but unmeasurable actuality of the soul. Psychotherapy turns inward in rejection of social structures and the economic system as sources of individual failure and unhappiness. So too, has the American public.

The Effectiveness of Psychotherapy

Since the publication of *The Benefits of Psychotherapy* (Smith et al. 1980) an increasing number of research papers have attempted to address the field's general effectiveness by summarizing the enormous primary literature of treatment outcomes. By and large, the summaries—meta-analyses, systematic reviews, along with less rigorous box-score tabulations and intuitive summaries—conclude that psychotherapy is effective but less so than the basic outcome research they summarize. The reviews often select for summary only the stronger, more scientifically credible research and occasionally raise points of skepticism. More often they defend the field in spite of the weaknesses of its data. Yet, after employing a truly scientific standard of clinical research—randomized controlled trials along with other research protections—there remains little if any credible evidence to sustain the field's promises of treatment effectiveness. Debilitating meanders from credible scientific practice undercut the best of the research. Researcher bias, other demand characteristics of the research situation itself, nonexistent and compromised controls, attrition, predisposing characteristics of the patients, and additional violations of scientific protocol typically account for the results more than treatment itself.

Exact replication of research is rare and the few outcome studies that seem to be the least biased of the lot may have simply selected fortuitous samples. Indeed, without neutral research situations, that is, research conducted by those without professional or personal stakes in the outcomes, replications simply transmit symmetrical biases through similar demand characteristics of the research situation. It is stunning that no test of psychotherapy's effectiveness has been conducted by independent researchers. None.

Summary assessments of psychotherapy prior to Smith et al. (1980) were often surprisingly critical about its effectiveness. However, their methods were often as impaired as the primary research they evaluated. Eysenck (1952), Eysenck and Rachman (1965) concluded that psychotherapy was no more effective than controls and occasionally even less effective. However, his reviews excluded pertinent research but included faulty controls; some of the analyses were problematic. Rachman (1970) stated that only one of the twenty-three studies reviewed credibly demonstrated positive outcomes. Bergin (1971) found that psychotherapy was only moderately successful; however, his review contained studies without controls and many with other methodological pitfalls.

In contrast, a host of weak subsequent reviews attempted to bury doubts about the effectiveness of psychotherapy (Meltzoff and Kornreich 1970; Luborsky et al. 1975; Gurman and Kniskern 1978; the Office of Technology Assessment 1980; and others). Notably, the succeeding revisions of Bergin's essay (Bergin and Lambert 1978; Lambert et al. 1984; Lambert and Bergin 1994) were buoyant, having discovered nonspecific factors across many therapies.

> Interpersonal and nonspecific or nontechnical factors still loom large as stimulators of patient improvements… These considerations imply that psychotherapy is laden with nonspecific factors or placebo factors…but these influences, when specified, may prove to be the essence of what provides therapeutic benefit. Instead of "controlling" for them in research designs by adopting a spurious parallel with medical placebos, we may be dismissing the active ingredients we are looking for. (Bergin and Lambert 1978, pp. 179–180).

However, these nonspecific factors if in fact they are the essence of successful psychotherapy do not require advanced training in psychotherapy. "Trust, warmth, acceptance and human wisdom" are decidedly not franchised to the field and could be provided at lower cost and perhaps with even greater effect by the loving embrace of naturally empathetic people (ibid.). The essential claims of clinical practice depend on the rare skills of insight provided through long clinical education and mentorship. Yet Dawes (House of Cards 1996) asserts but fails to offer credible evidence that the level of training relates to outcomes. The Bergin essays and the field generally ignore the social alternative to psychotherapy; caring probably needs to be embedded in long processes of socialization in order to produce well-adjusted and productive citizens. The short-term provision of caring through psychotherapy has little demonstrated value.

A placebo by definition must be devoid of therapeutic value but convincing for subjects to believe that they are receiving treatment. Any test of clinical value is fatally impaired without a placebo control. Yet, then and now, the field pleads for a special dispensation from rigor in research—in particular the deployment of placebos, the blinding of evaluators and patients to group assignment, and objective measurement—but yet arrogates the authority of the clinical trial.

Smith et al.'s (1980) seminal meta-analysis attempted to correct the pitfalls of the earlier summary assessments by employing more rigorous methods and a far more comprehensive inclusion of presumably rigorous primary clinical research. They concluded that psychotherapy was enormously effective. "The average person who would score at the 50th percentile of the untreated control population, could expect to rise to the 80th percentile with respect to that population after receiving psychotherapy" (ibid., p. 88). The thirty percentage point advantage covers sixty percent of the maximum 50 percentage point gain. Moreover, patients receiving some form of cognitive therapy were better off than 99% of controls after therapy.

However, the Smith et al. (1980) meta-analysis was itself diminished by serious flaws. Contrary to its claims for applying rigorous scientific standards, the review included many studies that were not randomized. Indeed, repeating Bergin's antipathy to randomized controls, the meta-analysis included studies without controls but only pre/post-comparisons, with waitlist controls, with comparison groups as well as analogue studies and studies whose findings did not reach statistical significance. Randomized controls were sneered at as "'textbook' standards...learned as dicta in graduate school." A reanalysis confined to the randomized studies in Smith, Glass, and Miller, reduced positive outcomes from 30 percentage points to twelve percentage points (Prioleau et al. 1983). A later review of randomized studies confirmed this finding; restricting the analysis to only randomized studies reduces the benefits of psychotherapy to only a sixteen percentage point advantage (Lambert et al. 1993). Smith, Glass, and Miller's own comparison of placebos with other controls reduced the benefits to only about nine percentage points. Yet the placebo studies themselves were porous in other regards, usually related to measurement, blinding, and attrition.

Further problems of psychotherapeutic research generally probably reduce the likely benefits of psychotherapy even further. Rosenthal and Rubin (1978) estimated the size of "expectancy" bias, that is, the degree to which the experimenters' preferences alone rather than therapy itself account for reported outcomes. They concluded on the basis of 345 studies of the phenomenon that expectancy bias was widely prevalent and in "psychophysical judgments" was enormous, distorting reported outcomes by a mean of 26 percentage points. This would explain almost all of the gains of psychotherapy reported by Smith et al. (1980). It also opens the question of patient deterioration in psychotherapy that may be routinely obscured by the subtle insistences of researchers that affect the self-report of symptoms.

In addition, most psychotherapeutic outcome research is conducted under optimal conditions by presumably the most skilled clinicians. Studies rarely include randomly selected community practitioners but most often university-based faculty and clinical staff who are more closely supervised and perhaps even more skilled than the customary solo practitioner. The studies are usually conducted under the unusual conditions of demonstration projects: highly skilled practitioners with great interests in the outcomes evaluated by similarly motivated researchers. Successful demonstrations of effective therapy confer large professional benefits of position, prestige, and income. The absence of protection against bias is a compelling issue.

A further speculation likely reduces the gains of Smith et al. (1980). The meta-analysis did not actually create a pooled data set from the separate studies. Instead it averaged their effect sizes. Thus, the reported averages are like a distribution of sampled means more than a distribution of individual cases and the standard deviations are like standard errors. As a result, the underlying distributions of effect sizes increase enormously and the outcomes of psychotherapy become wildly unpredictable.

A large number of similar reviews shored up the findings of Smith et al. (1980) and largely by repeating its convenient errors (Epstein 1993, 2006). The research avows a commitment to science but then goes on to include flawed research amenable to a large number of biases as well as research designs that cannot test the true effects of psychotherapy. Much of the problem resides with subjective measures since the measurement of symptoms and outcomes typically rely on patient self-report. Truly objective tests in the manner of urine and hair analyses for drug use are rare.

Three large areas of contemporary psychotherapeutic clinical practice—post-traumatic stress disorder, depression, and substance abuse—are analyzed in the next two chapters. The three therapies collectively stand as a representative sample of psychotherapy generally. The analyses rely on the state of the art of psychotherapy outcome research. They draw on the most comprehensive meta-analyses and systemic reviews. A few instances of the most credible primary research that the reviews identify are further analyzed to evaluate the scientific credibility of the reviews' conclusions about effective treatment. Thus, the following discussions of psychotherapy, while necessarily limited, test the clinical value of the field by analyzing a sample of the best reviews that contain the best primary research—the most rigorous tests of effectiveness in three crucial areas of practice. In each area, the field claims to have developed credible evidence of important treatment gains. Yet in each area and indeed throughout psychotherapy and more generally in the social clinic, there have been no decisive tests of effectiveness. Instead, the field has substituted its own consensus for credible science. Few observations offer worse criticism of a community of scholars but unfortunately a criticism that has long outlived its bite.

References

Bausell, R. B. (2007). *Snake Oil Science: The Truth About Complementary and Alternative Medicine*. New York, NY: Oxford University Press.

Bergin, A. E. (1971). The Evaluation of Therapeutic Outcomes. In S. L. Garfield & A. E. Bergin (Eds.), *Handbook of Psychotherapy and Behavior Change*. New York: Wiley and Sons.

Bergin, A. E. & Lambert, M. J. (1978). The Evaluation of Therapeutic Outcomes. In S. L. Garfield & A. E. Bergin (Eds.), *Handbook of Psychotherapy and Behavior Change*. New York: Wiley and Sons.

Crews, F. (1993). The Unknown Freud. *New York Review, 30*(19), 55–66.

Crews, F. (2017). *The Making of an Illusion*. New York: Metropolitan Books.

Dawes, R. M. (1994). *House of Cards: Psychology and Psychotherapy Built on Myth*. New York: Free Press.

Eisenberg, D. M., Davis, R. B., & Ettner, S. L., et al. (1998). Trends in Alternative Medicine Use in the United States: Results of a Follow-Up National Survey. *JAMA, 280*(18), 1569–1575.

Eisenberg, D. M., Kessler, R. C., Foster, C., Norlock F. E., Calkins D. R., & Delbanco T. L. (1993). Unconventional medicine in the United States. *NEngljMed, 328*, 246–252.

Epstein, W. M. (1993). *The Dilemma of American Social Welfare*. New Brunswick, NJ: Transaction Publishers.

Epstein, W. M. (2006). *Psychotherapy as Religion: The Civil Divine in America*. Reno, NV: University of Nevada Press.

Epstein, W. M. (2017). *The Masses Are the Ruling Classes: Policy Romanticism, Democratic Populism, and Social Welfare*. New York, NY: Oxford University Press.

Eysenck, H. J. (1952). The Effects of Psychotherapy: An Evaluation. *Journal of Consulting Psychology, 16*, 319.

Eysenck, H. J., & Rachman, S. (1965). *The Causes and Cures of Neuroses*. San Diego, CA: R. R. Knapp.

Gardner, M. (1998). *Martin Gardner's Table Magic*. Mineola, NY: Dover Publications.

Grunbaum, A. (1984). *The Foundations of Psychoanalysis: A Philosophical Critique*. Berkeley, CA: University of California Press.

Gurman, A. S., & Kniskern, D. P. (1978). Behavioral Marriage Therapy: II. Empirical Perspective. *Family Process, 17*, 139–148.

Horwitz, A. V., & Wakefield, J. C. (2007). *The Loss of Sadness*. New York: Oxford University Press.

Kirk, S. A., & Kutchins, H. (1992). *The Selling of DSM: The Rhetoric of Science in Psychiatry.* New York, NY: Aldine De Gruyter.

Lambert, M. F., & Bergin, A. E. (1994). The Effectiveness of Psychotherapy. In A. E. Begin & S. L. Garfield (Eds.), *Handbook of Psychotherapy and Behavior Change.* New York: Wiley and Sons.

Lambert, M. J., Christensen, E. R., & DeJulio, S. S. (1984). The Assessment of Psychotherapy Outcome. *Psychological Bulletin, 83*(1), 23–62.

Lambert, M. J., et al. (1993). *Psychotherapy versus Placebo Therapies: A Review of the Meta-analysis Literature.* Poster presented at the annual meeting of the Western Psychological Association, Phoenix Arizone, 1993.

Luborsky, et al. (1975). Comparative Studies of Psychotherapies: Is It True that Everyone has Won and All Must Have Prizes? *Archives of General Psychiatry, 32,* 995–1008.

Macmillan, C. (1997). *Freud Evaluated: The Completed Arc Cambridge.* MA: MIT Press.

Meltzoff, J., & Kornreich, M. (1970). *Research in Psychotherapy.* New York: Atherton.

Mohr, D. C., Ho, J., Hart, T. L., Baron, K. G., Berendsen, M., Beckner, V., et al. (2014). Control Condition Design and Implementation Features in Controlled Trials: A Meta-Analysis of Trials Evaluating Psychotherapy for Depression. *Translational Behavioral Medicine Journal, 4,* 407–423. https://doi.org/10.1007/s13142-014-0262-3.

Norcross, J. C., VandenBos, G. R., & Freedheim, D. K. (Eds.). (2011). *History of Psychotherapy: Continuity and Change* (2nd ed.). Washington, DC, USA: American Psychological Association.

Nugent, W. R. (2017). Variability in the Results of Meta-Analysis as a Function of Comparing Effect Sizes Based on Scores From Noncomparable Measures: A Simulation Study. *Education and Psychological Measurement, 77*(3), 449–470.

Office of Technology Assessment. (1980). The Implication sof Cost Effectiveness Analysis of Medical Technology. Background Paper #3: *The Efficacy and Cost Effectiveness of Psychotherapy.* Washington, DC: United States Congress.

Prioleau, L., Murdock, M., & Brody, N. (1983). An Analysis of Psychotherapy Versus Placebo Studies. *Behavior and Brain Sciences, 6,* 275–310.

Rachman, S. (1970). *The Effects of Psychological Treatment.* Oxford: Paragon Press.

Ravetz, J. (1971). *Scientific Knowledge and Its Social Problems.* Oxford: Clarendon Press.

Rieff, P. (1966). *Triumph of the Therapeutic: Uses of Faith After Freud.* New York: Harper and Row.

Rosenthal, R., & Rubin, D. B. (1978). Interpersonal Expectancy Effects—The First 345 Studies. *Behavioral and Brain Sciences, 1,* 377–386. https://doi.org/10.1017/S0140525X00075506.

Singh, S., & Ernst, E. (2008). *Trick or Treatment: The Undeniable Facts About Alternative Medicine.* New York, NY: Norton.

Smith, M. L., Glass, G. V., & Miller, T. I. (1980). *The Benefits of Psychotherapy.* Baltimore, MD: Johns Hopkins University Press.

Wallerstein, R. S. (1995). *The Talking Cures: The Psychoanalyses and the Psychotherapies.* New Haven: Yale University Press.

3

Psychotherapy for Post-traumatic Stress Disorder

In conformity with the American Psychiatric Association's *Diagnostic and Statistical Manual (5th edition)* the National Center for Post-Traumatic Stress Disorder of the US Department of Veterans Affairs defines post-traumatic stress disorder (PTSD) as a serious reaction lasting at least one month to a traumatic event that is experienced either personally as a witness or victim or through a close friend or relative. The traumatic events include death, violence, rape, and assault as examples. The reactions to a traumatic event can include sleeplessness, intrusive thoughts, flashbacks, emotional distress, physical reactions, irritability, aggression, difficulty concentrating, destructive behaviors, and many others that impair normal functioning (https://www.ptsd.va.gov/professional/PTSD-overview/dsm5_criteria_ptsd.asp, July 25, 2017, n.p.). The Clinical Practice Guidelines of the US Veterans Administration "recommends individual trauma-focused psychotherapies, particularly Prolonged Exposure (PE), Cognitive Processing Therapy (CPT) and Eye Movement Desensitization and Reprocessing (EMDR) as the most effective treatments for PTSD.... CPT, PE, and EMDR have shown great success in outcome research" (https://www.ptsd.va.gov/professional/treatment/overview/overview-treatment-research.asp, July 25, 2017, n.p.). In

© The Author(s) 2019
W. M. Epstein, *Psychotherapy and the Social Clinic in the United States*,
https://doi.org/10.1007/978-3-030-32750-7_3

support of the success of these treatments, the VA cites Foa et al. (2005), Resick et al. (2002), Shapiro (1989a, b), and Rothbaum et al. (2005).

Yet three of the four studies, while among the most credible in the literature (the fourth is a case study, see below) and apparently sufficient for government to sanction particular clinical interventions are inadequate to substantiate the VA's claims of successful psychotherapeutic treatments for PTSD. Foa et al. (2005) tested prolonged exposure (PE) with and without cognitive restructuring (CR) at academic and community clinics. "PE includes four components, in the following order: education-rationale, breathing retraining, behavioral exposures, and imaginal exposures" (Resick et al. 2002, p. 867). PE with cognitive restructuring

> was identical to PE alone with two exceptions. Session 3 was devoted to presenting the idea that posttrauma symptoms are maintained in part by trauma related thoughts and beliefs and to practicing CR. Specifically, participants were taught to identify and challenge erroneous and unhelpful beliefs.... Second, all subsequent sessions included 30-45 min [sic] imaginal exposure followed by 15-25 min of CR. (Foa et al. 2005, p. 957)

The study enrolled women "with chronic PTSD resulting from rape, nonsexual assault, or childhood sexual abuse," employed a waitlist control and followed patients for up to one year after therapy (ibid., p. 954). Treatments lasted up to twelve sessions. The research concluded that prolonged exposure was superior to wait-list; that those who completed therapy did better than those who began treatment including those who dropped out; and that cognitive restructuring did not improve outcomes.

At the outset, it is not at all certain that the patient's symptoms were caused by their reports of violence. After all, all the information about backgrounds comes from the patients themselves while the alleged traumas took place an average of nine years before enrollment in treatment. Moreover, the patients typically suffered from other psychological and psychiatric problems along with their diagnosis of PTSD. Still and all, whether in fact PTSD was treated is probably a secondary concern to whether patients in distress were helped by therapy. In the event, there was not much positive gain. The basic effect size improvement for no treatment (the waitlist) was 29 percentage points while prolonged exposure and prolonged exposure with cognitive restructuring, the two treatment conditions, only outperformed no treatment group by 11 and 12 percentage points, respectively. Among subsamples of those who completed treatment, prolonged exposure patients and prolonged exposure with cognitive restructuring patients both improved over nontreatment by 18%. Such as they are, the gains appeared to be stable during the one-year follow-up although attrition continued to increase. However, the waitlist was apparently terminated after the active treatment period thus depriving the research of nontreatment comparisons during the follow-up year.

Even these modest findings are ambiguous because of deficiencies in the research. Attrition was a considerable problem, 34% for prolonged exposure and 41% for prolonged exposure with cognitive restructuring. Curiously only one of the 26 participants assigned to the wait-list dropped out. The authors adjusted for attrition by carrying forward the most recent patient symptom scores that are often higher than their initial scores. The choice of carrying forward the most recent observations probably exaggerates the reported therapeutic effects since many if not most patients experience an initial rush at the beginning of therapy when they are most hopeful to gain remission from their suffering. This positive mood probably results in reporting diminished symptoms. Indeed, the early portions of therapy may have the same effects as a placebo. Yet the alternative intention to treat logic of handling attrition by carrying forward the *initial* clinical scores of patients who were lost to the analysis might well have wiped out any short-term or long-term benefit of treatment.

More problematic, there was no placebo control nor were patients and raters blinded to the assignments. The absence of these precautions creates the possibility, even the likelihood, of exaggerated measures of success. Moreover, waitlist patients may exaggerate their conditions to remain eligible for treatment while a variety of unaddressed biases may have encouraged treated patients to exaggerate their recovery. The latter biases are created by the treatment relationship itself in which pleasant therapists gain the benefits of grateful patients who may feel obliged to report clinical gains as a reward for their therapists' attentions. These deficits in research protocol are enough to seriously diminish any enthusiasm over the small and questionable net benefits of exposure therapy that Foa et al. (2005) reported.

Resick et al. (2002) reported that cognitive processing therapy and prolonged exposure were "highly efficacious" in treating PTSD in female rape victims. Twelve sessions of each treatment were provided during six weeks. In the end, the study found that in the full samples treated patients are from 24 percentage points to 39 percentage points better off than untreated patients, depending on the outcome measure. Completers, depending on the measure, are generally more than 45 percentage points better off than controls. These are huge findings since the maximum percentage point improvement is only fifty points (going from the initial mean of 50 percentage points to the maximum of 100 percentage points).

Once again, the outcome measures relied on patient self-report. The "average length of time since the rape was 8.5 years…with a range of 3 months to 33 years" (ibid., p. 868). Moreover, 31% were taking psychotropic medication while, in addition women, also apparently suffered from other serious psychological and psychiatric problems. Both the deeply troubled patient population and the great amount of time since the initial trauma raise serious questions about the reliability of patient self-report. Reliability is further taxed by the enduring problems of false memories that may be induced by the patient's social situation as well as by reporting conditions, in this case, the research situation itself. The research lacked a placebo control. Neither patients nor evaluators were blind to patient assignment. And quite to the point, demand characteristics may have been subtly introduced into the research situation that encourages patients to report treatment gains. Moreover, the principal author and presumably others are clinical psychologists with apparently great stakes in the effectiveness of the treatments they are evaluating. They collected outcome measures from patients. The research was funded by the National Institute of Mental Health, a federal agency that promotes psychotherapy.

Resick et al. (2002) mentioned problems of attrition: about 23% of those who enrolled but 31% counting those who dropped out after assignment to treatment. To compensate for attrition, they carry forward the most recent observations instead of the original assessments, as in Foa et al. (2005), above, a choice that probably increases the appearance of effective treatment. They also attempt to compensate for "missing data due to drop out by estimating time trend lines for each individual based on available data for that individual as well as information about the parameters of the entire sample" (ibid., p. 873). This highly dubious procedure substitutes the known for the unknown without any ability to test the assumption that they are substantially equivalent.

Resick et al. (2002) insist that the analysis of those who completed treatment is "very important from a clinical standpoint" since, they claim, it answers the question of the therapy's effectiveness when a patient goes through the entire therapeutic regimen. Yet the logic of completer analyses is quite dubious since it attributes the cause of the improvement to the therapy rather than characteristics of the patient, that is, a problem of selection bias. However, in light of substantial attrition, the heightened benefits of completing treatment may be due to a self-selection bias that predisposes certain patients to stay in treatment rather than to the treatment itself. Furthermore, the study's reliance on follow-up data is typically compromised by terminating the waitlist condition at the end of treatment. Yet the study does not translate the amount of gain into its clinical significance. Its statistics focus on relative gain—the degree to which means differ, not the degree to the mean differences, that is, the reported improvements in the treated groups, are clinically important.

In the end, the huge gains of Resnick et al. (2002) are challenged by the study's serious deficiencies: attrition, the absence of a placebo controls, the absence of rater and patient blinding, the likelihood of unreliable patient self-report including false memories, and the failure to isolate the research from the institutional stakes of the researchers, their funding sources and probably the Veterans Administration in creating subtle demands for positive patient self-reports. Indeed, psychotherapy research in general is greatly undercut by the near universal absence of neutral evaluators, neutral evaluation situations, and reliable instrumentation of both diagnosis and outcome measures.

The VA cites Shapiro (1989a) and Rothbaum et al. (2005) in support of the effectiveness of eye movement desensitization and reprocessing (EMDR) in treating PTSD.

> EMDR involves having the patient imagine a scene that represents the worst part of the trauma, focusing on the sensations of distress in her body, and increasing negative thoughts that match the picture. The patient simultaneously follows the therapist's finger moving back and forth approximately 18 in. in front of her, a minimum of 20 times each repetition. (Rothbaum et al. 2005, p. 610)

Employing a randomized design, EMDR was compared with PE and a waitlist control. Participants were female victims aged about 34 years who had been raped more than three months prior to entry into the study. The mean time in the three groups since the rape ranged from about ten to fourteen years. Therapies were provided by "three doctoral psychologists trained in both therapies" (ibid., p. 610). Patients received nine sessions of either therapy; 35% of the sample had only a PTSD diagnosis; the remainder had one or two comorbid conditions.

Sixty of the 74 women enrolled in the study completed treatment and only 3 of those treated were lost to the six-month follow-up. The authors argue that "intention to treat analyses provide no consequentially different results and are not included" in the published report (ibid., p. 611).

The pre-post gains for both treated groups were very large, 47 percentage points out of a possible 50 percentage points. However, comparison to the waitlist reduced the gain to a moderate 21 percentage points. Presumably the unpublished intention to treat analysis further reduces the moderate gains of treatment. Other considerations reduce the credibility of the research and its reported gains even further. The authors claim that the "independent assessors" were blind to the treatment condition. However, it is unlikely that they were blind to the waitlist condition. Moreover, no description is provided of the independence of the assessors. Being formally independent of the research is not the equivalent of lacking stakes in its outcomes. Thus, the use of graduate students and others as assessors who are active in the psychotherapy field fails as a warrant for independence. Finally, measures of symptoms were self-reported and thus likely to be reactive to the research situation by reflecting gratitude for therapy, appreciation of therapist concern, and other sources of bias rather than the actual state of the patient's PTSD symptoms.

Shapiro (1989a) cited by the VA in support of the effectiveness of EMDR in treating PTSD is a case study which states that "the procedure can be extremely effective in only one session as indicated by a previous controlled study and a case history presented here" (ibid., p. 21). To say the least, case studies are hardly important proofs of outcomes or even credible clinical statements without objective verification of outcomes. In the case study, the therapist is evaluating her own treatment. To cite so prominently such a questionable study as definitive proof of general effectiveness raises questions about the VA's judgment. It is possible that the VA meant to cite Shapiro (1989b). Yet even this controlled study is quite deficient.

To test the effectiveness of EMDR against PTSD, Shapiro (1989b) randomized 22 patients—five males and eleven females—diagnosed by their therapists as suffering from PTSD to either a treatment group or a placebo group that became a delayed treatment group. Most of the patients appeared to have been assault and rape victims; one and possibly a few more may have been veterans of the US military. Five of them appear to have been "mental health professionals who desired relief from traumatic memories" (ibid., p. 202). Treatment took place in only one session that continued until patients reported the remission of symptoms. All subjects were evaluated before treatment, post-treatment, one month, and three months later. There was no attrition. The reported results were spectacular: All subjects benefited enormously to the point of remission. Results were maintained at follow-up. "The evidence clearly indicates that a single session of the EMDR procedure is effective in desensitizing memories of traumatic incidents and changing the subjects' cognitized assessments of their individual situations" (ibid., p. 216).

However, Shapiro was again the author of the study, the sole provider of treatment in the experiment, and the sole assessor of results to whom patients reported their symptoms as well as the developer of the EMD procedure itself. She argues at length but unconvincingly that experimenter bias, patient expectancies, and demand characteristics played little if any part in creating the results. Simply one of these roles compromises the independence of evaluation and should disqualify participation in the research. Moreover, the reliability of the instrumentation that measured symptoms is not discussed while no standardized process seems to have been employed to diagnose PTSD. It is also worth wondering how many patients reported remission so as to terminate treatment. Shapiro (1989b) may be superior to a case study but not by much.

Yet the Veterans Administration considers these four trials and a case history to provide the most credible evidence of the effectiveness of psychotherapy for PTSD and presumably with military veterans. "These treatments have been tested in numerous clinical trials, in patients with complex presentations and comorbidities, in comparison to active control conditions, and with long-term follow-up designs" (https://www. ptsd.va.gov/professional/PTSD-overview/dsm5_criteria_ptsd.asp, July 25, 2017, n.p.). It is more than a little strange that only one of these five studies contains any military veterans (and possibly only one in Shapiro 1989b). The overwhelming number of these patients are female with PTSD subsequent to rape or other forms of assault.

Besides prolonged exposure, cognitive processing therapy and EMDR, the VA also recommends other therapies—exposure therapy, brief eclectic therapy, narrative exposure therapy, and written narrative exposure therapy—but with less enthusiasm since apparently less rigorous research provides only "sufficient evidence" of effectiveness. As for the variety of additional therapies—e.g., Seeking Safety, hypnosis, brief psychodynamic therapy, and others—"at this time, there are insufficient data [to] conclude whether these treatments are helpful (or harmful) to individuals with PTSD" (https://www.ptsd.va.gov/professional/treatment/overview/overview-treatment-research.asp, July 25, 2017, n.p.).

The best of the recent reviews—meta-analyses and systematic reviews—of PTSD generally follows a pattern that does not improve on the VA's base of clinical authority. The recent reviews report considerable effectiveness for uncontrolled, pre-posttreatment comparisons, much less effectiveness for waitlist comparisons and, echoing Prioleau et al. (1983), only modest positive outcomes if any in studies that compare treatment groups to placebo controls.[1] And then again, "Several including those that provided more positive results, had strong methodological characteristics" (Roberts 2012, p. 15). Yet, the positive results were inconsistent and relatively weak while the methodological characteristics are strong only in comparison with highly compromised research. Most frequently the primary research summarized in the reviews compares different treatments to each other or to treatment as usual and less often compares treatments to wait-list controls and rarely to placebos.

The reviews frequently document methodological problems that seriously undercut the credibility of the research. Nonetheless, they proceed to assert clinically important prowess for a variety of psychotherapeutic interventions to handle PTSD. Forneris et al. (2013) identified only 19 studies of interventions to prevent PTSD among the selective Cochrane Collaboration base of research that met their inclusion criteria. They concluded that "brief trauma-focused cognitive behavioral therapy was more effective than supportive counseling" but then cautioned that "evidence about relevant outcomes was unavailable for many interventions or was insufficient owing to methodologic shortcomings" and that "evidence is very limited regarding best practices to treat trauma-exposed individuals" (ibid., p. 635 passim).

Mendes et al. (2008) reviewed the 23 most scientifically credible evaluations of cognitive behavioral therapy's effects on PTSD. They reached the happy conclusion that "cognitive behavioral therapy, exposure therapy and cognitive therapy are equally effective" (ibid., p. 242) but acknowledged that these results are based only on the analysis of those who completed therapy. The intention to treat analyses addressing dropouts found no statistically significant and thus no clinically significant advantages for any among the therapies covered in the research.

---

[1]Roberts et al. (2015) note a rare exception of stronger research producing larger effect sizes.

Moreover, comparisons with controls—waitlists in this review—that are necessary to estimate the basic effectiveness of therapy were not possible because large differences between the groups presumably due to attrition prevented meaningful comparisons. Thus, significant differences among the therapies depended on the bias of studying only the self-selected group of those who completed therapy while tests of basic effectiveness were prevented by the absence of relevant controls. In the absence of appropriate controlled comparisons, Mendes et al. (2008) should also have addressed the possibility, even the likelihood, that all positive reported outcomes were due to natural remission, biases in reporting and evaluation, small fortuitous samples, and others shortcomings of the research.

Making a point of deep skepticism, Ehlers et al. (2010) argue that the literature has not demonstrated that "treatments for PTSD are more effective than natural recovery" (p. 269). Natural recovery is not adequately tested by delayed treatment waitlist controls for reasons discussed in this section. Placebos are required over a long enough period to test natural processes. However, the belief in the efficacy of current therapies erects legal and ethical barriers to the employment of long-term controls. Still, together with Van der Kolk's argument for the necessity of a caring community, almost all recovery from PTSD might be accounted for by natural processes coincidental with fortuitous social supports as discussed below. Indeed, positive effect sizes in analyses that include adjustments for attrition are so modest, small, and often nonexistent that if all of the biases that exaggerate the reports of positive outcomes are considered, a cautious estimate of the effects of therapy might be forced to consider harm as a routine outcome of psychotherapy for PTSD.

Even the very best of the most highly screened base of research is quite inadequate to the task of assessing the effects of psychotherapy on PTSD. Out of an initial pool of 897 studies contained in the Cochrane Library's authoritative Database of Systematic Reviews only 14 met Roberts et al.'s (2015) inclusion criteria of methodological rigor. The Cochrane Library collects the highest quality research in a number of fields including psychotherapy. Yet even this very small group of research was judged as seriously compromised: "all findings were judged as being of low/very low quality" (ibid., p. 25). Their review confirmed the common observation that the joint occurrence of PTSD and substance abuse "are common, difficult to treat, and associated with poor prognosis" (ibid., p. 25). However, they still retrieve the very qualified finding from a weak pool of research that "a trauma-focused component *alongside* intervention for substance abuse disorder can help reduce PTSD symptom severity for individuals" with both problems (ibid., p. 34). Yet even these findings are acknowledged as small and in the context of weak research with high attrition they seem to be pointless. Unfortunately, the authors' attention to treatment completers begins to suggest a false inference (defying the logic of the intention to treat rule) that the completion of therapy would have helped those who dropped out. The intention to treat rule counts drop outs as failures by way of reducing the possible bias of self-selection. That is, those who complete treatment may be among the most amenable for cure and may in fact not need it. Completers are probably quite different than dropouts—after all they had the resilience or motivation to complete therapy. Thus, attributing their experience to drops is not legitimate. In the event, dropouts exceeded 30% in all but one study and reached 72% in another.[2]

In their meta-analysis of early psychological interventions for acute PTSD, Roberts et al. (2012) analyzed fifteen of the very best studies and included two more that reported long-term follow-up. Treatments began within three months of the traumatic event. The analysis concluded that

> Trauma-focused cognitive behavior therapy had greater effect than waiting list/usual care and supportive counselling at reducing traumatic stress symptoms in individuals who were symptomatic at entry into the study... The only evidence to support any other form of treatment was

---

[2]After repeatedly concluding that "the quality of evidence of the findings was graded as low to very low," Roberts et al. (2015) paradoxically state that "most studies were of good methodological quality" (ibid., p. 31) but then go on in the same paragraph to mention routine problems of blinding patients and assessors and the fact that "the level of drop-out was high across all studies" (ibid.).

for cognitive restructuring, which was also demonstrated to have a greater effect than a waiting list intervention on the primary outcome measure but less effective than Trauma-focused cognitive behavior therapy. (ibid., p. 14)

The authors of the meta-analysis point to a variety of problems in the base of their studies that reduces confidence in even these limited findings. Samples were often very small; only 6 of the 15 studies adequately blinded patients to their assignments; only 10 of the 15 incorporated blind assessment; there was great variety in the "clinical populations, especially with regards to the severity of symptoms at entry to the studies" with the result that findings between studies may not have been routinely comparable (ibid., p. 13). Their general assessment of methodological impediments in the covered research is telling.

> As with all psychological treatment trials there are issues with the control groups. This is particularly important in early intervention research where a reduction in symptoms over the duration of the trial would be expected *given the natural course of the traumatic stress reactions*. The development of a psychological treatment placebo is very difficult, if not impossible, as is blinding of participants and therapists. (emphasis added ibid., p. 15)

This concession is an acknowledgment that the best of the research may be inadequate to the task of testing the effectiveness of treatments. Nonetheless, in an earlier meta-analysis, Roberts et al. (2012) included 15 of the most credible primary tests of the effectiveness of psychotherapy for PSTD with co-occurring substance abuse. They concluded that "there was evidence to support the use of trauma focused cognitive behavioral therapy...although there were a number of potential biases in identified studies which means the results should be treated with some caution" (ibid., p. 2).

Yet, the 6 most scientifically sophisticated studies that Roberts et al. (2012) identified fail to sustain even their cautious optimism. The meta-analysis judged that Bryant et al. (2005), Ehlers et al. (2003), Bugg et al. (2009), Van Emmerik et al. (2008), Bisson et al. (2004), and Zatzick et al. (2004) provided adequate support for their separate findings with a low risk of bias. Nonetheless, each of the six was seriously flawed, offering little if any credible evidence that psychotherapy is an effective treatment for PTSD.

Bryant et al. (2005) found that six sessions of cognitive behavioral therapy with and without supportive hypnosis was superior at the end of treatment to supportive counseling in addressing trauma subsequent to nonsexual assault and motor vehicle accidents. However, even by employing a convenient adjustment for attrition (bringing forward the most recent measure instead of the pretreatment measure) differences evaporated after three years. There was no nontreatment, placebo, or delayed treatment control. All data were self-reported to presumably "independent clinicians."

Bisson et al. (2004) treated PTSD subsequent to physical injury with four sessions of cognitive behavioral therapy. After 13 months the treated group was less distressed than the nontreated control on two of six measures. Attrition was again handled by carrying forward the most recent score rather than the initial score. All measures except one were self-rated; however, all data were self-reports. More than 80% of both groups was considered to have only a "minor" reaction to trauma. The authors report statistical significance but acknowledge that the largest improvements took place in both groups as a function of time; "the treatment effect was modest" and seemingly not clinically substantial. But "time" in this context is a metaphor and perhaps the more important research question would pursue the conditions—family and community support, individual resilience and others—that seem to have had a more important effect on reactions to trauma than treatment. In short, results were episodic, perhaps even clinically unimportant while the data were collected in a manner that failed to discourage report bias. The small findings seem to estimate research enthusiasm more than clinical treatment.

The other four evaluations of treatment effectiveness for PTSD that Roberts et al. (2012) judged to be the most scientifically credible were also invalidated by similar problems and others as well. Bugg et al. (2009) tested "writing as a self-help intervention for patients at risk of developing PTSD." However, the risk was never demonstrated; the intervention was trivial; attrition topped 50% without intention to treat adjustment; self-selection bias was not handled; there were no adequate controls and the improvements in both groups were likely due to natural healing if in fact there was a risk of trauma to begin with. Van Emmerik (2008) compared structured writing therapy and cognitive therapy to a waitlist control. No differences in outcomes were reported between the two therapies while both appeared to confer modest benefits in comparison with the waitlist controls. However, attrition was very high, reaching 47% at follow-up and not random; intention to treat adjustments was not made; more distressed patients seemed to drop out, and thus the treatment samples were not representative of the problem. Zatzick et al. (2004) tested the effectiveness of collaborative care against usual care for acutely injured trauma survivors. Collaborative care incorporated case management with drug therapy and psychotherapy over one year. The total professional time, mostly case management, provided to collaborative care patients appears to be about 14 hours over a period of one year. During the one year of the study, there were no apparent or statistically significant differences between the incidence of PTSD among the collaborative care patients or the usual care patients. There was however a large increase in the rate of reported alcoholism among the usual care patients. All but one of the measures were based on self-report. In addition, none of these three studies employed independent raters; blinding was not certain; self-reports may have been unreliable and differential between controls and treated groups; the clinical meaning of the measured improvements even when statistically significant was usually neither clear nor dramatic; and recruitment procedures often produced questionably representative samples.

Yet Ehlers et al. (2003) stand out from even the best of the research included in the Kitchiner et al. (2012) meta-analysis: very low attrition, the likelihood of representative samples, careful procedures, attempts at neutral evaluation, relatively large outcomes clearly related to clinical significance, and interpretations attentive to points of skepticism toward their own findings. Ehlers et al. found that cognitive therapy was much more effective in treating trauma subsequent to a motor vehicle accident than either a self-help booklet or repeated assessment.

Yet, this careful study still fails as a definitive test of psychotherapy for PTSD. Its samples were small, only about 25 and restricted to

England. Rater blinding was at best only partial since clues to assignments would often become obvious during clinician ratings. Patient blinding was not maintained; patients were quite aware of their assignment to cognitive therapy or to one of two control conditions (self-help and repeated assessments). As a result, demand characteristics based on the researchers' stake in cognitive therapy may have exerted an influence over patient self-reports of symptoms (clinician assessments were still based on patient reports of symptoms). Patients in the two controls were also "informed that they would be offered [cognitive therapy] 9 months later if they still needed help with their symptoms" which may have encouraged them to exaggerate reports of their symptoms (ibid., p. 1025). Moreover, the research sample did not appear to be severely traumatized at pretreatment; the samples were only moderately anxious and depressed and barely qualified as disabled. Its representativeness of trauma victims of motor vehicle accidents may have been compromised by recruitment procedures that may have attracted patients relatively motivated for cure and perhaps even amenable to the rationalistic procedures of cognitive therapy; prospective subjects were required to respond to a leaflet describing PTSD and the availability of treatment by actively seeking further information. Finally, the research only concerned itself with therapy for trauma subsequent to a motor vehicle accident. Trauma subsequent to violence may pose greater challenges for recovery.

In the end, the best of the best primary research included in Roberts et al. (2012), one of the most selective meta-analyses, is not very good at all. They are inadequate tests of the effectiveness of psychotherapy for PTSD and incapable of dispelling the suspicion that treatment is ineffective and possibly even harmful.

Ehring et al. (2014) conducted a meta-analysis of psychotherapeutic effectiveness for PTSD in adult survivors of childhood abuse. Sixteen randomized studies met their inclusion criteria. They provided between six and 25 sessions of treatment. Sample sizes ranged from 11 to 77. Only 5 of the 16 studies incorporated all six of the study characteristics that Ehring et al. considered hallmarks of high-quality research. Ehring et al. reported an average 39 percentage point improvement of PTSD symptoms in pre-posttreatment; a 26 percentage point improvement for treated patients compared with waitlist patients; and a substantial fall off to 19 percentage point improvement when treated patients were compared with treatment as usual or placebo controls. The authors interpret these results as medium to large effects. However, subtracting the effect sizes of pre-posttreatment for controls from that of treated groups reduces the net gain of treatment to only 14 percentage points (patients who are treated are better off than 14% of those who are not). Follow-up improvement was large for uncontrolled groups.

Ehring et al. (2014) did not compute follow-up effects for controlled studies, claiming that the four controlled studies that followed their patients did not provide sufficient data to conduct similar analyses. It is understandable that few controlled studies conducted follow-up assessments since most control groups provide treatment after the experimental group is treated. Both in this event and when the delay of treatment is longer, many control patients seek alternative treatment or are lost to the analysis. Nonetheless, with such a large amount of natural remission reported in control groups, the absence of follow-up in controlled studies is itself a challenge to demonstrating the efficacy of treatment. It is also worth considering that Ehring et al. incorporated a restrictive definition of dropout—having attended no treatment session after random assignment—that minimizes the size of attrition but may still pose a threat to the representativeness of treatment samples. The same definition could not be applied to wait-list, treatment as usual and placebo controls. Yet, in spite of serious reported deviations from optimal research procedures, the authors still conclude without much hesitation that "psychological interventions for PTSD in adult survivors of childhood abuse are efficacious" (ibid., p. 653).

More problematic, as Ehring et al. (2014) acknowledge, "only five studies met all six methodological quality criteria assessed in this meta-analysis" (ibid., p. 649). Yet, while each reports important treatment gains for a variety of therapies, serious pitfalls compromise the credibility of findings in even this elite group. Resick et al. (2008) report large gains of 12 hours of psychotherapy for PTSD in women who were victims of interpersonal violence. However, attrition reached 43% and the gains are greatly exaggerated if their intention to treat adjustment brought forward the most recent clinical measure instead of the original one as in Resick et al. (2002, above). The research lacked a control. However, the large gains at the six month follow-up of the untreated group that had dropped out before the first session of therapy (often about half as much as the reported gains for those who completed treatment) cut against the author's claims that controls were not needed—"there have been ample studies of chronic PTSD that indicate little change over time without active intervention" (Resick et al. 2008, p. 253). The contention hides behind weak research; it is also obviously contradicted within their own study. Moreover, those who completed treatment did no better than the total group that include patients who had dropped out at a variety of times.

The other four among the five most methodologically credible studies of PTSD effectiveness against childhood sexual abuse that Ehring et al. (2014) cite are similarly flawed. McDonagh et al. (2005) compared the effectiveness of cognitive behavioral therapy in treating chronic stress disorder with problem-centered therapy and a waitlist. Their conclusion that patients who received cognitive behavioral therapy fared as well as patients assigned to problem-solving behavior and the waitlist is undercut by their procedures. Samples were small and the dropout rate for the cognitive behavior condition was 42% while those who dropped out were more traumatized than those who completed therapy. Thus, the interventions were measured against a more amenable group for recovery. The representativeness of their treatment sample is further impaired by their initial screening procedure for subjects which again seemed to select those who were less traumatized and troubled. Not surprisingly, the waitlist patients made substantial gains measured by the most common measure of PTSD (the Clinician-Administered Posttraumatic Stress Disorder Scale). Finally, the small measured differences in outcomes between treatment groups and the waitlist were statistically significant in 7 of 8 comparisons only against a probability standard of .10. The eighth comparison was significant against the standard criteria of .05 employed in the overwhelming majority of similar studies. The fact that The Journal of Consulting and Clinical Psychology—among the most influential journals in clinical psychology—published McDonagh et al. (2005) says much about the weakness of the field itself and its strained reach for supportive evidence. Cloitre et al. (2010),

Chard (2005), and Van der Kolk (2007) are similarly impaired: small and questionably representative samples, large attrition, dubious choices to adjust for attrition, absence of neutral measurement, little attention to patient report biases, absence of adequate controls (sometimes lacking even a waitlist), lack of follow-up nontreatment comparisons, and others.

In all, Ehring et al.'s (2014) five most methodologically sound studies failed to employ methods to handle the likelihood of researcher biases including demand characteristics as well as of patients' faulty and biased self-reports. Treatments were invariably short, rarely lasting more than 12 hours over three months. The studies also frequently employed self-serving analytic procedures that illegitimately boosted the appearance of effectiveness. The most credible research identified in one of the most careful meta-analyses provides little confidence in the ability of psychotherapy to treat PTSD among survivors of childhood sexual abuse with short and relatively superficial interventions.

The best reviews of the outcome research of psychotherapeutic treatments for PTSD are equivocal, not nearly as positive as the VA claims. Guarded as they are, the best of the outcome reviews still overstates the credibility of the primary research to often conclude that cognitive behavioral therapy is probably the most successful. Nonetheless, the most credible primary research that they cite is too impaired to sustain even their temporizing conclusions. Typically, the most selective of the reviews (including Swan et al. 2017; Forman-Hoffman 2003; Cusack et al. 2016; Visser et al. 2015; Dinnen et al. 2015; Banks et al. 2015; Gerger et al. 2013; Barrera et al. 2013; Dossa and Hatem 2012; Van Dam 2012; Haugen et al. 2012; Crumlish and O'Rourke 2010; among others) often reach wary conclusions about the literature's scientific credibility but invariably mute their analytic skepticism in order to squeeze a few drops of effectiveness out of bruised fruit. Analysts who are not committed to psychotherapy, that is, neutral critics, might interpret the same primary evidence as a profound challenge to the clinical claims that any form of psychotherapy provides effective treatment for PTSD.

The best of the research covered by the reviews is deeply flawed—researcher and institutional biases, lack of blinding, large attrition, questionable patient self-report, and others. Moreover, while the best of the research randomizes their samples into treatment and control groups, few introduce placebo controls and even fewer are able to conduct follow-up assessments against controls. Even more problematic, none of the samples are randomly drawn from the population with PTSD; as a result, the representativeness of the samples and the meaning of results are always difficult if not impossible to interpret. The patients who end up in the primary research are often referred from clinics and have lengthy histories of psychotherapy, many respond to advertisements. In these ways, research samples may well be relatively motivated for cure and thus more amenable for treatment compared to those with PTSD who are not in treatment and do not appear in the research sample. Their motivation may also increase the likelihood of false self-reports of symptoms: exaggerating persistence on waitlists and underreporting severity in treatment samples, both of which would inflate estimates of effectiveness. Furthermore, the primary research pays little attention to the possibility that positive results when they occur may be fortuitous artifacts of the common small samples involved in psychotherapy. Few studies report harm in treatment. In the end, there is little if any credible evidence that psychotherapy is an effective treatment for PTSD and little concern that it may be routinely harmful.

It is worth considering that the VA and NIMH, as agencies of government that presumably bear the obligation for objective and neutral assessment in protection of the health of the nation, are simply carrying forward the stakes of the treatment community and apparently the priorities of the society. The VA offers very little critical scrutiny of the research. In fact, the VA funds and houses much of the deficient research. The VA's medical system incorporates the social clinic while the society's priorities, expressed in the annual Federal budget, obviously prizes social efficiency over successful treatment. This tradeoff is quite understandable insofar as successful treatment following Van der Kolk (2015) involves the great expense of protracted care. In contrast, many of the favored treatments involve only a handful of short (usually one hour) sessions with a therapist.

Van der Kolk argues that

In order to recover, mind, body, and brain need to be convinced that it is safe to let go. That happens only when you feel safe at a visceral level and allow yourself to connect that sense of safety with memories of past helplessness....After an acute trauma, like an assault, accident, or natural disaster, survivors require the presence of familiar people, faces and voices; physical contact; food; shelter and a safe place and time to sleep. It is critical to communicate with loved ones close and far and to reunite as soon as possible with family and friends in a place that feels safe. Our attachment bonds are our greatest protection against threat. (ibid., p. 212)

Quite distinct from psychotherapy, this caring alternative provides the material conditions that presumably promote recovery—warm social contact, food, shelter, and safety. Yet it is also important to point out that this caring alternative to psychotherapy for PTSD has not been tried or tested and the rare examples Van der Kolk cites in support of his theory are not at all compelling. The uncertain contrast between children who stayed with their parents in London during World War II blitzkrieg and those sent "to the countryside for protection" is at best suggestive (ibid., p. 213). Worse, his reliance on the common belief that "traumatized human beings recover in the context of relationships: with families, loved ones, AA meetings, veterans' organizations, religious communities, or professional organizations" is not sustained by the citation of any research. In fact, there is no credible research to sustain the therapeutic virtues of any of these elements. Indeed, recovery in these relationships if in fact it occurs remains plausibly due to natural healing. Nevertheless, the common assumption of supportive caring as a necessary condition to address trauma and unbearable stress seems so humane and so much an article of social parity that it should in fact inspire interventions when other remedies for PTSD as well as other emotional and mental problems fail.

The policy choice is stark and difficult: either continue with ineffective treatments or try something different although considerably costlier and also uncertain. More importantly, the reality of this dilemma that will probably continue reveals an important theme in American society and politics. The nation would rather continue the soothing fiction of psychotherapeutic treatment than incur large public costs in behalf of traumatized, deserving groups. The costs are multiplied greatly by attending to the needs for care of other obviously deserving citizens: foster children, poor children generally, the millions of totally and permanently disabled, the elderly poor, the technologically displaced, and many others. The caring function might also be enlarged under assumptions of social discrimination to include the economically displaced and disadvantaged. Yet American society has routinely rejected a generous social welfare policy.

References

Banks, K., Newman, E., & Saleem, J. (2015). An Overview of the Research on Mindfulness-Based Interventions for Treating Symptoms of Posttraumatic Stress Disorder: A Systematic Review. *Journal of Clinical Psychology, 71,* 935–963. https://doi.org/10.1002/jclp.22200tyPress.

Barrera, T., Mott, J., Hofstein, R., & Teng, E. (2013). A Meta-Analytic Review of Exposure in Group Cognitive Behavioral Therapy for Posttraumatic Stress Disorder. *Clinical Psychology Review, 33,* 24–32. https://doi.org/10.1016/j.cpr.2012.09.005.

Bisson, J. I., Shepherd, J. P., Joy, D., Probert, R., & Newcombe, R. G. (2004). Early Cognitive-Behavioural Therapy for Post-Traumatic Stress Symptoms After Physical Injury. *British Journal of Psychiatry, 184,* 63–69. https://doi.org/10.1192/bjp.184.1.63.

Bryant, R. A., Moulds, M. L., Guthrie, R. M., & Nixon, R. D. (2005). The Additive Benefits of Hypnosis and Cognitive-Behavioral Therapy in Treating Acute Stress Disorder. *American Psychological Association, 73,* 334–340. https://doi.org/10.1037/0022-006X.73.2.334.

Bugg, A., Turpin, G., Mason, S., & Scholes, C. (2009). A Randomised Controlled Trial of the Effectiveness of Writing as a Self-Help Intervention for Traumatic Injury Patients at Risk of Developing Post-Traumatic Stress Disorder. *Behaviour Research and Therapy, 47*(1), 6–12. https://doi.org/10.1016/j.brat.2008.10.006.

Chard, K. M. (2005). An Evaluation of Cognitive Processing Therapy for the Treatment of Posttraumatic Stress Disorder Related to Childhood Sexual Abuse. *Journal of Consulting and Clinical Psychology, 73,* 965–971.

Cloitre, M., et al. (2010). Treatment for PTSD Related to Childhood Abuse: A Randomized Controlled Trial. *American Journal of Psychiatry, 167*(8), 915–924.

Crumlish, N., & O'Rourke, K. (2010). A Systematic Review of Treatments for Post-Traumatic Stress Disorder Among Refugees and Asylum-Seekers. *The Journal of Nervous and Mental Disease, 198*, 237–251. https://doi.org/10.1097/NMD.0b013e3181d61258.

Cusack, K., Jonas, D. E., Forneris, C. A., Wines, C., Sonis, J., Cook Middleton, J., et al. (2016). Psychological Treatments for Adults with Posttraumatic Stress Disorder: A Systematic Review and Meta-Analysis. *Clinical Psychology Review, 43*, 128–141. https://doi.org/10.1016/j.cpr.2015.10.003.

Dinnen, S., Simiola, V., & Cook, J. M. (2015). Post-Traumatic Stress Disorder in Older Adults: A Systematic Review of the Psychotherapy Treatment Literature. *Aging & Mental Health, 19*, 144–150. https://doi.org/10.1080/13607863.2014.920299.

Dossa, N. I., & Hatem, M. (2012). Cognitive-Behavioral Therapy Versus Other PTSD Psychotherapies as Treatment for Women Victims of War-Related Violence: A Systematic Review. *The Scientific World Journal, 2012*, 1–19. https://doi.org/10.1100/2012/181847.

Ehlers, A., Bisson, J., Clark, D. M., Creamer, M., Pilling, S., Richards, D., et al. (2010). Do All Psychological Treatments Really Work the Same in Posttraumatic Stress Disorder? *Clinical Psychology Review, 30*, 269–276. https://doi.org/10.1016/j.cpr.2009.12.001.

Ehlers, A., Clark, D. M., Hackmann, A., McManus, F., Fennell, M., Herbert, C., et al. (2003). A Randomized Controlled Trial of Cognitive Therapy, a Self-Help Booklet, and Repeated Assessments as Early Interventions for Posttraumatic Stress Disorder. *Archive of General Psychiatry, 60*, 1024–1032.

Ehring, T., et al. (2014). Meta-Analysis of Psychological Treatments for Posttraumatic Stress Disorder in Adult Survivors of Childhood Abuse. *Clinical Psychology Review, 34*(8), 645–657.

Foa, E. B., Hembree, E. A., Cahill, S. P., Rauch, S. A., Riggs, D. S., Yadin, E., et al. (2005). Randomized Trial of Prolonged Exposure for Posttraumatic Stress Disorder With and Without Cognitive Restructuring: Outcome at Academic and Community Clinics. *Journal of Consulting and Clinical Psychology, 73*, 953–964. https://doi.org/10.1037/0022-006X.73.5.953.

Forman-Hoffman, V. L. (2003). Comparative Effectiveness of Interventions for Children Exposed to Nonrelational Traumatic Events. *Pediatrics, 131*(3), 526–539.

Forneris, C. A., Gartlehner, G., Brownley, K. A., Gaynes, B. N., Sonis, J., Coker-Schwimmer, E., et al. (2013). Interventions to Prevent Post-Traumatic Stress Disorder: A Systematic Review. *American Journal of Preventative Medicine, 44*, 635–650. https://doi.org/10.1016/j.amepre.2013.02.013.

Gerger, H., Munder, T., & Barth, J. (2013). Specific and Nonspecific Psychological Interventions for PTSD Symptoms: A Meta-Analysis with Problem Complexity as a Moderator. *Journal of Clinical Psychology, 70*(7), 601–615.

Haugen, P. T., Evces, M., & Weiss, D. S. (2012). Treating Posttraumatic Stress Disorder in First Responders: A Systematic Review. *Clinical Psychology Review, 32,* 370–380. https://doi.org/10.1016/j.cpr.2012.04.001.

Kitchiner, N. J., et al. (2012). Systematic Review and Meta-Analyses of Psychosocial Interventions for Veterans of the Military. *European Journal of Psychotraumatology, 3,* 1–16. http://dx.doi.org/10.3402/ejpt.v3i0.19267.

McDonagh, A., et al. (2005). Randomized Trial of Cognitive-Behavioral Therapy for Chronic Posttraumatic Stress Disorder in Adult Female Survivors of Childhood Sexual Abuse. *Journal of Consulting and Clinical Psychology, 73*(3), 515–524.

Mendes, D. D., Mello, M. F., Ventura, P., De Medeiros Passarela, C., & De Jesus Mari, J. (2008). A Systematic Review on the Effectiveness of Cognitive Behavioral Therapy for Posttraumatic Stress Disorder. *International Journal of Psychiatry in Medicine, 38,* 241–259. https://doi.org/10.2190/PM.38.3.b.

Prioleau, L., Murdock, M., & Brody, N. (1983). An Analysis of Psychotherapy Versus Placebo Studies. *Behavior and Brain Sciences, 6,* 275–310.

Resick, P. A., Nishith, P., Weaver, T. L., Astin, M. C., & Feuer, C. A. (2002). A Comparison of Cognitive-Processing Therapy with Prolonged Exposure and a Waiting Condition for the Treatment of Chronic Posttraumatic Stress Disorder in Female Rape Victims. *Journal of Consulting and Clinical Psychology, 70,* 867–879. https://doi.org/10.1037/0022-006X.70.4.867.

Resick, P. A., et al. (2008). A Randomized Clinical Trial to Dismantle Components of Cognitive Processing Therapy for Posttraumatic Stress Disorder in Female Victims of Interpersonal Violence. *Journal of Consulting and Clinical Psychology, 76*(2), 243–258.

Roberts, N. P., Kitchiner, N. J., Kenardy, J., & Bisson, J. I. (2012). Early Psychological Interventions to Treat Acute Traumatic Stress Symptoms (Review). *Cochrane Database of Systematic Reviews,* 1–81. http://dx.doi.org/10.1002/14651858.CD007944.pub2.

Roberts, N. P., Roberts, P. A., Jones, N., & Bisson, J. I. (2015). Psychological Interventions for Post-Traumatic Stress Disorder and Comorbid Substance Use Disorder: A Systematic Review and Meta-Analysis. *Clinical Psychology Review, 38,* 25–38. https://doi.org/10.1016/j.cpr.2015.02.007.

Rothbaum, B. O., Astin, M. C., & Marsteller, F. (2005). Prolonged Exposure Versus Eye Movement Desensitization and Reprocessing (EMDR) for PTSD Rape Victims. *Journal of Traumatic Stress, 18,* 607–616. https://doi.org/10.1002/jts.20069.

Shapiro, F. (1989a). Efficacy of the Eye Movement Desensitization Procedure in the Treatment of Traumatic Memories. *Journal of Traumatic Stress, 2,* 199–223.

Shapiro, F. (1989b). Eye Movement Desensitization: A New Treatment for Post-Traumatic Stress Disorder. *Journal of Behavioral Therapy and Experimental Psychiatry, 20,* 211–217.

Swan, S., Keen, N., Reynolds, N., & Onwumere, J. (2017). Psychological Interventions for Post-Traumatic Stress Symptoms in Psychosis: A Systematic Review of Outcomes. *Frontiers in Psychology, 8,* 1–14.

Van Dam, V., et al. (2012). Psychological Treatments for Concurrent Posttraumatic Stress Disorder and Substance Use Disorder: A Systematic Review. *Clinical Psychology Review, 2*(3), 202–214.

Van der Kolk, B. A. (2007). A Randomized Clinical Trial of Eye Movement Desensitization and Reprocessing (EMDR), Fluoxetine, and Pill Placebo in the Treatment of Posttraumatic Stress Disorder: Treatment Effects and Long-Term Maintenance. *Journal of Clinical Psychiatry, 68*(1), 37–46.

Van der Kolk, B. (2015). *The Body Keeps the Score: Brain, Mind, and Body in the Healing of Trauma.* New York, NY: Penguin Books.

Van Emmerik, A. A., Kamphuis, J. H., & Emmelkamp, P. M. (2008). Treating Acute Stress Disorder and Posttraumatic Stress Disorder with Cognitive Behavior Therapy or Structured Writing Therapy: A Randomized Controlled Trial. *Psychotherapy and Psychosomatics, 77,* 93–100. https://doi.org/10.1159/000112886.

Visser, E., et al. (2015). The Course, Prediction, and Treatment of Acute and Posttraumatic Stress in Trauma Patients: A Systematic Review. *Journal of Trauma and Acute Care Surgery, 82*(6), 1158–1183.

Zatzick, D., Roy-Byrne, P., Russo, J., Rivara, F., Droesch, R., Wagner, A., et al. (2004). A Randomized Effectiveness Trial of Stepped Collaborative Care for Acutely Injured Trauma Survivors. *Archives of General Psychiatry, 61,* 498–506.

4

Psychotherapy for Depression and Addiction

Substantively as well as symbolically, psychotherapy for depression and addiction repeats the clinical record of post-traumatic stress disorder. Psychotherapy persists in spite of its clinical ineffectiveness to affirm deeply held social values, in particular personal responsibility, but also as a soothing fiction that accompanies widespread indifference to mental health problems and the nation's unwillingness to adjust priorities. Unfortunately, alternative treatment strategies to the social clinic, however humane, that involve supportive care and prevention are extremely expensive, uncertain, and unpopular.

Depression

The primary clinical literature of depression conforms to the general pattern of psychotherapy's outcome research; it reports buoyant estimates of the effectiveness of psychotherapy. Similar to the meta-analyses in other areas of psychotherapy, the meta-analyses of psychotherapy for depression are somewhat forthcoming about the weakness of the primary studies. Yet, in the manner of unrepentant confession,

W. M. Epstein, *Psychotherapy and the Social Clinic in the United States*,
https://doi.org/10.1007/978-3-030-32750-7_4

the meta-analyses cling to important conclusions about the effectiveness of psychotherapy for depression even after pointing to pitfalls in the tests of effectiveness that invalidate the authority of the research.

On the basis of seven randomized trials, presumably the most credible tests in the literature, the meta-analysis by Pu et al. (2017) concluded that interpersonal psychotherapy was superior to controls in treating depression among adolescents. Patients receiving interpersonal psychotherapy were 27 percentage points better off than controls, a considerable improvement. However, the quality of the research was assessed as only moderate and publication bias was likely—that is, negative findings were excluded from the base of studies. Only one of the seven studies (Mufson et al. 1999) employed a placebo control, and all but one study employed samples with fewer than 37 patients. No intention to treat analysis was reported, and follow-up periods were short except in one study that reported data for 18 months subsequent to the end of treatment.

The meta-analysis by Kolovos et al. (2017) summarized the outcomes of psychotherapeutic treatment-as-usual controls in studies of psychotherapy for major depression. Presumably treatment-as-usual contains the full range of psychotherapeutic interventions and provides a baseline of expectations for the field. The study found from separate analyses that at least six months from beginning treatment 33% of patients recovered, 27% showed at least 50% improvement in their symptoms, 31% improved more than chance would predict, and 12% deteriorated. Yet many of the studies in the base were methodologically impaired. The true comparisons for treatment-as-usual are with waitlist controls or ideally with placebo controls since depression and even major depression are seasonal—the bad feelings come and go. On this score, Kolovos et al. (2017) cite Whiteford et al. (2013) whose meta-analysis reported that 23% of depressed subjects receiving no treatment at all were free of diagnosed major depressed at 13 weeks after the initial assessment. Thus, Kolovos et al. adjust their findings to estimate that treatment-as-usual produced only a 10% remission rate. Moreover, this modest finding may be inflated by methodologically impaired studies at risk of a variety of biases. It is also worth wondering whether some portion of the deterioration rate was attributable to treatment itself.

Cuijpers et al. (2016) conducted a meta-analysis of personalized psychotherapy for adult depression. The analysis of 41 randomized studies concluded that only cognitive behavioral therapy produced positive outcomes of sufficient clinical importance and statistical significance. Compared to other therapies, cognitive behavioral therapy improved outcomes for older adults by 11 percentage points, for those with comorbid addictive behaviors by 12 percentage points and for college students by 18 percentage points. As the authors acknowledge, "the risk of bias in most of the studies was considerable…. Only 2 studies (5%) met all quality criteria."

In a meta-analysis of 44 randomized trials, Karyotaki et al. (2016) calculated the odds of psychotherapy improving outcomes for depression. They found that patients who underwent psychotherapy were 1.92 times likelier to achieve long-term improvement than patients in control groups. Long term was defined as at least six months after randomization. However, long-term follow-up comparisons with controls were typically not possible since most control group patients received treatment after the psychotherapy groups' treatment was completed. Unfortunately, the odds ratio says little about the clinical size of the improvement or its importance. Thus, remission and recovery when it occurred may have been achieved with less depressed patients making modest gains. Karyotaki et al. (2016) report neither the pretreatment nor posttreatment depression scores of subjects. They also fail to discuss the size of attrition or adequacy of the intention to treat procedures employed to handle attrition in the few studies that bothered to do so. Nonetheless, the authors note routine and considerable risks of bias in the base of studies with only 16 of the 44 studies considered adequate. Only one study employed a placebo control.

In an additional variety of well-conducted meta-analyses, Cuijper and colleagues argue for the general effectiveness of psychotherapy in treating depression despite the methodological deficiencies of the primary research (Cuijpers et al. 2008, 2009, 2010, 2014, 2016; and others). Cuijpers (2017) summarized previous meta-analyses that reviewed in total about 500 randomized tests of the effectiveness of psychotherapies for adult depression: "all therapies are effective and there are no significant differences between treatments" (p. 7). The meta-analyses typically found substantial reductions in reported symptoms for major depression and somewhat less for mild depression but also substantial improvement in control group subjects. Psychotherapy also improved the outcomes of pharmacotherapy for depression. Many of the meta-analyses also concluded that cognitive behavioral therapy and interpersonal therapy were superior to other therapies and controls.

Yet many meta-analyses commented throughout about substantial problems with risk of bias and other problems in the base of the research. For example, of 25 studies included in Cuijpers et al. (2009) only three met their minimal quality criteria; 10 studies did not blind assessors; 9 of the studies ignored attrition. Still, it was quite likely that the evaluators who were reportedly blinded by research procedures were not blind at all to the patient's group assignment (e.g., when patients speak about their therapists or therapy during evaluation sessions). Attrition bedevils the research.

> Drop-out rates for the treatments were reported in 34 [of 53] studies. The other studies either contained no data on drop-out rates or gave only overall drop-out rates (not specified for each of the conditions). The methods of calculating drop-out differed considerably. In some studies, clients who did not participate in any of the treatment sessions were included in the drop-out rate, whereas other studies did not include them. Furthermore, the number of sessions that had to be completed by clients varied considerably in the studies, and the difference between drop-out from the intervention and drop-out from the study was not always reported. (Cuijpers et al. 2008, p. 917)

Cuijpers et al. (2010) compared high-quality studies with other randomized controlled trials in treating depression. In a base of 115 randomized controlled trials, only 11 met all 8 quality criteria of the meta-analysis. The high-quality studies improved the outcomes of depressed patients by only 9 percentage points compared with 27 percentage points among the other studies. Cuijpers et al. (2010) concluded that "the effects of psychotherapies have been overestimated because of the low quality of many trials and due to publication bias," that is, the suppression by authors and by publications of negative or weak findings that fail to sustain the effectiveness of psychotherapy (ibid., p. 7). Cuijpers et al. (2010) detailed other large differences between the high-quality and weaker studies. Most telling, the quality of the research was significantly associated with reported effectiveness; weaker studies reported greater success; the strongest studies reported very modest gains, if any. However, the so-called stronger studies in this review, other similar reviews, and the field itself are rarely if ever strong. The high-quality studies are only superior in comparison with frankly inadequate research. They too are marred by considerable risks of bias and other problems.

Six of the most scientifically credible primary studies of psychotherapy's effectiveness in treating depression are discussed below. From among the huge available pool of research, the better meta-analyses selected only a relatively small number of studies that most closely conformed to standard criteria of science: randomized controlled trials and a variety of other techniques to reduce risks of bias. The meta-analyses then often identified the most credible among the selected few. Yet even these elite primary studies—the best of the best outcome evaluations—fail to sustain the modest claims of the meta-analyses. Verduyn et al. (2003) that were listed among the best research by Karyotaki et al. (2016) are one of the rare examples of psychotherapeutic research that employs a placebo control. Mufson et al. (1999), a highly rated study in the meta-analysis by Pu et al. (2017), received 278 citations by November 2017, an enormous number, in the Social Sciences Citation Index of the Web of Knowledge. It employed a "clinical monitoring" control that Pu et al. considered a placebo.

In their meta-analysis of the best 41 primary evaluations of personalized psychotherapy for depression, Cuijpers (2017) found that only Markowitz et al. (1998) and Milgrom et al. (2005) met all of the quality criteria for research. Only 11 studies within a base of 115 randomized controlled trials met all of the Cuijpers et al. (2010) quality criteria. Of these 11, six employed an ambiguous "care as usual control"; the other five employed placebo controls among which DeRubeis et al. (2005) employed relatively large samples. The sixth study, Johnson et al. (2016) retrieved from an independent search of the Web of Science and PsycInfo, is among the best of the current research of psychotherapy for depression but too recent to be included in a published meta-analysis. It employs a randomized design but no nontreatment control. It is about as sophisticated as the previous five studies. The debilitating pitfalls of the very best attempts to measure the effectiveness of psychotherapy for depression say much about both the failed authority of the field's claims to clinical expertise and its lack of progress toward achieving the credibility of science.

Verduyn et al.'s (2003) randomized controlled trial of cognitive behavioral therapy for depression among pairs of mothers and children, conducted in the Manchester, England area, is quite unusual for a few reasons. It employed both a placebo control and a nontreatment control in order to estimate natural remission as well as placebo effects. The placebo control entailed "mother and toddler groups." They were

> run by a health visitor together with an experienced clinical psychologist. These sessions were designed as an attention placebo and run at the same frequency as the active treatment groups, using the same staffing ratio. They had the same facilities available and included informal, non-directed group discussion of problems raised by the mothers and separate play opportunities for the children. The format was similar to many community-based support groups for mothers with young children, but no advice was given on parenting or other problems. (ibid., p. 344)

Even rarer, Verduyn et al. screened the community to identify and recruit subjects who were seriously depressed and had children. A community sample presumably avoids a sample of patients who seek treatment and are thus disproportionately motivated to be cured. The overwhelming number of studies of all psychotherapeutic interventions recruits samples from clinics or through public advertisements. The two controls allowed for follow-up comparisons, another unusual feature of the study, which were conducted six months and twelve months subsequent to treatment. In addition, more than two-thirds of the mothers were diagnosed with major depression while one-third of them were comorbid with other psychiatric problems.

The research found that children and parents receiving cognitive behavior fared no better than either the placebo control or the nontreatment control. Each improved a modest amount while there was no statistically significant difference between the placebo control and the nontreatment control. Thus, the findings estimate the degree of natural remission perhaps due to the seasonality of depression, changes in life circumstances, or other factors.

While the study conformed to other necessary requirements of scientific research—notably blinding of assessors—all of its findings are undercut by enormous attrition and the study's failure to conduct an intention to treat analysis. Only 39% of patients in the psychotherapy group completed "a substantial number" of the 16 planned sessions. Still, as an estimate of the effects of cognitive behavior on those who complete or nearly complete treatment, it casts doubt on the effectiveness of cognitive behavioral therapy among presumably the most motivated. The loss of assessment data at one-year follow-up (censoring) was modest in the treatment and placebo groups but 46% in the nontreatment group. Furthermore, as the authors acknowledge, there were recruitment problems that contributed to attrition and also undercut the demographic representativeness of final samples. Because many of the sampled patients had previously experience psychotherapy for depression, the samples may have been little different from customary samples drawn from clinics. In the end, Verduyn et al. apparently failed to sustain the value of cognitive therapy for its sample of depressed patients—a rare finding. However, more commonly, it also failed as a true test of treatment.

Mufson et al. (1999) evaluated the effectiveness of interpersonal psychotherapy for depressed adolescents. Research patients were randomized to either the interpersonal psychotherapy group that received 12 weeks of treatment or to the control group that received "clinical modeling" during the same period. Clinical modeling entailed brief sessions once per month with an option for a second session. The therapists who provided clinical modeling "were given a brief treatment manual instructing them to refrain from advice giving or skills training and to use the sessions to review depressive symptoms, school attendance, assess suicidality, and just listen supportively" (ibid., p. 574). The study reported considerable gains for interpersonal psychotherapy.

However, considerable deficiencies in the research cast doubt on the findings. Samples were small—24 subjects in each group—and attrition was enormous in the clinical monitoring group—13 of the 24 (54%) subjects dropped out, some of whom experienced serious clinical symptoms such as suicidality and psychosis. The study's intention to treat analysis relied on a format that carried forward the subject's most recent score rather than the initial score. This procedure may have minimized depression in the treated group—the tendency of patients to report initial improvement in treatment—while increasing the report of depression in the control group that experienced serious symptoms after randomization.

Furthermore, it is difficult to accept that those who rated outcomes were either neutral judges or blind to the assignment of patients. The evaluators were authors of the research or professional psychotherapists. Indeed, depressive symptoms and other outcome measures that were scored by evaluators through interviews with subjects using the Hamilton Rating Scale of Depression consistently produced more favorable reports of improvement than by patients through self-administered questionnaires of the Beck Depression Inventory. For example, evaluator scoring produced significant differences in the completer sample but self-administered questionnaires did not. Moreover, it is not surprising that the therapists themselves—"the treating clinicians"—scored subjects in the treatment group "as significantly less depressed...than control patients" (ibid., p. 576). They were essentially asked to rate their professional competence.

Finally, clinical modeling may not constitute either an adequate placebo or even an adequate control. It is difficult to assess the degree to which clinical modeling actually may have provided an active intervention that inadvertently induced extreme behaviors by reviewing depressive symptoms and assessing suicidality. Indeed, the nonspecific factors considered generic to psychotherapy, notably supportive listening, may have themselves contributed to anxiety among the control patients. In contrast, a true placebo should engage subjects in the expectation of recovery—the promise of treatment—but without any of the factors associated with the psychotherapeutic process itself. Thus, hampered by small samples, great and differential attrition, uncertain elements of control, lack of blinding, and imperfect measurement, Mufson et al. (1999) failed to provide a credible test of the effectiveness of psychotherapy for depression.

Markowitz et al. (1998) evaluated psychotherapy for "depressive symptoms" in HIV-positive patients. They randomized subjects to four groups: two psychological treatments—interpersonal psychotherapy and cognitive behavioral therapy—supportive therapy (presumably a placebo control) and supportive therapy that also provided imipramine, an antidepressant drug. The study reported that all groups improved over time with the intention to treat analyses showing less improvement than completer samples. The authors conclude that "depressive symptoms appear treatable in HIV-positive patients. Interpersonal psychotherapy may have particular advantages..." (ibid., p. 452). However, considering supportive therapy as a placebo largely wipes out the gains of the other three conditions. Measured by the Hamilton Rating Scale of Depression, the supportive therapy intention to treat group gained more than six points by the end of treatment. The comparable cognitive behavioral therapy group gained less. The two other treatment groups performed marginally better—interpersonal therapy up only four points and drug treatment only three. The same pattern is repeated using the Beck Depression Inventory. All of the comparative gains are clinically trivial. If supportive therapy is not considered a placebo, then the study has not adjusted therapeutic effects by the seasonality of depression, that is, the effects of natural healing which is likely to be substantial, especially among a patient population that does not exhibit severe depression. Without a placebo control, the study simply failed to measure the effects of treatment.

Markowitz et al. (1998) acknowledged "numerous limitations" of their research: small samples, subjects with relatively low depression ("forty-seven percent of subjects lacked [measured] mood disorders, although all were deemed clinically depressed by supervising psychiatrists," p. 456). They might also have added to their list of limitations apparently low-reliability scores among their raters, lack of follow-up, raters with a professional stake in outcomes, high attrition rates, and an undefined procedure for measuring the intention to treat sample.

Utilizing a randomized design, Milgrom et al. (2005) measured the effectiveness of three psychotherapeutic interventions—group-based psychotherapy, group-based counseling, and individual care—for postnatal depression against routine primary care. They found that "psychological intervention per se was superior to routine care in terms of reductions in both depression and anxiety following intervention" (ibid., p. 529). However, attrition was substantial and the intention to treat analysis apparently carried forward the most recent "observed" scores of depression rather than initial scores. The control of routine primary care may be an adequate nontreatment control for psychotherapy. However, it is not an adequate placebo control to address patient report bias—the degree to which patients receiving free psychotherapy from an engaging therapist may feel an obligation to exaggerate recovery—and other subtle signals from therapists and the therapeutic environment that again encourage patients to minimize their enduring symptoms. This is a particularly germane consideration since the gains of therapy over routine primary care that Milgrom et al. assess as clinically and statistically significant amounted to only seven points on the 30-point Beck Depression Inventory. The authors comment on the "high prevalence of postnatal depression" (n.p.) and presumably the high natural rates of recovery that again underscore the desirability of a true placebo control and follow-up. The study's follow-up to assess the durability of outcomes was undercut by an enormous loss of data with only 57 of 192 cases reporting. The authors also note that "poor social support is a known risk factor for postnatal depression," and thus, the research might have prudently employed a control group of social support that compared psychological interventions with less professionalized care. In the end, it is not at all clear whether the small reported gains against postnatal depression ensued from psychotherapy or from the exaggerated reports of grateful patients and other nontherapeutic artifacts of clinical treatment.

DeRubeis et al. (2005) tested the effectiveness of psychotherapy for moderate to severe depression in adults. Patients were assigned to 16 weeks of cognitive therapy, 16 weeks of drug therapy, or eight weeks of pill placebo. The authors conclude that "cognitive therapy can be as effective as medication for the initial treatment of moderate to severe major depression, but the degree of effectiveness may depend on a high level of therapist experience or expertise" (p. 409). However, the differences between treated groups and the pill placebo at eight weeks (the limit of the pill placebo treatment) were very small, only about three points measured on the Hamilton Depression Rating Scale, and thus of questionable clinical value. Moreover, cognitive therapy enjoyed no statistically significant advantage over the pill placebo at eight weeks. While the pill placebo was discontinued at eight weeks for ethical reasons, it is worth considering that natural remission rates may have continued for the remaining eight weeks of therapy, wiping out any advantage for drug therapy or cognitive therapy. The research did not employ a placebo for therapy nor even a nontreatment control.

Other problems diminish the credibility of the research. Follow-up evaluations were not conducted to test the durability of effects. The authors' concluding comment—"pharmacotherapy and cognitive therapy outperformed placebo"—is misleading unless they ignore their own statistical analysis that found no statistically significant advantage for cognitive therapy at eight weeks. The placebo comparisons were only available until week eight at which time only drug therapy outperformed the placebo. Furthermore, the finding about therapist skill—measured as years of experience but that are not actually detailed in the study—is at best speculative based as it is on analyses of the morbidity of the separate samples. This sidebar on the research, given undue prominence, still needs to be formally tested especially since the literature often reports that therapist training and presumably skill have little influence on psychotherapeutic outcomes (Strupp and Hadley 1979; Smith et al. 1980).

Johnson et al. (2016) compared the value of group interpersonal psychotherapy with group cognitive behavioral therapy in treating major depression subsequent to "miscarriage, stillbirth or early neonatal death" (p. 845). "The main purpose of this pilot study was to adapt interpersonal psychotherapy to treat major depressive disorder following perinatal loss" and to test its clinical effectiveness. Twenty-five subjects were randomized to the two treatment conditions that provided 12 group and 2 individual sessions of therapy during a twenty-week period. The study did not utilize a nontreatment control. Subjects were recruited through intensive advertisement and clinical referrals. Assessments were made during treatment and at three and six months subsequent to treatment.

The results tend to favor interpersonal therapy over the interpersonal psychotherapy group although many of the major outcomes were not statistically significantly different between the two treatment conditions: treatment satisfaction, post-traumatic stress recovery in the small subset of patients with the problem, and others. However, there were no statistically significant differences in a number of major outcomes: time to recovery of major depressive disorder, depressive symptom scores among others.

Major pitfalls impair the findings of Johnson et al. (2016). Samples were small, and attrition was high: 28% in the interpersonal psychotherapy group and 40% in the cognitive behavioral therapy group. The research does not indicate whether the intention to treat analysis carried forward initial scores or the most recent scores. Attendance was poor in both groups and many in the cognitive behavioral therapy group and almost half of the total sample began other forms of therapy during the study period in violation of the research protocol. The authors frequently report trends, that is, findings that were not statistically significant, in the spirit that their small samples and thus low power to distinguish differences somehow embellish weak findings. However, it is not legitimate to infer the outcomes of large samples from the outcomes of small samples. This tendency to favor their frank hypothesis and apparent commitment to group interpersonal psychotherapy undercuts the neutrality of the research. The commitment to specific forms of psychotherapy, running through almost all of the psychotherapeutic research, is the vehicle for a variety of biases created by demand characteristics, in particular, response bias but others as well. While the research notes that one of the two assessors was blind to assignment and the other not, it fails to provide any comparison of their scores. Most telling, the absence of a nontreatment control vitiates any ability to assess the degree of natural remission and thus the true effects of psychotherapy for depression. In the end, small samples, large attrition, self-reported outcome measures, low attendance in treatment, uncertain intention to treat analyses, the absence of a nontreatment control, and uncertain blinding of assessors undercut any faith in the accuracy and clinical relevance of the reported outcomes. Indeed, the research fails to dispel the suspicion that therapy had little effect if any at all.[1]

The best of the best studies of psychotherapy for depression is weak science. They fail as true tests of treatment while they routinely appear to exaggerate the effectiveness of psychotherapy. Hardly, any of the studies adequately adjusted or controlled for the seasonality of depression by employing true placebos or credible estimates of natural remission and seasonality. The retreat to the claim that the nonspecific factors included in placebos are actually important components of psychotherapy is self-defeating leading to the deprofessionalization of the field. After all, if a supportive environment and a patient listener commonly lead to lower depressive symptoms, then interventions that require years of graduate preparation might defer to untrained people who exude compassion and have the patience to listen to troubled people down on themselves. It would seem more reasonable to construct placebos around those generic factors of caring and to test the ability of psychotherapy to improve on simple human kindness and patience. As it is, the placebo controls in the research are inadequate.

A host of biases bedevils the studies. Blinding is often breached, and evaluators are not neutral. Attrition is often enormous, and intention to treat adjustments seems to be more convenient than fair carrying

---

[1]Johnson, the lead author of Johnson et al. (2016) was queried by this author for further information: How was intention to treat handled—carrying forward initial or recent scores—and what if any were the scoring differences between the blind rater and the assessor who was not blind. In return, Johnson emailed "No carryforward - used general linear models that accommodate missing data." A further query was sent: "What were the assumptions of the linear models? What data was used to substitute for the missing data? And the comparison of the blinded and unblinded raters? I could not find the answers in the paper. Did I miss something?" No response. If the undisclosed linear model in any way extrapolated the initial ratings of patients who dropped out, it probably exaggerates the effectiveness of the intervention since many if not most patients in psychotherapy report initial gains. Those gains, probably emerging in large part from the hope of recovery, may be ephemeral especially in those who drop out. Further, it is beyond strange that a study would report differences in blinding but not report an analysis of its effects. The absence leads to two suspicions: first that the differences were real with the blinded rater providing scores that undercut the effectiveness of the intervention and second that both the absent evaluation and the use of a linear model for intention to treat analyses were conscious attempts to enhance the reported effectiveness of the interventions.

forward most recent symptom scores or applying "linear models" rather than initial scores. The situations of the research are optimal, employing presumably the most adept therapists in situations of great accountability rather than those representatives of common community care. Demand characteristics are not handled; recall that Mufson et al. (1999) reported substantial differences in reported symptoms of depression depending on whether they were obtained from interviews by therapists or through self-administered questionnaires. Moreover, Cristea et al. (2017) noted that papers that included a statistician among its authors reported far smaller positive effects than papers with authors who were psychotherapists. Moreover, most of the meta-analyses note that the size of positive findings in the primary research decrease with the rigor of the studies. The incentives for report bias are different in delayed treatment controls (the most commonly employed) compared with treated samples. The difference exaggerates reported effectiveness. Finally, sampling problems may produce subject samples that are not representative of patient populations or the demographic incidence of depression. Samples often contain those most amenable for cure, that is, those who actively seek a cure for their depression. The samples also seem to contain many patients who have been through previous episodes of psychotherapy for their depression. These patients accustomed to therapy may be inured to the cycle of depression that includes therapy and perhaps too the ceremony of reporting improvement without actually experiencing any real improvement in the long run. Indeed, some patients may become addicted to therapy.

In short, the research does not dispel the likelihood that psychotherapy for depression fails to improve on the processes that account for natural remission. Indeed, the enormous degree of bias and the small degree of reported success in the best conducted research may even mask and obscure the routine harm caused by psychotherapy for depression.

The Palpacuer et al.'s (2016) meta-analysis concluded that "the effects of psychotherapies compared to the waiting list control condition failed to remain significant after adjusting for nonspecific factors" (p. 95). The apparent influence of the nonspecific factors of the psychotherapy treatment situation itself—"number of treatment sessions, length of fol-low-up, therapeutic allegiance of the investigator" and others, notably empathy—rather than the essential therapeutic core of talk therapies may imply that simple mute caring over time—a warm lap, a listening ear, and perhaps the expectation of feeling better—dispel gloom better than skilled therapy. Although this is not the specific conclusion that Palpacuer et al. (2016) prefer since they appear to consider nonspecific factors as implicit to all psychotherapies, it seems a logical conclusion to their research particularly if those factors are generic to human empathy. In terms of their study, controls that incorporate nonspecific factors are live treatment controls; on the other side of the debate, they are place-bos for psychotherapy. As placebos, they diminish the effectiveness of psychotherapy.

There has not been a scientifically credible test of the effective-ness of psychotherapy for depression, let alone one that is decisive. Nevertheless, the field has reached a consensus that it is effective even with the support of those who argue that outcomes are more modest. Yet a consensus reached without credible proof by those with the most to gain is hardly convincing. The fact that their position is enhanced by broad public support only serves to underline the essentially social and political stakes in psychotherapy. The failure of its clinical reality sus-tains alternative reasons for the long persistence of the social clinic. The design of an adequate test of psychotherapy for depression and more generally most psychotherapeutic interventions may be impossible. Yet professional consensus—the literature as it is—offers a misleading sub-stitute that confuses the biases of self-interest and social convenience with objective fact.

It is worth emphasizing that the obligation of proof rests with clinical practice if it is to be taken at its word as evidence-based and scientific. However, the burden of proof is shifted to the skeptic when practice, clinical or otherwise, is institutionalized within the society. This shift seems to have occurred with the social clinic that persists as a totem of popular folklore, mores, and myth rather than as an engineered cure for psychic distress and behavioral deviance.

Drug Addiction

Psychotherapy offers no apparent cure for drug addiction. The variation in reported addiction rates from year to year, suspect in itself, may be due more to generational learning and changing fashions in social attitudes to illicit drug use than to any form of treatment. The small amount of remission and true long-term abstinence reported in psychotherapy trials are likely determined by rare patient motivation and their situations rather than treatment itself. Yet the problems of assessing the prevalence, incidence, and social effects of addiction as well as the pervasive methodological pitfalls of the studies undercut any claim of abstinence, remission, or harm reduction that is systematically related to psychotherapeutic treatment of any kind. For that matter, medical attempts at drug substitution do not seem to have fulfilled their initial promise.

With a few exceptions, the meta-analyses of psychotherapy for addiction often agree on a few points. The research is weak with high risks of bias, and the value of psychotherapeutic interventions is modest if even that. The paucity of trials is notable especially in light of popular perceptions that addiction is a serious social threat. However, it is not surprising considering the serious problem of attrition, that is, the difficulty of engaging addicts in a course of treatment of any length.

Magill and Ray (2009) are among the most positive of the meta-analyses and the least critical of the pitfalls in the research. Their meta-analysis of 53 randomized studies of cognitive behavioral therapy for "adult substance abuse disorder" concluded that cognitive behavioral therapy was effective "across a large and diverse sample of studies and under rigorous conditions for establishing efficacy" (ibid., pp. 516, 521). It was most effective in treating marijuana use although positive effects declined rapidly after treatment. Yet the overall effect was negligible conferring an advantage of only six percentage points. Outcomes subsequent to treatment were even lower. Psychotherapy was not effective against alcohol abuse. The meta-analysis does not discuss the extent of abuse in its base of research. However, most of the research relied on patient self-reports of "days abstinent" and the percentage of days abstinent that are unverified and amenable to the biases of memory, in particular the hopeful gloss that distorts addicts' perceptions of reality. By itself, this vitiates the value of the reported outcomes. Indeed, such a large plausible exaggeration of positive outcomes in research with very small positive gains begs attention to the possibility that treatment may have been routinely harmful.

Li et al. (2015) analyzed the ten best trials that evaluated the effectiveness of motivational interviewing in reducing illicit drug use in adolescents. Motivational interviewing is a psychotherapeutic intervention

> designed to elicit and strengthen the intrinsic motivation for, and commitment to, a specific goal through holding a person-centered conversation… The clinician must understand and use the underlying skills of motivational interviewing (partnership, acceptance, compassion and evocation) throughout the four processes model of motivational interviewing, by focusing, evoking and planning. (ibid., p. 795)

They found that motivational interviewing was consistently ineffective in reducing adolescent use of illicit drugs although "it may influence intentions to change" (ibid.). Nonetheless, their analysis of publication bias—the suppression of negative findings in the literature and by researchers—undercuts even this tenuous finding.

Stanton and Shadish (1997) located 15 studies for their meta-analysis of family or couples psychotherapy for substance abuse that met their three inclusion criteria: abuse or addiction to one or more illicit drugs, two or more comparison conditions, and random assignment. Family psychotherapy and couples psychotherapy were compared with individual counseling, group therapy, or treatment-as-usual. Presumably all the subjects in the 15 studies had families or partners that entered treatment with them. Stanton and Shadish (1997) found that family therapy was superior to individual therapy, peer group therapy, and family psychoeducation for both adults and adolescents. The intention to treat analysis of total attrition reported generally modest statistically significant advantage of about 13 percentage points. Many of the gains persisted at follow-up. They claimed that the quality of the studies was generally "very good." In contrast to the general experience of enormous attrition in drug therapy, often over 50%, the authors point out that family therapy was able to retain more than 70% of patients. The authors conclude that the results of other therapies "can be improved by the addition of family therapy or couples therapy."

Yet there are numerous problems with the base of research in the Stanton and Shadish meta-analysis that undercut its credibility and applicability to the general problem of treating addiction. The research is only "very good" in comparison with the generally deplorable quality of evaluations of psychotherapy for addiction. In the first instance, the quality scores in the meta-analysis did not include sources of bias, notably ignoring whether raters were blind to the group assignment of subjects. Ratings were made by those with apparently strong stakes in the outcomes. Second, most of the studies did not incorporate objective tests (urine or blood analysis) of substance abuse but relied on patient self-reports. Third, none of the studies employed nontreatment controls (waitlists or placebos), citing the American Psychiatric Association's position that it is unethical to deny treatment (ibid., p. 172), apparently under the assumption that treatment is effective. Fourth, the severity of the addiction was neither noted nor accounted for against outcomes. Fifth, psychotherapy offered in demonstration situations that employ experienced therapists under scrutiny is not representative of the common context of therapy in the community. Sixth, the samples are unlikely to be representative of the underlying addict population.

Consequently, Stanton and Shadish's (ibid.) claim that family and couples therapies add value to other therapies in treating addiction is not sustained by either the meta-analysis or the base of studies. The research samples represented amenable addicts, those both motivated for treatment who had the support of families. This is clearly not the situation for addicts under duress to seek treatment without the support of families or the far greater number of addicts without the motivation to seek treatment. Family therapy and couples therapy are neither a credible solution to the addiction problems of motivated subjects with social support let alone a general prescription for addressing addiction. Still and all, the presence of social supports, in this instance of family, is unappreciated as a necessary element in recovery. It is largely ignored in the psychotherapy literature that prizes its dubious transformative magic over the simple luck of being with caring people when one gets into trouble.

It is notable that one of the two studies with very large positive findings, Joanning et al. (1992), is seriously impaired by high attrition, lost data, the failure to utilize intention to treat analyses, and most importantly the frequent use of subjective reports of drug use. The other study with enormous positive findings (McLellan et al. 1993) has not been credibly sustained in a comprehensive meta-analysis (see Amato et al. 2011 below).

Thus, an informed skepticism discounts Stanton and Shadish's (ibid.) modest findings by a variety of likely biases in evaluating outcomes, by the absence of nontreatment controls to estimate natural remission, by the unusual circumstances of treatment itself, and by the likelihood that the subjects and situations were unrepresentative of patients and treatment situations.

A final caution: Fals-Stewart, the lead author of Fals-Stewart et al. (1996) included as one of the 15 studies in Stanton and Shadish, was accused of fabricating data in 2004. "A University at Buffalo Inquiry Panel found the data fabrication charges to be warranted and recommended that a formal investigation be undertaken." A principal investigator and professor at the University of Buffalo's Research Institute on Addictions, he was subsequently arrested on "multiple felony charges (attempted grand larceny, perjury, identity theft, offering a false instrument and falsify business records) and was found dead at his home" (https://writedit.wordpress.com/2010/03/04/one-that-wont-make-it-to-ori/, November 25, 2017, n.p.). The scandal emerged years after Stanton and Shadish selected studies. Nonetheless, data falsification is obviously a concern in clinical research that increases skepticism toward weak research with positive outcomes. Still, the addiction literature persists in citing the work of Fals-Stewart without caveats to sustain its claims of effectiveness.[2]

---

[2]Note, too, the winter study with Fals-Stewart as coauthor that did not experience any attrition but also scheduled urinalyses.

Klimas et al. (2012) conducted a systematic review of randomized controlled trials and case-controlled studies that evaluated psychosocial interventions, i.e., psychotherapies, to reduce alcohol consumption among concurrent alcohol and illicit drug users, an admittedly narrow but still prevalent concern. They identified only four studies that met their inclusion criteria but noted their poor quality with many risks of bias. The studies compared treatments but none employed a nontreatment control. Klimas et al. only draw the general conclusion that there is little evidence to sustain the superiority of one treatment over another. In light of the substantial threats of bias in the research—subjective measures of outcomes, lack of blinding, even lack of randomization, and others—and nontreatment comparisons, there is little evidence if any to sustain the effectiveness of any treatment.

Mayet et al. (2005) located five randomized studies that looked at a variety of psychosocial treatments for opiate abuse and dependence. Four of the five control conditions mirrored nontreatment although it was apparent that the subjects were aware that they were not receiving psychosocial services. The fifth condition received an intensive alternative to psychosocial treatment. Few of the outcomes were positive and then not clearly important (e.g., the reenrollment of a few high-risk patients); all of the positive gains evaporated at follow-up. Yet even these tenuous outcomes are suspect since attrition was huge—in three studies 39, 48, and 80% at the end of treatment and even higher at follow-up. Many of the studies failed to employ intention to treat analysis. At times, relapse was tested by self-report rather than urine tests. Only one study provided inpatient treatment but failed to follow-up afterward. Sample sizes were very small. "Despite the wide use of psychosocial interventions used alone in clinical practice, there are very few experimental studies that examine the effectiveness for opioid dependence" (ibid., p. 9). Yet those few cases provided inadequate tests of outcomes. Indeed, risk of bias was so strong, and the outcomes so marginal that the possibility persists psychosocial interventions are actually harmful.

One of the most thorough reviews, Amato et al. (2011) analyzed 35 randomized studies that test the value of psychosocial interventions in improving outcomes for opioid addicts in drug (e.g., methadone) maintenance treatment. The psychosocial interventions included acceptance and commitment therapy, biofeedback, cognitive behavioral therapy, contingency management approaches, information-motivation-behavioral skills model, subliminal stimulation, supportive-expressive therapy, short-term interpersonal therapy, customized employment support, enhanced methadone services, enhanced pharmacy services, relational psychotherapies mothers groups, and twelve-step facilitation therapy (ibid., p. 10). Their findings challenge the effectiveness of retention in treatment and opiate use during treatment: "Present evidence suggests that adding psychosocial support does not change the effectiveness of retention and opiate use during treatment" (ibid., p. 2). Still and all, the base of research as in other reviews was commonly impaired raising the question of whether outcomes measure objective conditions or simply reflect the biases of the researchers.

Many of the studies were at risk of bias, and high attrition was consistent although not uniformly high but generally handled through intention to treat analyses. However, one study stands out in this review as well as in the Stanton and Shadish meta-analysis, above. McLellan et al. (1993) found that "methadone alone may only be effective for a minority of eligible patients. The addition of basic counselling was associated with major increases in efficacy; and the addition of on-site professional services was even more effective" (ibid., p. 1953). As computed by Stanton and Shadish, methadone maintenance patients receiving counseling in the McLellan et al.'s study were as much as 44 percentage points better off (50 percentage point improvement is the maximum) than those who only received methadone treatment. However, attrition was enormous in the minimum service group (60% and largely accounted for by "protective transfers," switching persistent drug abusers to standard treatment) but surprisingly low in the two treatment conditions (less than 10%). While both groups receiving treatment had better outcomes on a variety of measures than the low service group, the two groups rarely differed from each other. That is, the standard service group often performed as well as the enhanced service group measured against baselines with few statistically significant differences between them. In the critical area of "drug factor," the standard services group performed better than the enhanced services group although the difference was not statistically significant nor was the difference between these groups and the minimal service group. As the authors prudently state, "because only ten subjects (31%) completed the minimal methadone services condition the data need to be interpreted with caution" (ibid., p. 1958). Moreover, McLellan et al. did not report on the abuse during treatment of other illicit drugs and alcohol, a common substitute for opiates and cocaine.

The large positive findings in McLellan et al. (1993) concern differences at 12 weeks when only about 20% of the two groups receiving services were opiate positive compared with 69% of the minimal service group. While the authors state that the presented data are based on 92 male veterans...who were contacted at twenty-four weeks" (p. 1955), their data at that time are apparently based on only 70 respondents (see chart, p. 1958). Apparently no intention to treat analysis was performed. In the end, the most impressive findings occur at 12 weeks but are undercut by a variety of issues with data. Those findings were not corroborated in Amato et al. (2011). Be that as it may, the McLellan et al. (1993) have been cited, usually appreciatively, 588 times as of December 2017 in the Web of Science. Perhaps their samples were fortuitous outliers; perhaps the research is impaired by unacknowledged biases of research enthusiasm; in any event, they have not been corroborated by credible research.

Amato et al. rated the quality of Hayes et al. (2004) as even stronger than McLellan et al. (1993). However, in contrast with McLellan et al. (1993), Hayes et al. evaluated the effectiveness only of acceptance and commitment therapy and of twelve-step facilitation while the intention to treat analyses found no statistically significant positive gains for psychotherapy during methadone treatment for opiate addicts either at posttreatment or follow-up. A few of the completer analyses were marginally significant. Also in contrast with minimal attrition in McLellan et al.'s treatment groups, attrition was notably high, approximately 40%, in the two treatment conditions in Hayes et al. The contrasts highlight the near uniqueness of McLellan et al. Furthermore, Hayes et al. have only been cited 80 times in the Web of Science, perhaps a reflection of the drug treatment community's disappointment with its findings that psychotherapy is not effective in improving the outcomes of methadone treatment.[3]

And so it is with other well-regarded and well-published meta-analyses and systematic reviews of psychotherapy to reduce drug addiction that should not be so well regarded. Even after acknowledging the poor quality of the primary studies, Benishek et al. (2014), Goodman et al. (2013), and Waldron and Turner (2008) among others still accept weak research on the way to generally positive conclusions about the effectiveness of psychotherapy in handling drug addiction. Attrition, the lack of neutral evaluation, of relevant controls, of follow-up, and of appropriate methods to handle potential biases among many other pitfalls including the Fals-Stewart enhancement bedevil the base of research and thus weaken the value of compliant meta-analyses.

Why even bother with psychotherapy for addiction? The plausible answer falls into the category of "something must be tried" especially when it is inexpensive, when the culture takes pleasure in affirming personal responsibility and when drug addiction is a modern fairy tale of retribution for sin and, in rare cases, redemption. The importance of alternatives to psychotherapy such as supportive family and caring, attentive communities are unappreciated in explaining the prevention of illicit drug use and of remission, rare as it is. Yet the cost to create a social milieu that both discourages drug addiction and facilitates a healing conformity is beyond political tolerances and outside of social priorities. As social interventions, they are also undefined and untested even while their necessity is implied by a number of program evaluations and discussed as alternatives to psychotherapy in the final chapter.

Legalization of opioids as well as other addictive drugs is a plausible alternative to psychotherapy that may in fact be effective in reducing the incidence of addiction, reducing its medical costs as well as the social costs of policing, incarceration, and crime. Switzerland, Portugal, parts of England, and even occasional efforts in the United States have legalized drugs and witnessed impressive gains: few and routinely functional

---

[3]As an aside, the fact that both objective tests for drug use agreed with subjective reports in Hayes et al. provides no warrant to employ subjective tests without objective corroboration.

addicts, hardly any associated crime, lower medical costs, and large rates of recovery (Hari 2015). A Swiss psychiatrist explains its success, detailing the supportive services after the state legalized heroin. The Swiss program provided heroin-assisted treatment only for "refractory opioid addicts with exiting severe somatic and/or mental problems" (Rehm et al. 2005, p. 137).

Most addicts here, he says come with an empty glass inside them; when they take heroin, the glass becomes full, but only for a few hours, and then it drains down to nothing again. The purpose of this program is to gradually build a life for the addict so they can put something else into that empty glass: a social network, a job, some daily pleasures. If you can do that, it will mean that even as the heroin drains, you are not left totally empty. Over time, as your life has more in it, the glass will contain more and more, so it will take less and less heroin to fill it up; And in the end, there may be enough within you that you feel full without any heroin at all... Users can stay on this program for as long as they want, but the average patient will come here for three years and at the end of that time, only 15 percent are using every day. (Hari 2015, p. 221)

Yet enthusiasm about the Swiss experiment is dampened by a number of failures in research method. Hari presents data from related studies that document the very large benefits of the Swiss program. However, some of the outcomes, presented in footnotes, are not all that dramatic. For example, "over a three-year period, of the 353 patients leaving the heroin program studied in *Prescription of Narcotics for Heroin Addicts...* (Uchtenhagen et al. 1999) 83 left to choose an abstinence based therapy" (Hari, p. 349). This represents only a short-term abstinence rate of 24% of those who volunteered for the program. Presumably there were more, perhaps many more, "refractory" addicts who did not volunteer for the program; according to Ribeaud (2004), "only about 1,000 out of the estimated 30,000 habitual heroin users in Switzerland are targeted by the heroin maintenance program" and apparently enrolled (p. 164). Thus, the 353 addicts studied in Uchtenhagen signal an enormous attrition of about 65%; excluding a small number for other reasons only reduces attrition to 52% (Ribeaud 2004). Further, choosing an abstinence-based therapy is decidedly not the same as being abstinent. Ribeaud (2004) found enormous drops in criminal activity among those who stayed with the program. Yet similarly decreased criminal activity was reported for those who dropped out of the program after one year raising questions about the contribution of the program itself to the outcomes. Additionally, the absence of a randomized comparison group discourages fundamental skepticism toward the reported outcomes in all of the related research—the degree to which they were true effects of the interventions or simply a result of self-selection within the studied groups.

A six-year follow-up study by Guttinger et al. (2003) replicated some of the earlier findings but continued to employ questionable methods. Guttinger et al. reported that 31% were terminated from the study for failure to adhere to protocols. In contrast, patients who voluntarily terminated treatment and those still in treatment reported enormous decreases in "daily illegal uses of substances" along with small decreases in homelessness (that was already at very low levels) but enormous decreases in illegal income. However, the patients' reliance on social benefits and unemployment both increased. The most troubling finding is that few in the program reported substantial changes in their social contacts and maintained contact with currently addicted friends. Moreover, the very large failure rate suggests that at least a portion of the positive findings may be due to patient motivation independent of the program. More troubling, all of the Guttinger et al.'s data are self-reported including current drug use that was "not validated by urinalysis." The absence of objectively verified outcomes, the highly screened sample, the enormous attrition, and the absence of a randomized control throw considerable doubt on the accuracy of the data, in particular those concerning drug use and illegal income. Furthermore, data concerning the direct effects of legalization as well as the success of the supportive programs were produced in the unusual conditions of a demonstration and by program advocates, that is, those with apparent commitments to the program and presumably great stakes in positive outcomes.

Still, the potential of legalization and supportive care under more routinized conditions is inviting despite the troubling imperfections in the research. Hari's all-too-credulous presentation of the Swiss experience does not help his intriguing argument. The social effects of quasi-legalization and full legalization for more occasional and recreational users and on previous nonusers—whether it increases use and the attendant problems or not—remain unclear. Yet compared with the devastation of current addictions, attempting some combination of decriminalization and support programs seems compelling.

The impediments to adopting legalization and supportive services—job training, jobs, and others—that reintegrate addicts into society are erected by social convictions. Addiction and its vilification reinforce cherished social values of individualism and sin in the United States. They also reinforce noxious stereotypes of race and ethnicity. On its part, the social clinic, as ever, entertains popular preferences with ceremonies of personal responsibility.

References

Amato, L., Minozzi, S., Davoli, M., & Vecchi, S. (2011). Psychosocial Combined with Agonist Maintenance Treatments Versus Agonist Maintenance Treatments Alone for Treatment of Opioid Dependence. *Cochrane Database of Systematic Reviews*, 1–93. http://dx.doi.org/10.1002/14651858.CD004147.pub4.

Benishek, L. A., Dugosh, K. L., Kirby, K. C., Matejkowski, J., Clements, N. T., Seymour, B. L., et al. (2014). Prize-Based Contingency Management for the Treatment of Substance Abusers: A Meta-Analysis. *Addiction, 109,* 1426–1436. https://doi.org/10.1111/add.12589.

Cristea, I. A., Gentili, C., Pietrini, P., & Cuijpers, P. (2017, February 3). Is Investigator Background Related to Outcome in Head to Head Trials of Psychotherapy and Pharmacotherapy for Adult Depression? A Systematic Review and Meta-Analysis. *PLoS One, 12,* 1–18. http://dx.doi.org/10.1371/journal.pone.0171654.

Cuijpers, P. (2017). Four Decades of Outcome Research on Psychotherapies for Adult Depression: An Overview of a Series of Meta-Analyses. *Canadian Psychology, 58*(1), 7–19.

Cuijpers, P., Cristea, I. A., Weitz, E., Gentili, C., & Berking, M. (2016). The Effects of Cognitive and Behavioural Therapies for Anxiety Disorders on Depression: A Meta-Analysis. *Psychological Medicine, 46*, 3451–3462. https://doi.org/10.1017/S0033291716002348.

Cuijpers, P., Dekker, J., Hollon, S. D., & Andersson, G. (2009). Adding Psychotherapy to Pharmacotherapy in the Treatment of Depressive Disorders in Adults: A Meta-Analysis. *Journal of Clinical Psychiatry, 70*, 1219–1229. https://doi.org/10.4088/JCP.09r05021.

Cuijpers, P., Karyotaki, E., Weitz, E., Andersson, G., Hollon, S. D., & Van Straten, A. (2014). The Effects of Psychotherapies for Major Depression in Adults on Remission, Recovery and Improvement: A Meta-Analysis. *Journal of Affective Disorders, 159*, 118–126. https://doi.org/10.1016/j.jad.2014.02.026.

Cuijpers, P., Van Straten, A., Andersson, G., & Van Oppen, P. (2008). Psychotherapy for Depression in Adults: A Meta-Analysis of Comparative Outcome Studies. *Journal of Consulting and Clinical Psychology, 76*, 909–922. https://doi.org/10.1037/a0013075.

Cuijpers, P., Van Straten, A., Bohlmeijer, E., Hollon, S. D., & Andersson, G. (2010). The Effects of Psychotherapy for Adult Depression Are Overestimated: A Meta-Analysis of Study Quality and Effect Size. *Psychological Medicine, 40*, 211–223. https://doi.org/10.1017/S0033291709006114.

DeRubeis, R. J., Hollon, S. D., Amsterdam, J. D., Shelton, R. C., Young, P. R., Salomon, R. M., et al. (2005). Cognitive Therapy vs. Medications in the Treatment of Moderate to Severe Depression. *Archives of General Psychiatry, 62*, 409–416. https://doi.org/10.1001/archpsyc.62.4.409.

Fals-Stewart, W., Birchler, G. R., & O'Farrell, T. J. (1996). Behavioral Couples Therapy for Male Substance-Abusing Patients: Effects on Relationship Adjustment and Drug-Using Behavior. *Journal of Consulting and Clinical Psychology, 64*, 959–972.

Goodman, J. D., McKay, J. R., & DePhilippis, D. (2013). Progress Monitoring in Mental Health and Addiction Treatment: A Means of Improving Care. *Professional Psychology: Research and Practice, 44*, 231–246. https://doi.org/10.1037/a0032605.

Guttinger, F., et al. (2003). Evaluating Long-Term Effects of Heroin-Assisted Treatment: The Results of a 6-Year Follow-Up. *European Addiction Research, 9*(2), 73–79.

Hari, J. (2015). *Chasing the Scream*. New York: Bloomsbury.

Hayes, S. C., Wilson, K. G., Gifford, E. V., Bissett, R., Piasecki, M., Batten, S. V., et al. (2004). A Preliminary Trial of Twelve-Step Facilitation and Acceptance and Commitment Therapy with Polysubstance-Abusing Methadone-Maintained Opiate Addicts. *Behavior Therapy, 35,* 667–688. http://dx.doi.org/10.1016/S0005-7894(04)80014-5.

Joanning, H., Thomas, F., Quinn, W., & Mullen, R. (1992). Treating Adolescent Drug Abuse: A Comparison of Family Systems Therapy, Group Therapy, and Family Drug Education. *Journal of Marital and Family Therapy, 18,* 345–356. https://doi.org/10.1111/j.1752-0606.1992.tb00948.x.

Johnson, J. E., Price, A. B., Kao, J. C., Fernandes, K., Stout, R., Gobin, R. L., et al. (2016). Interpersonal Psychotherapy (IPT) for Major Depression Following Perinatal Loss: A Pilot Randomized Controlled Trial. *Archives of Women's Mental Health, 19,* 845–859. https://doi.org/10.1007/s00737-016-0625-5.

Karyotaki, E., Smit, Y., De Beurs, D. P., Henningsen, K. H., Robays, J., Huibers, M. J., et al. (2016). The Long-Term Efficacy of Acute-Phase Psychotherapy for Depression: A Meta-Analysis of Randomized Trials. *Depression and Anxiety, 33,* 370–383. https://doi.org/10.1002/da.22491.

Klimas, J., Field, C. A., Cullen, W., O'Gorman, C. S., Glynn, L. G., Keenan, E., et al. (2012). Psychosocial Interventions to Reduce Alcohol Consumption in Concurrent Problem Alcohol and Illicit Drug Users. *Cochrane Database of Systematic Reviews,* 1–43. http://dx.doi.org/10.1002/14651858.CD009269.pub2.

Kolovos, S., Van Tulder, M. W., Cuijpers, P., Prigent, A., Chevreul, K., Riper, H., et al. (2017). The Effect of Treatment as Usual on Major Depressive Disorder: A Meta-Analysis. *Journal of Affective Disorders, 210,* 72–81. https://doi.org/10.1016/j.jad.2016.12.013.

Li, L., Zhu, S., Tse, N., Tse, S., & Wong, P. (2015). Effectiveness of Motivational Interviewing to Reduce Illicit Drug Use in Adolescents: A Systematic Review and Meta-Analysis. *Addiction, 111,* 795–805. https://doi.org/10.1111/add.13285.

Magill, M., & Ray, L. A. (2009). Cognitive-Behavioral Treatment with Adult Alcohol and Illicit Drug Users: A Meta-Analysis of Randomized Controlled Trials. *Journal of Studies on Alcohol and Drugs, 70,* 516–527. http://dx.doi.org/10.15288/jsad.2009.70.516.

Markowitz, J. C., Kocsis, J. H., Fishman, B., Spielman, L. A., Jacobsberg, L. B., Frances, A. J., et al. (1998). Treatment of Depressive Symptoms in Human Immunodeficiency Virus-Positive Patients. *Archives of General Psychiatry, 55,* 452–457. https://doi.org/10.1001/archpsyc.55.5.452.

Mayet, S., et al. (2005). Psychosocial Treatment for Opiate Abuse and Dependence. *Cochrane Database of Systematic Reviews* (1): CD004330.

McLellan, A. T., Arndt, I. O., Metzger, D. S., Woody, G. E., & O'Brien, C. P. (1993, April 21). The Effects of Psychological Services in Substance Abuse Treatment. *Journal of the American Medical Society, 269,* 1953–1959. http://dx.doi.org/10.1001/jama.1993.03500150065028.

Milgrom, J., Negri, L. M., Gemmill, A. W., McNeil, M., & Martin, P. R. (2005). A Randomized Controlled Trial of Psychological Interventions for Postnatal Depression. *British Journal of Clinical Psychology, 44,* 529–542. https://doi.org/10.1348/014466505X34200.

Mufson, L., Weissman, M. M., Moreau, D., & Garfinkel, R. (1999). Efficacy of Interpersonal Psychotherapy for Depressed Adolescents. *Archives of General Psychiatry, 56,* 573–579. http://dx.doi.org/10-1001/pubs. ArchGenPsychiatry-ISSN-0003-990x-56-6-yoa8163.

Palpacuer, C., Gallet, L., Drapier, D., Reymann, J., Falissard, B., & Naudet, F. (2016). Specific and Non-specific Effects of Psychotherapeutic Interventions for Depression: Results from a Meta-Analysis of 84 Studies. *Journal of Psychiatric Research, 87,* 95–104. https://doi.org/10.1016/j. jpsychires.2016.12.015.

Pu, J., Zhou, X., Liu, L., Zhang, Y., Yang, L., Yuan, S., et al. (2017). Efficacy and Acceptability of Interpersonal Psychotherapy for Depression in Adolescents: A Meta-Analysis of Randomized Controlled Trials. *Psychiatry Research, 253,* 226–232. http://dx.doi.org/10.1016/j.psychres.2017.03.023.

Rehm, J., et al. (2005). Mortality in Heroin-Assisted Treatment in Switzerland 1994–2000. *Drug and Alcohol Dependence, 79*(2), 137–143.

Ribeaud, D. (2004). Long-Term Impacts of the Swiss Heroin Prescription Trials on Crime of Treated Heroin Users. *Journal of Drug Issues, 34,* 163–194. https://doi.org/10.1177/002204260403400108.

Smith, M. L., Glass, G. V., & Miller, T. I. (1980). *The Benefits of Psychotherapy.* Baltimore, MD: Johns Hopkins University Press.

Stanton, M., & Shadish, W. R. (1997). Outcome, Attrition, and Family-Couples Treatment for Drug Abuse: A Meta-Analysis and Review of the Controlled, Comparative Studies. *Psychological Bulletin, 122,* 170–191. https://doi.org/10.1037/0033-2909.122.2.170.

Strupp, H. H., & Hadley, S. W. (1979). Specific vs. Nonspecific Factors in Psychotherapy: A Controlled Study of Outcome. *Archives of General Psychiatry, 36,* 1125–1136. http://dx.doi.org/10.1001/archpsyc.1979. 01780100095009.

Uchtenhagen, A., Dobler-Mikola, A., Steffen, T., Gutzwiller, F., Blattler, R., & Pfeifer, S. (1999). *Prescription of Narcotics for Heroin Addicts: Main Results of the Swiss National Cohort Study*. New York, NY: Karger.

Verduyn, C., et al. (2003). Maternal Depression and Child Behaviour Problems: Randomised Placebo-Controlled Trial of a Cognitive-Behavioural Group Intervention. *British Journal of Psychiatry, 183*, 342–348.

Waldron, H. B., & Turner, C. W. (2008). Evidence-Based Psychosocial Treatments for Adolescent Substance Abuse. *Journal of Clinical Child & Adolescent Psychology, 37*, 238–261. https://doi.org/10.1080/15374410701820133.

5

Psychotherapy and Society

The critical analysis of psychotherapy, the core intervention of the American social clinic, indicts each link in the chain of American social welfare policy making: the inability of the social clinic itself to achieve the remission or prevention of mental and emotional disorders; the community of scholars that fails to offer scientifically credible tests of its outcomes; and the American culture that endorses the affirming myths of the social clinic thus encouraging the distortions of its research community and the fecklessness of its interventions.

The previous analyses of psychotherapy for PTSD, depression, and addiction are more broadly sustained as generally accurate of psychotherapy. While the skeptical position is well published and scientifically credible (e.g., Moloney 2013; Zilbergeld 1983; Eisner 2000; Dineen 1996; Epstein 2006), it has been largely ignored by the field's community of scholars and the society itself. The general failure of psychotherapy suggests the plausibility of alternatives—caring rather than curing—usually remain untried and untested because of cost. The literature itself often provides hints that systemic interventions may be necessary to prevent or treat mental and emotional problems. Even schizophrenia seems to be engendered by social deficits—persistent

© The Author(s) 2019   **83**
W. M. Epstein, *Psychotherapy and the Social Clinic in the United States*,
https://doi.org/10.1007/978-3-030-32750-7_5

abuse particularly in childhood, trauma and other gross adequacies of socialization—more often than the linear result of innate predispositions or deviant character. Indeed, character itself is better understood as nurtured by environment than as romantic self-invention.

Research methods are designed as walls to protect the integrity of science. Many decades of psychotherapy research indicate that every wall erected by its research methods has been stormed by higher ladders of bias, professional self-promotion, ambition, fraud, and incompetence. The bias is not simply individual nor the insidious effect of a conspiracy. Rather it conforms to the most critical assessments of the field as a self-protective industry (e.g., Moloney 2013; Throop 2009; Dineen 1996; Rieff 1966) but also one that enjoys widespread popular enthusiasms in spite of its failures of treatment. Compared with the avalanche of articles and books touting psychotherapy, there is barely a trickle that question its effectiveness and benefits and those are given little notice.

It is intriguing that reported outcomes have apparently improved over the decades even as the length of therapeutic treatments has grown shorter. Yet the quality of the field's critical tests of outcomes has not changed much in spite of the greater deployment of randomized controlled trials. At the same time, the amount of skepticism seems to have decreased with very few within the field or even outside of it criticizing the quality of research and its improbable estimates of clinical effectiveness. Yet even the very best of the primary research is too compromised to certify psychotherapy's ability to cure, prevent, or rehabilitate. Randomized controlled trials often seem more dutiful than sincere combined as they often are with a great number of methodological deficiencies that overwhelm any advantage that randomized procedures confer.

The meta-analyses are not merely the reluctant recipients of weak research. They have been seriously criticized and not least for misapplying statistical techniques that routinely violate basic assumptions and end up inflating effect sizes (Nugent 2017). Yet their reliance on patently inadequate research creates misleading conclusions that routinely exaggerate the value of psychotherapy. Combining the data of separate analyses to increase statistical power and thus the ability to detect subtle differences is only legitimate to the extent to which the combined data are true. However, the underlying data gleaned from the primary research are routinely unreliable and distorted. As a result, the meta-analyses are inaccurate and misleading.

Moreover, the usefulness of increased statistical power is lost when few of the meta-analyses are able to interpret the clinical significance of small and modest statistically significant effects. Statistical significance is a necessary but insufficient criterion for clinical importance. The distinction between statistical differences—in this case effect sizes—and their clinical meaning has long been recognized. The statistician Cohen who provided the rule of thumb for interpreting Hedges effect sizes as small medium or large, cautioned that the context of the research should govern interpretation. Thus, weak, porous research such as the body of psychotherapy outcome studies should require far higher effect sizes to substantiate any claim to important findings. Because of their deficiencies, systematic reviews and conspicuously meta-analyses are inadequate substitutes for definitive tests of effectiveness. Indeed, their prevalence and increasing popularity without true tests is a notice of a bankrupt scholarly community.

The enduring success of the social clinic and psychotherapy belies the rational core of cultural affections and social policy making. It pays tribute to embedded social preferences, in this case the remarkable romantic commitments of American theology and ideology, rather than evidence that national discourse is progressing toward either rational understanding or rational ends. The attainment of explicit goals tied to treatment gives way to the implicit preferences of an enduring culture—the triumph of the therapeutic over the rational or even the reasonable, populism rather than liberal democracy, perhaps even schadenfreude displacing empathy.

The embedded preferences of the culture for the psychotherapeutic social clinic are translated by the community of scholars and practitioners into the research distortions of the field, its false testimonies to effective treatment. The biases themselves are mediated through the therapeutic relationship between therapist and patient. The process of building the therapeutic relationship entails reducing the defenses of the patient and creating trust, indeed, deep belief that often approaches true belief, in the value of therapy. It must be pleasurable and supportive or patients will be reluctant to continue. Thus, a successful therapeutic relationship eludes the patient's natural skepticism building on his or her needs for assurance of psychic growth, insight, self-discovery, compassion, wisdom and often changed behaviors. Patients who achieve a successful therapeutic relationship and patients who simply develop a stake in psychotherapy and reliance on the psychotherapist have lost the ability to evaluate their progress. Neither the patient nor the therapist is competent, reliable judges of progress in therapy. Without objective, neutral and independent evaluation, no test of psychotherapy's effectiveness is credible. The community of psychotherapists have failed in this task.

The freedom of expression assured to Americans becomes an obligation in a community of scholars to challenge orthodoxy in its field. The most credible and thus highest status fields are scientific whose challenges are grounded in methods of coherent objectivity, that is, rational tests. Psychotherapy's community of scholars, in pursuit of greater status, have violated this obligation by creating a self-serving literature based on pseudo-science. It is done with knowing impunity by a cherished social institution beyond the reach of the rational. The constituency for a scientific practice of therapy is small and thus the pressure is very weak for a responsible practice of research in the field.

A scholarly enterprise that progresses toward knowledge employs a process of definitive tests of theory. Without definitive tests, progress is impossible and change takes place as a result of social acceptance. Yet this is not clinically scientific but rather social, speaking more to questions of satisfaction, myth, and style than to basic clinical concern with cure, treatment, and prevention.

Ideally, each area of psychotherapeutic practice would be able to cite definitive tests of psychotherapeutic effectiveness. These tests would employ randomized procedures, reliable measures, appropriate controls, notably placebos and nontreatment situations, neutral measurement, patient and assessor blinding, long-term follow-up, and other methodological protections that assure that effectiveness is tested. None of the studies included in the meta-analyses and systematic reviews conform to these criteria. Deviations from scientifically credible standards are characteristically great even among the best of the research: measures that rely on uncorroborated patient self-report, breaches of randomization, high attrition and problematic intention to treat procedures, uncorrected reactivity to the research including demand characteristics, and the inability to employ credible placebos.

Accordingly, the conclusions that the field reaches about treatment effectiveness even when based on the most thoroughgoing and selective reviews of the primary research characteristically rely on a very unsatisfactory process of balancing the evidence of a very weak base of research. This has long been the situation of psychotherapeutic treatment: little if any credible evidence that psychotherapy is successful, substantial grounds to interpret this persistent absence as evidence of ineffectiveness, and some suspicion that treatment may be routinely harmful.

There are other concerns that deepen pessimism about psychotherapy. The research is typically conducted not in field situations but in demonstration situations, usually under university auspices. It has little relevance to the more common situation of practice in the community where the majority of psychotherapy is delivered by social workers and others with weak clinical preparation while the demonstrations are customarily conducted by psychologist and psychiatrists with many more years of quality training. The long-term observation that the level of therapist training makes little difference in the outcomes (Strupp and Hadley 1979; Smith et al. 1980) should be paired with the conclusion that psychotherapy does not appear to be effective. Moreover, the researchers are among those with great professional stakes in effectiveness while few studies if any adequately employ methods to counteract plausible bias, notably the demand characteristics or the research situation, including expectancy effects (Orne 1962a, b; Rosenthal and Rubin 1978). Presumably greater neutrality in the psychotherapy research would produce lower estimates of effectiveness. Credibility would seem to require that the research be turned over to neutral investigators. Indeed, the desirability of neutrality is given great impetus by findings that positive effect sizes decrease in research that includes a statistician among its authors (Cristea et al. 2017; Peron et al. 2013); Singh et al. (2013) "found a substantial and statistically significant authorship effect"—that the interests of authors distorted findings—earlier documented by Gorey (1996). The pattern of shrinking effect sizes as the quality of research increases goes back to Smith et al. (1980) and Prioleau et al.'s (1983) reanalysis that reduced their huge positive findings to uncertain clinical importance by focusing on the more rigorous research. Thus, the findings of clinical effectiveness, modest and overstated as they are, probably exaggerate outcomes and suppress what may be the routine harms of careless treatment, of unconcerned and poorly prepared practitioners, and of the implicit threats of poorly understood procedures.

A less flattering way to look at the very imperfect research is to see that a community of self-promoting researchers were only able to create very modest and episodic evidence of success from amenable, grateful patients with often questionable diagnoses. Under the assumption that therapy is effective, many studies discard nontreatment controls and simply compare one form of treatment to another. In this way, the literature often becomes a squabble among professionals more than a serious issue of service.

The neutrality of the researchers is often assumed to be adequately protected by the instruments and processes of the research itself. Yet these assumptions are often violated and not least of all because many of the researchers and those involved as professionals in the research have themselves been in therapy and have become profoundly protective of the belief that they have benefited from treatment if not actually transformed through the experience. Indeed, the therapeutic community and notably including its academics often display a fervid dedication to its virtues that suggests a religious cult more than a community of scientific scholars. While therapists and even former patients may have a role in the design of clinical research, their abiding control of design and evaluation subverts neutrality and opens numerous opportunities for bias.

Ahola et al. (2017) concluded that scheduled waiting and thus delayed treatment controls contain active treatment components. Yet a more plausible interpretation of their own findings leads to the more plausible skepticism that the gains of scheduled waiting represent natural remission and placebo effects. Still, Ahola et al. cut against other research, equally speculative because of design flaws, that finds that patients on waiting lists maintain symptoms perhaps to stay eligible for care. The possibility remains that the outcomes in all of these studies are tributes to demand characteristics—patient reports induced subtly by researchers to sustain their hypotheses—more than careful bias-free research. The issue of nonspecific factors is not settled. However, the possibility of large positive therapeutic gains created without highly trained psychotherapists and their expensive social clinics turns attention back to less expensive alternatives and to the social conditions that engender mental and emotional distress (Strupp and Hadley 1979).

There are so many unanswered questions of bias along with other crippling problems in the research that simple statistical tests of significance that address the probability of random results are probably inadequate. The variety of effect size measures often obscure the important issues of clinical meaning. Apparently large changes in reported symptoms may not easily convert into important and lasting gains against disabling mental conditions. Rather than sheltering behind statistical elegance, effective outcomes of psychotherapeutic research need to be large and obvious so as to quell skepticism rooted in all the little ways that practitioners with the support of the culture manufacture comforting evidence of successful clinical practice.

A small but substantial literature within the field has recognized its research problems, notably bias of one sort or another, that undercut the scientific authority of claims for effective psychotherapy (in addition to previous references, Dal-Re et al. [2017]; Dragioti et al. [2017]; Leichsenring et al. [2017]; Sugarman [2016]). However, they have had little effect on psychotherapeutic practice which is accepted more as a social institution than an engineered clinical intervention valued for its production functions in handling mental and emotional problems. The problem of establishing scientific authority is broader than psychotherapy. In particular, Armstrong and Green (2017) claim that "fewer than one-percent of papers" published in social science fields "follow the scientific method." However, the lack of scientific credibility seems unrelieved and entrenched in psychotherapy.

Especially due to the debilitating ambiguities of the outcome research, the reported modest improvements in symptoms are not equivalent to remission or cure, that is, whether the gain is clinically substantial or only statistically significant. Simple improvement may have little clinical meaning and large reported gains that produce enormous effect sizes may represent only modest clinical gains, if even that (as in Resick et al., above). The absence of definitive tests of psychotherapeutic effectiveness is due in part to the unanswered problem of whether reported gains are real or are the result of the absence of rater and patient blinding, unadjusted attrition, misdiagnoses, or accurate patient self-reports. The instrumentation of psychological diagnoses and symptoms is still in a rudimentary stage of development (Kirk and Kutchins 1992). In the end, the literature is more an indicator of professional and social stakes in relatively inexpensive, short-term treatment and less a credible estimate of the outcomes of psychotherapy or even sincere evidence of the society's willingness to address disabling mental and emotional problems.

It is not a purist excess to insist on scientific research in clinical practice even if it may be impossible to design and then conduct a flawless study. Despite the arguable elusiveness of the ideal test for the effectiveness of psychotherapy, deviations from dispositive research mark the areas of ambiguity, uncertainty, and ignorance. Crucially, it may be impossible to construct a placebo for psychotherapy that convinces the subject that it is real therapy. Moreover, the assumption that psychotherapy is effective largely prevents the deployment of any control except a delayed treatment control and thus largely eliminates the possibility of extended follow-up.

Yet the consistent failures and refusals in the literature of psychotherapy to handle plausible sources of bias and the extent of consistent natural remission and other forms of self-healing suggest both an institutional unwillingness as well as methodological barriers. The most notable source of bias that could be addressed is the fact that the overwhelming amount of evaluative research is conducted by psychotherapists, those with the greatest stakes in demonstrating their field's potency. Yet the most notable point of skepticism begins with the nature of therapy itself and the implausibility of talking people out of ingrained, habitual, customary behaviors that are often sustained by tacit social values.

Psychotherapy's ambitions to earn clinical prestige on the same scientific grounds as the medical clinic may face intractable barriers. Definitive tests of psychotherapy's effectiveness are impeded in the first instance by the failure to develop objective tests of mental and emotional conditions—the problems of reliable diagnosis. In this case, "intersubjectivity" is not an adequate substitute for the objective since the research situation itself, replete with practitioner, patient and institutional biases, conspire to engineer misleading reliabilities. Without reliable objective measures, there is little point to the research. Yet even if this problem is set aside by the continued acceptance of subjective measures, that is, patient self-report, the meaning of the field subtly morphs from a clinical presence similar to the medical clinic to what it actually is now—a social entity contingent on broad acceptance rather than objective effectiveness, an institution that expresses the romantic core of American mores, an enduring folkway, an engine of soothing myth.

The political point of the social clinic's mythic content places psychotherapy in competition with political ideologies focused on systemic failures rather than flawed character or genetic determination. Social conditions may be the sustaining causes of mental and emotional impairments except when patients are motivated through therapy to act on their own behalf. However, the psychotherapy literature has not demonstrated its influence on personal agency while the isolation of psychotherapy from the lived conditions of patients may explain much of its ineffectiveness. When change is coincidental with therapy, it may more credibly be attributed to patent maturation, the seasonality of the condition itself, or the corruption of the research. An agnostic attitude toward reports of psychotherapeutic effectiveness rests on the failure of the psychotherapy literature to include appropriate controls for treatment, neutral evaluation, or independent researchers. Skepticism is also nourished by the many voluntary patients whose conditions may actually be prolonged by the therapy itself. After all, the one sure skill of the therapist rests on establishing trust and a warm relationship with patients. However, the comforting retreat that therapy offers from the patient's harsh reality may prolong symptoms in order to justify continued but temporary serenity.

The research seems more than simply oblivious but rather evasive of the threats posed to its scientific credibility. It looks more like the factional studies of political disputes, the false sophistication of commercial advertisement, conformity with social institutions, and avowals of faith. In the end, the therapy industry has turned clinical research into hype. Nonetheless, psychotherapy fails to relieve social and individual problems. Absent effective psychological practice, the social clinic masks an abiding loyalty to romantic cultural norms, notably the extreme individualism of American society and culture.

Psychotherapy Versus Care

Throughout the primary literature of psychotherapy, the question remains open whether the reported gains in remission, typically modest if not small, are simply coincidental with the patient's present and past environment—the amounts of social and psychological support—or the result of treatment itself. The necessity of long-term family and community caring or substitutes for it as either alternatives to treatment or its necessary accompaniment emerges as a subtheme in the literature that tests psychotherapy's outcomes. Van der Kolk (2015) pointed to caring support as necessary for the resolution of PTSD. The meta-analysis by Palpacuer et al. (2016) hints at the same possibility of caring as a defining condition of recovery from depression. Stanton and Shadish (1997) offer clues that the degree of previous caring may predict recovery from addition. More than a condition of successful psychotherapy for addiction, caring may exist as the primary reason for recovery in spite of psychotherapy. Indeed, personal resilience, perhaps the psychological money banked by longtime family and community support, may best explain the purported outcomes of psychotherapy.

The British psychologist David Smail inspired the critical psychology movement in Britain. He worked out and justified on ethical, philosophical, and political grounds a "psychology of distress" inspired by egalitarian commitments and the ineffectiveness of traditional psychotherapy that ignored the societal determinants of mental and emotional distress. The psychology of distress and thus Smail's clinical practice grew from four principles. First, the process of demystification "cleared the conceptual undergrowth obscuring the client's view of his or her immediate predicament" (Smail 2005, p. 81). Demystification taught patients the true systemic causes of their discomforts thus presumably reducing the patient's guilt and shame but suffering from "an external reality highly resistant to individual influence and totally imperviousness to wishfulness" (ibid., p. 81). Rescuing subjectivity, the second pillar of the psychology of distress, is the patient's recognition through clinical practice "that we are, as subjective individuals, *all* uniquely, chaotically and (at least potentially) creatively *peculiar*" (ibid., p. 82, emphasis in original). The third pillar, the rehabilitation of character, excluded personal change as a goal of therapy and instead argued that "what clients have to change, if they can, is not themselves, but their world…The role for therapeutic psychology is to record, celebrate and wonder at the extraordinary diversity of human character and to reject…making moulds for people" (ibid., p. 84). The fourth pillar, reinstating the environment, is the essential assumption of the psychology of distress and the basis for its clinical practice.

> How environmental influence works, how it interacts with embodiment, how some social relations become crucial while others glance off apparently unnoticed, constitute questions of enormous subtlety and difficulty and provide material for generations of study. (ibid., p. 85)

Smail was trained in conventional psychotherapy that performs a heroic role and relies on the romantic possibility of self-invention, that is, the ability of patients to cure themselves through insight into their emotional motives and development. Yet he came to define a role for the psychotherapist in convincing patients to see themselves as the subject of their lives rather than as the object of social imperatives. Psychotherapy became for Smail a professionally guided rebellion of the patient's own self-will against the cruel objectifying powers of socialization.

> There are no ways that we ought to be other than those which we determine for ourselves. The abandonment of our myths, even though it may free us of the anxiety which arises from self-deception, will not bring us peace of mind, but it may enable us to engage with a real world which we have allowed to get dangerously out of hand. (Smail, p. 223)

Aside from clever wordplay that damages language, insistence on an alternative reality of the subjective does not come along with proof of the alternative reality. An alternative reality—a series of untested assumptions about the metaphysics of human existence—fails to work out a successful series of techniques to handle depression, anxiety and other problems that Smail attributed to the objectification of the individual as a social and economic commodity. Importantly though, it acknowledges both the failure of clinic psychotherapy to achieve its avowed treatment goals and the improbability of the social clinic as a political influence to modify society. Smail saw this problem.

> Whatever clarity may have been gained through having broken free of the conceptual restraints placed on our understanding of human distress by the disciplinary structures, greedy individualism and meshed interests of a hierarchy of power, we are still no nearer to knowing how to change our lives or to escape the influences we may now see as damaging us. (Smail 1993, p. 391)

Smail came to see the failure of psychotherapy as inevitable without deep changes in social and economic structures, a sad realization for a social clinician. He saw the alternative as caring which entailed structural reforms.

> Attention to the conditions which make possible a public life would do much to alleviate what too many of us experience as purely private gain… Rather than attempting to normalize the infinite range of differences between people and to "pathologise" the extraordinary tenacity with which they live out their experience, we should be attending to those very conditions which make culture historically transmissible and the future open to forms of social evolution which cannot now even be guessed at. (ibid., pp. 406, 407)

Smail had almost given up on psychotherapy by the end of his life and he never detailed a clinical practice that grew out of the principles of the psychology of distress. In fact, he never came to grips with the ignorance that he acknowledged in its guiding principles—"we are still no nearer to knowing.....:" To do so would reduce his theories to ideology and deprive them of philosophical and humanistic grandeur. He wanted to trust both the contention that "we cannot, I think, escape the clinic" and the contention that distress was caused by the structural imperfections of society. Caring resolved the conflict but alas at the price of psychotherapy.

Smail's caring was politically inspired and relied on social enlightenment, the assumption that recognition of the societal sources of mental and emotional distress would largely by themselves prove liberating. Yet enlightenment in this sense, including much of critical psychology, is as ideologically driven as what it replaces. Again there are problems in the fundamental construction of the idea, notably the apparent reality that social mores, the source of psychological distress and social enchainment, are the consensual product of members of a social system rather than an unwanted imposition by conspirators or illegitimate elites. A solution that predicates itself on revolutionary shifts in human consciousness is little better than prayer, especially by coming along with little in the way of methods to achieve its goals beyond belief in a new order. Yet, even while refusing or incapable of defining its program elements, Smail's caring was refreshed with a deep suspicion of psychology, social work, and the other professionalized forms of the social clinic. Still and all, any dependence on tradition, folk knowledge, the wisdom and goodness of the masses, hopefulness, and other simple naïve fictions that substitute for credible supports for theory seems to have produced much of the situation that Smail deplores. Few argue that Eden was realized in the feudal ages, the English village or the pioneer's frontier in the United States. Striving for truth—the defining purpose of Smail's critical psychology—would seem to require some of the rational arts and not just the blurry invocation of reason, goodness and a sense of human possibility.

Nonetheless, Smail's turn to the political and the active is a far cry from the typical bog of psychotherapy's rhetorical exhortations with largely passive patients. It recognizes the social roots of psychotherapy, its role as myth, in perpetuating the very problems it proclaims to treat. Yet Smail avoids the likelihood that myths are consensual affirmations of popular values. In the end, critical psychotherapy comes to the conclusion that the best that psychotherapy can do is ask sufferers not to take it out on themselves. The amelioration of psychic pain—although without much evidence that even this compromised goal is achieved—is not much of a justification for a profession of mental healing and behavioral change. The social clinic remains the practice of "magic and interest," on the one hand devoid of credible demonstrations of effectiveness and on the other beholden to long-dominant social institutions (Smail 1993, p. 316) "...Psychology has been used to mystify an understanding of the reasons for our conduct, and therapy to stifle our often anguished protests at the injustices of our world, all in the interest of the smooth running of a society which threatens to destroy us" (ibid.). Care "in commitment to the other" that rejects the control of psychotherapy requires a considerable social investment in nurturing education, family support, and social welfare that protects and indemnifies people against the vagaries of life and the economy (ibid., p. 416).

Smail's attention to enduring systemic inadequacies also cast doubt on the initial hope of humanistic psychology that societal change would ever occur through psychotherapy or clinical practice. However, the patient's awareness of economic and social inequalities and injustices is inadequate in itself to provide troubled people with more than transitory relief from guilt, shame, and anxiety if even that. Critical psychology for all its emphasis on the social and economic genesis of unhappiness and dysfunctional emotional adaptation never commanded the resources to provide the material supports that its theories pointed to. It also never expressed its theories with the modest recognition that they were as ideological and as untested as those it criticized.

Depression is quite understandable as a consequence of depressing situations in which many are caught: poor parents with children, the work-ready unemployed, the socially disabled, marginalized groups of citizens. Impossible situations and unattainable social demands create unsustainable anxieties. Yet, "quite understandable" is quite different than demonstrably true. This distinction may be moot in politics; it is not in the construction of theory that claims rational truth. Deprived of evidence to sustain effective treatment, traditional psychotherapy becomes political ideology and the social clinic is best seen as an institution that promotes the soothing fictions of myth. Yet Smail never gave up on clinical practice and he never detailed a clinical practice that grew out of the principles of the psychology of distress.

Smail's critical psychology provides no respite care for the beleaguered, no housing for the homeless, no income for the poor and unemployed, no job retraining for the economically displaced, redundant and obsolete, no protection against economic catastrophe, no surrogate families for orphans. Nor does the American social welfare system provide adequate surrogates for systemic failures. More generally, no form of the social clinic, including clinical social work, community psychology and psychiatry as well as less formalized practices, has the resources to compensate for the systemic refusal to provide needed material supports. These alternatives to psychotherapy, or perhaps better said, substantial material augmentations of clinical practice have been routinely denied by American social welfare policies. Ideas are not transformative without the social will to follow them. In rejecting supportive social services—caring—the United States announces its approval of great inequality. Not coincidentally, there is little credible evidence that any form of psychotherapy including practice based on the psychology of distress has achieved the less instrumental and very modest goals of simply making people feel good in the long term, that is, less anxious about themselves and their situations.

On his part, Smail condemned the "interest of any powerful minority that has been able to shape society to its own considerable material benefit" by way of lessening the anxiety of patients who felt responsible for their own situations. Yet the goodness, wisdom, and innocence of the masses—a founding tenet of the revolutionary left that runs through much of Smail's writing—seemed to crumble for Smail and conspiratorial theory in general as popular sentiments increasingly expressing themselves in both Britain and the United States in support of seemingly self-defeating policies and predatory political forces. It is not at all easy to be both a humanist who practices psychotherapy and a leftist critic of society.

Paul Moloney, one of Smail's prominent disciples, took an important step further to clearly accept the failure of psychotherapy and to place it without hesitation in the mores of society—"that all feeling, ideation and expression might be rooted in the material and social world" (Moloney 2013, p. 199). This combination has rarely occurred in the United States and perhaps because of cultural differences. Moreover, Moloney derived the therapy industry from reigning principles of market society. He argued that it followed commercial dictates for profit and professional status rather than humanistic imperatives rebelling against soulless capitalism.

The critics of psychotherapy have rarely attributed its failures to embedded social preferences and even less commonly have given up on the possibility of a successful clinical practice of talk therapy. Stuart (1973) criticized psychodynamic psychotherapy but advocated behavioral therapies. Szasz (1974) an unusual critic of psychotherapy for constraining individual freedom and by extension a critic of society thought that it was effective and perhaps necessary in the same way as Catholic confession. Similar to Szasz, Masson (1988) was concerned about the costs of successful psychotherapy—constraints on personal expression and individual growth—more than its actual clinical record. Dryden and Feltham (1992), Gross (1978) and Eysenck and Rachman (1965) pointed to many failures of psychotherapy but argued that in some areas, usually related to anxiety and depression, it was often successful. Perhaps the best of the critiques, Zilbergeld (1983) argued that although psychotherapy was generally a clinical failure, cognitive therapy for depression and behavioral therapy for phobias were successful. Dawes (1994) insisted that psychotherapy was effective but only in the hands of highly trained clinicians with doctorates from recognized programs. Lilienfeld et al. (2003) draw a distinction between therapy endorsed by scientific evidence and alternative psychotherapy. However, they have not given the evidence a thoughtful parsing. In fact, no form of psychotherapy whether similar to faith healing or standard clinical practice has scientific evidence to sustain it. The differences lie in the strangeness of technique more than in the outcomes. The argument by Lilienfeld et al. (2003) reduces the issue to a quibble over style—ponytails or buzz cuts—more than the substance of effective treatment.

However, the criticisms relied on hermeneutic expositions of texts more than on analyses of clinical data. Few of them critically analyzed the clinical literature, such as it has been. Many relied on frankly inadequate research. Eisner (2000) was a notable exception, however his coverage of the clinical literature was incomplete, and as with the others he accepted case studies that typically channeled evidence from the couch through the therapists themselves. The critical literature of psychotherapy's outcomes is more a squabble among competing schools of thought than a thoughtful debate informed by scientifically credible evidence. With a bit of droll humor, all of their criticisms of alternative schools may be accurate.

The possible harm of psychotherapy persists as the most disturbing subtheme of the critical literature. Tests of psychotherapy's effectiveness typically occur as demonstration research in optimal settings of surveillance and accountability, usually under the auspices of the university and thus often employing presumably the most skilled clinicians. In contrast most psychotherapy is delivered in community settings, often provided by solo practitioners, without the same conditions of accountability and by practitioners with less training. Masson (1988), Gross (1978), and Zilbergeld (1983) have argued that the common practice of psychotherapy is often destructive. Crews (1993, 2017) extended the comment to Freud.

Barlow's (2010) thoughtful essay documents tentative evidence of harm but also notes a general inattention to the phenomena. The literature focuses on measures of effectiveness but has largely ignored deterioration as an outcome of psychotherapy: "methodologies suitable for ascertaining positive effects often obscure negative effects" (ibid., p. 13). Dimidjian and Hollon (2010) address the issue of appropriate methods to document the negative effects of psychotherapy. Yet neither article estimates the incidence of harm. The critics, even those who document recurring harm, do not question the clinical role of psychotherapy but rather only the form that it takes. They assume that psychotherapy is effective. The degree of effectiveness becomes a question of skill and training. The harm of psychotherapy is not a pressing issue; only a tiny literature documents its negative effects and this is done imperfectly. As late as 2016, the plea was still unfulfilled that "psychotherapies should be assessed for both benefit and harm" (Scott and Young 2016, p. 208).

The harshest critics remain loyalists to the field. And the harshest criticism of the social clinic is probably correct; mental and emotional problems are embedded in society and not amenable to isolation for clinical treatment. There are even hints within the clinical literature that rather than psychotherapy the caring function and even surrogates for failed institutions, notably the family, are at least necessary and perhaps even decisive in preventing and treating mental and emotional problems. More broadly, structural reforms are persistently inviting.

Writing in 1992, Rollo May, an eminent humanistic psychologist, put his finger on the field's most enduring social function and the source of its soothing fictions.

> ...We in America have become a society devoted to the individual self. The danger is that psychotherapy becomes a self-concern fitting what has recently been called the narcissistic personality.... [W]e have made of psychotherapy a new cult, a method in which we hire someone to act as a guide to our success and happiness. Rarely does one speak of duty to one's society – almost everyone undergoing therapy is concerned with individual gain, and the psychotherapist is hired to assist in this endeavor. (Norcross et al. 2011, p. xxvi)

Rollo May and the humanistic psychologists along with Britain's critical psychologists initially looked to psychotherapy as a prosocial, anti-authoritarian response to the social and political depravities of the twentieth century. Their disenchantment with traditional psychotherapy was profound but their alternative notions of clinical practice contained a basic flaw. May and other reformers assumed incorrectly that psychotherapy could be clinically effective, that with some modification, it would be capable of engineering success and happiness. Yet psychotherapy is in fact immensely effective but only as a symbol of extreme individualism, the soothing fiction and the defining core of romanticism that the human will conquers all. The reckless pursuit of goodness is not good; it is the tyranny of social enchainment as triumphant individualism.

References

Ahola, P., et al. (2017). Effects of Scheduled Waiting for Psychotherapy in Patients with Major Depression. *Journal of Nervous and Mental Disease, 205*(8), 611–617.

Armstrong, J. S., & Green, K. C. (2017). *Guidelines for Science: Evidence and Checklists Scholarly Commons.* https://papers.ssrn.com/sol3/papers.cfm?abstract_id=3055874.

Barlow, D. H. (2010). Negative Effects from Psychological Treatments. *American Psychologist, 65,* 13–19. https://doi.org/10.1037/a0015643.

Crews, F. (1993). The Unknown Freud. *New York Review, 30*(19), 55–66.

Crews, F. (2017). *The Making of an Illusion.* New York: Metropolitan Books.

Cristea, I. A., Gentili, C., Pietrini, P., & Cuijpers, P. (2017, February 3). Is Investigator Background Related to Outcome in Head to Head Trials of Psychotherapy and Pharmacotherapy for Adult Depression? A Systematic Review and Meta-Analysis. *PLoS One, 12,* 1–18. http://dx.doi.org/10.1371/journal.pone.0171654.

Dal-Re, R., Bobes, J., & Cuijpers, P. (2017). Why Prudence Is Needed When Interpreting Articles Reporting Clinical Trial Results in Mental Health. *TRIALS, 18*(March) Article Number: 143.

Dawes, R. M. (1994). *House of Cards: Psychology and Psychotherapy Built on Myth.* New York, NY: Macmillan.

Dimidjian, S., & Hollon, S. D. (2010). How Would We Know If Psychotherapy Were Harmful. *American Psychologist, 65,* 21–33. https://doi.org/10.1037/a0017299.

Dineen, T. (1996). *Manufacturing Victims.* Montreal: Robert Davies Publishing.

Dragioti, E., et al. (2017). Does Psychotherapy Work? An Umbrella Review of Meta-Analyses of Randomized Controlled Trials. *Acta Psychiatrica Scandinacica, 136*(3), 236–246.

Dryden, W., & Feltham, C. (1992). *Psychotherapy and Its Discontents.* Buckingham: Open University Press.

Eisner, D. A. (2000). *The Death of Psychotherapy.* Westport, CT: Praeger.

Epstein, W. M. (2006). *Psychotherapy as Religion: The Civil Divine in America.* Reno, NV: University of Nevada Press.

Eysenck, H. J., & Rachman, S. (1965). *The Causes and Cures of Neuroses.* San Diego, CA: R. R. Knapp.

Gorey, K. M. (1996). Effectiveness of Social Work Intervention Research: Internal Versus External Evaluations. *National Association of Social Workers.* https://doi.org/10.1093/swr/20.2.119.

Gross, M. L. (1978). *The Psychological Society.* New York: Random House.

Kirk, S. A., & Kutchins, H. (1992). *The Selling of DSM: The Rhetoric of Science in Psychiatry.* New York, NY: Aldine De Gruyter.

Leichsenring, F., et al. (2017). Biases in Research: Risk Factors for Non-Replicability in Psychotherapy and Pharmacotherapy Research. *Psychological Medicine, 47*(6), 1000–1011.

Lilienfeld, S. O., Lynn, S. J., & Lohr, J. M. (2003). *Science and Pseudoscience in Clinical Psychology.* New York, NY: The Guilford Press.

Masson, J. M. (1988). *Against Therapy: Emotional Tyranny and the Myth of Psychological Healing.* New York: Atheneum.

Moloney, P. (2013). *The Therapy Industry: The Irresistible Rise of the Talking Cure, and Why It Doesn't Work.* London, UK: Pluto Press.

Norcross, J. C., VandenBos, G. R., & Freedheim, D. K. (Eds.). (2011). *History of Psychotherapy: Continuity and Change* (2nd ed.). Washington, DC, USA: American Psychological Association.

Nugent, W. R. (2017). Variability in the Results of Meta-Analysis as a Function of Comparing Effect Sizes Based on Scores From Noncomparable Measures: A Simulation Study. *Education and Psychological Measurement, 77*(3), 449–470.

Orne, M. T. (1962a). Implications for Psychotherapy Derived from Current Research on the Nature of Hypnosis. *The American Journal of Psychiatry, 118,* 1097–1103.

Orne, M. T. (1962b). On the Social Psychology of the Psychological Experiment: With Particular Reference to Demand Characteristics and Their Implications. *American Psychologist, 17,* 776–783. http://dx.doi.org/10.1037/h0043424.

Palpacuer, C., Gallet, L., Drapier, D., Reymann, J., Falissard, B., & Naudet, F. (2016). Specific and Non-specific Effects of Psychotherapeutic Interventions for Depression: Results from a Meta-Analysis of 84 Studies. *Journal of Psychiatric Research, 87,* 95–104. https://doi.org/10.1016/j.jpsychires.2016.12.015.

Peron, J., et al. (2013). Influence of Statistician Involvement on Reporting of Randomized Clinical Trials in Medical Oncology. *Anti-Cancer Drugs, 24*(3), 306–309.

Prioleau, L., Murdock, M., & Brody, N. (1983). An Analysis of Psychotherapy Versus Placebo Studies. *Behavior and Brain Sciences, 6,* 275–310.

Rieff, P. (1966). *Triumph of the Therapeutic: Uses of Faith After Freud.* New York: Harper and Row.

Rosenthal, R., & Rubin, D. B. (1978). Interpersonal Expectancy Effects—The First 345 Studies. *Behavioral and Brain Sciences, 1,* 377–386. https://doi.org/10.1017/S0140525X00075506.

Scott, J., & Young, A. H. (2016). Psychotherapies Should Be Assessed for Both Benefit and Harm. *British Journal of Psychiatry, 208*(3), 208–209.

Singh, J. P., Grann, M., & Fazel, S. (2013). Authorship Bias in Violence Risk Assessment? A Systematic Review and Meta-Analysis. *PLoS One, 8.* http://dx.doi.org/10.1371/journal.pone.0072484.

Smail, D. (1993). *The Origins of Unhappiness: A New Understanding of Personal Distress.* London: HarperCollins.

Smail, D. (2005). *Power, Interest and Psychology.* London: PCCS Books.

Smith, M. L., Glass, G. V., & Miller, T. I. (1980). *The Benefits of Psychotherapy.* Baltimore, MD: Johns Hopkins University Press.

Stanton, M., & Shadish, W. R. (1997). Outcome, Attrition, and Family-Couples Treatment for Drug Abuse: A Meta-Analysis and Review of the Controlled, Comparative Studies. *Psychological Bulletin, 122,* 170–191. https://doi.org/10.1037/0033-2909.122.2.170.

Strupp, H. H., & Hadley, S. W. (1979). Specific vs. Nonspecific Factors in Psychotherapy: A Controlled Study of Outcome. *Archives of General Psychiatry, 36,* 1125–1136. http://dx.doi.org/10.1001/archpsyc.1979.01780100095009.

Stuart, R. B. (1973). *Trick or Treatment.* Champaign, IL: Research Press.

Sugarman, M. A. (2016). Are Antidepressants and Psychotherapy Equally Effective in Treating Depression? *A Critical Commentary Journal of Mental Health, 25*(6), 475–478.

Szasz, T. (1974). *Myth of Mental Illness: Foundations of a Theory of Personal Conduct.* New York: Harper and Row.

Throop, E. A. (2009). *Psychotherapy, American Culture, and Social Policy: Immoral Individualism.* New York: Palgrave Macmillan.

Van der Kolk, B. (2015). *The Body Keeps the Score: Brain, Mind, and Body in the Healing of Trauma.* New York, NY: Penguin Books.

Zilbergeld, B. (1983). *The Shrinking of America: Myths of Psychological Change.* Boston: Little Brown.

Part II

Clinical Social Work

6

Precursors to Modern Social Work

Histories of social work and the social clinic face a number of barriers to fulfill the most basic tasks of description. Until quite recently, perhaps shortly after World War II, little information existed that accurately described let alone evaluated any social service program. The assessments tended to be case studies, administrative reviews, or budgets of income and expenditures. Little can be surmised about the extent of operations, the details of service, the number served and most important the effects of the services on recipients or more broadly on the culture itself. Aside from the episodic journalism of abuse and vain advertisements of philanthropic virtue, there are hardly any quality assessments of social work agencies and services. Yet even the more recent program evaluations, and notably those that did in fact attempt to address outcomes—Head Start, the Job Corps, and others—are themselves tortuously biased. Nonetheless, their methods, data, and conclusions can be untwisted to provide a general estimate of outcomes that usually reduce their modest claims to levels of ineffectiveness.

In light of more than one hundred years of organizations of social workers and social work practice, it is surprising that little data exist that accurately describe the distribution of social workers across areas

© The Author(s) 2019
W. M. Epstein, *Psychotherapy and the Social Clinic in the United States*,
https://doi.org/10.1007/978-3-030-32750-7_6

of practice. Social work is one of the few long-established occupations that cannot describe where social workers practice, what they do and how much they earn. Consequently, the social work literature, notably its textbooks and histories, usually fall back on case studies of practice—what social workers might be doing in a variety of settings—or descriptions of service based on a very limited number of examples. Yet impaired as they are, the few broad surveys of social work—the US Department of Labor's survey of occupations and two surveys of licensed social workers—lead to a few reasonable conclusions. The social clinic dominates the field and salaries for the most highly trained social workers are modest if not actually low.[1]

If social work and the social clinic are to be taken as modern professional activities with specified and measurable goals, then they bear the obligation to prove their ability to achieve those goals. The persistence of social work and the social clinic without credible proof of effectiveness suggests that they have become broadly consensual institutions dependent on popular satisfaction more than modern professions such

---

[1]Part of the problem of accurately describing the field concerns the various definitions employed by different sources of what constitutes a social worker. In its 2016 survey of occupations, the US Department of Labor counted about 631,000 self-identified social workers of whom only about two-thirds have any degree in the field; however, it provided little data that described practice (https://www.bls.gov/ooh/community-and-social-service/social-workers.htm#tab-6). A survey commissioned by the National Association of Social Workers and replicated a few years later are the most comprehensive and credible sources of information about social workers and social work practice but still inadequate. They only surveyed social workers licensed by various state boards (NASW Center for Workforce Studies 2010). The 2006 survey reported that licensed social workers only comprise about 50% of all social workers with social work degrees (ibid., p. 6) although they are apparently among the most educated in the field. The survey only achieved a response rate of 45%. Mental health was by far the most commonly reported primary area of practice containing 37% of respondents while social workers in many other areas of practice apparently employed a variety of clinical interventions (e.g., child welfare, addictions, school social work, and others). Average annual salaries were $37,650. The 2008–2009 replication of the survey largely repeated its findings although it with a response rate below 40%. The shortcomings of both surveys undercut their value. They addressed only a small portion of the field and achieved low response rates. They relied on respondent perceptions but failed to test the accuracy of the responses. The tasks and areas of practice the reports were poorly described. Salary data conflated full-time and part-time workers. As a result, basic knowledge of social workers and social work activities—the distribution of social workers across areas of practice and their activities through the years—is speculative at best.

as medicine and engineering justified by demonstrable achievement of service goals. Without proof of effectiveness, the truth of social work lies in its symbolic role rather than in its clinical presence, an issue of the national ethos rather than the justice or harms of socioeconomic stratification, inequality, or personal deviance.

The histories of social work frequently flatter the field for independence in choosing its own role. The less heroic reality sustains the common intuition that social institutions such as social work closely abide dominant and embedded social preferences. As such, social work practice opens a window into the preferences and priorities of the society. James Leiby had it about right:

> ...[T]he knowledge base, as social workers put it, is so confused at any point along the continuum that the prospect of pulling the insights together is dubious, and it is certainly true that the interventions and practice skills at any level do not seem to be very effective. But the burden of this history is that social welfare institutions and the profession of social work did not grow into their present prominence because of their theoretical elegance or practical success. They took form because a powerful and growing group in society – the urban business and professional class – was willing to support them. Its support was persistent, but never united or strong: it was a feeling that, despite confusions and frustrations, social work was on the right track. The right track was essentially the idea that if people were in trouble or need, someone ought to help, and that insofar as helping was organized – insofar as it took the form of a social agency – it ought to be rational, with a scientific elucidation of means and ends. (Lieby 1978)

However, Leiby's assumption running throughout his work that social work had an important role in delivering effective social services misses the field's most telling feature. Rather than the remission of social and personal problems, the field persists largely as a ceremonial affirmation of embedded social values—limited costs, individual responsibility, and administrative coherence. In the place of an advocate of social responsibility for individual failure, the right track implied an acceptance of a politically conservative practice tamed and limited by budgetary constraints, attention to individual deviance, and agency supervision that precluded social activism in pursuit of fairness and greater socioeconomic equality. These romantic expressions of an extreme personal agency are shared among the general population as well as the nation's commercial, social, and political elites. Reigning elites that appear to dominate social work practice and social policy in general do so but only as the intermediary of broadly consensual values that sanction both.

Early social work activities episodically included social and political organizing. They never dominated practice although a few social workers were prominent progressive social critics and activists. However, by the 1920s the social clinic was well on its way to capture the center of social work, marking the end of the field's brief and superficial challenge to institutionalized social values. The histories of social work share little of Leiby's strengths but bolster the field's illusions. Even when acknowledging the limitations of social work and the social clinic, the histories, with attention to the dynamics of decision making within social work organizations, do little more than document the field's accommodations. In turn, social work and the social clinic have attracted practitioners with compatible attitudes and compliant dispositions. The failures of the field and the centrality of the social clinic result from the irresistible momentum of American society.

The Orphan Trains

The orphanages and other childcare arrangements for poor and abandoned children of the nineteenth century were awful places failing to provide adequate food, clothing, shelter, or safety.

There were few public provisions for either children or the poor and those that existed were grossly underfunded. The orphan trains were an improvement, placing children with families rather than in large congregate settings. The program operated between the 1850s and 1920s and succeeded in placing perhaps as many as 250,000 poor children in rural western settings as well as a few destitute adults. The program is associated with Charles Loring Brace, the head of the New York Children's Aid Society. An early model of the modern social worker,

Brace drew his inspiration from religious conviction and a romantic faith in the general goodness of people as well as the individual's capacity for resilience and renewal.

Without either consistent or adequate public funding for the protection of needy children, the New York Children's Aid Society had little choice but to act more as an agent of actual social preferences or at least on behalf of the charitable impulses of their wealthy clients rather than as an advocate for the poor. Indeed, the humane impulses of donors may have been more kindly and caring than the prevailing inattention of the population to the needs of children and the destitute. Some placements did in fact provide the orphans with "spiritual and material salvation" but other placements did not. Most of the operation of the orphan trains and indeed most care for destitute children took place outside of legal supervision. The children lacked legal or public representation that acted on their behalf. They were largely dependent on the good intentions and skills of private charities. While the program provided some supervision over initial placements in attempting to settle the children with appropriate families, the coverage was desultory. Local committees judged the fitness of families applying for children. Neither the committees nor the poorly staffed program provided consistent surveillance.

The orphan trains paired a desire to address the incapacity or unwillingness of eastern states to attend to the needs of the poor with a shortage of farm labor and domestic help largely in the west. While most of the children were true orphans without parents or family, many had destitute parents.

Placing out was intended to improve the conditions of the children. Yet, they were apparently accepted primarily for their labor. The goal was for "homeless waifs [to find] themselves in comfortable and kind homes, with all the boundless advantages and opportunities of the Western farmer's life about them" (Holt 1992, p. 7). The reality may have been considerably different.[2]

---

[2]The reality of the orphan trains program is difficult to assess accurately. There is no systematic accounting of the children's situations nor of their outcomes. Most of the information is anecdotal. The historical reconstructions are dependent on the partial records of agencies such as the

Andrea Warren's *Orphan Train Rider: One Boy's Success* (1996) is surely not a unique tale but just as surely the Children's Aid Society did not have the data to assert in 1910 that "87 percent of the orphan train riders had 'done well'" (Warren, p. 60). Warren does not accept that estimate while Holt (1992) and O'Connor (2001a, b) are even more pessimistic about the program's conditions. After all, most of the legacy of the orphan trains is detailed in the incomplete manuscripts and records created by the agencies that constituted the program. In fact, there was little follow-up supervision of the children after placement and little commitment to rigorous accountability of the charitable heart especially during a time when the orphan train seemed to be a frank improvement over congregate care. No periodic census of orphan train children was taken and failures were probably underreported. In the end, most of the orphan train experience is simply lost.

Presumably incidents of abuse had drawn attention to orphan train children. The program was criticized for inadequate management, notably concerning the care with which it selected and monitored placements. That is, the orphan trains program itself fell under suspicion of child abuse (O'Connor, p. 227). It was also charged for "knowingly sending delinquents and undesirables west, with the express (sic) purpose of ridding New York of this element" (Holt, p. 120). The complaints against the program may have reflected unrelated political issues and insular fears of outsiders. Yet the Children's Aid Society was not prepared to rebut the charges, let alone refute them; it had neglected to institute a process of tracking the children and their placements. Just as likely, there were many more failures than the program was willing to acknowledge. Apparently, the opportunity to provide convenient labor for an expanding nation and to reduce the inconvenience and burden of urban poverty triumphed over the commitment to nurture and protect children without parents.

New York Children's Aid Society and interviews conducted with the few remaining and available orphan train children. Those interviews are unlikely to adequately represent children who experienced abusive placements, runaways, and others who did not settle into lives easily accessible to interviewers or who died as a result of their placements.

Placing out was perceived as respectable in its intent and motivation and could be presented to the general public as an example of what good could be done for thousands of unfortunate children. In the age of rugged American individualism, Social Darwinism and self-made men and women, the advertised results of the placing-out system gave validity to American ideals of success. That the emphasis was on children and not adults reflected the general consensus that few adults, tarnished by their years on city streets, could be saved. Grit and determinism were championed, and those who had been placed out become symbols for the ideals of the Protestant American work ethic. (Holt, p. 5)

Yet the assessment of the orphan train experience rests on very imperfect anecdotes and the degree to which prevailing social attitudes provided context for their interpretation. Much to the point, indentured service had a long tradition in the United States during which slavery was still prevalent and legal in the 1850s and workers had yet to realize an organized voice. The promise of a fireside home with loving surrogate parents was the soothing fiction of the orphan trains and placing out. The New York Children's Aid Society, the quintessential social work agency, pressed forward a humanistic face of compassion and reform while fulfilling the popular market imperatives of the society. The social agency's autonomy was limited to the manner in which it chose to serve popular values. It was not sanctioned in any form to change society but rather to fulfill popular social mandates—the often tacit imperatives of the popular will and the prevalent tolerance for theft of labor.

The impulse to provide surrogates for absent families was largely correct. Yet the delivery was inadequate without screening potential families and orphans and without subsequent visits by agency personnel to assure humane environments and decent treatment. Indeed, the imperfections of the placements are repeated in the current child foster care program even while the orphan trains may have provided a greater proportion of decent situations for the children than contemporary orphanages or even the present foster care program.

By the early 1900s, the ideas that sustained the orphan train—a mysticism of rural life and the resilience of children, among others—had changed in recognition that leaving children unsupervised in largely unknown situations was "the height of moral and social irresponsibility" (O'Connor, *Orphan Trains* 2001b, p. 307). Yet the reforms in record keeping, case finding, and clinical support that largely paralleled the professionalization of social work did not provide much routine improvement in care for the children. Essential surrogate services, expensive then and now, were not funded publically or provided privately by quality families willing to adopt or foster children in need. Again, the soothing fictions of agency responsibility for supervision and case finding hid the challenges of quality supportive care. The alternative, "a growing consensus…that the best way to help poor children was not to send them away but to work with their families, and within their communities, to maximize everybody's opportunity, safety and happiness" never reached a consensus sufficient to actually realize these goals (O'Connor, p. 307). Brace's legacy lies in recognition of the superiority of foster family care to placing children in large congregate setting but not in its realization. Indeed, social work propagated then as it does now, unattainable goals as though they were programmatic realities. It does so not out of malice but within a social mandate that constrains its practice.

At least in theory, Brace's idea of placing abandoned, neglected, and orphaned children in homes rather than in then commonly abusive penal institutions and orphanages was desirable. In practice, it may not have been much better. Phyllis Day (2006) summarizes the early history of the program with little sentimentality.

> For twenty years, haphazardly and without follow-up, often simply "taking" (kidnapping) children they felt were in need, agents loaded children on trains and shipped them to cities in the West, where they were "picked over" and chosen by families. Unfortunately, many families just wanted the extra help and badly mistreated the children. Many simply disappeared, either running away, getting lost, or dying.

While Loring Brace, the son of Charles Loring Brace and his replacement at the Children's Aid Society, improved the ability of the Children's Aid Society to monitor the program by implementing common management practices and at least the spirit of an emerging social work profession to collect relevant measures of program outcomes, the continuing experience of the orphan trains may not have changed much. However, the lack of adequate child fostering did not result from deficient program management or the immaterial spirit of a newly emerging social work. The problem of care was a problem of American priorities. Too few quality adults stepped forward to foster the children; the charitable sector failed to compensate with adequate resources for quality placements; and government refused to foot the costs of humane care. In short, the society's indifference to the plight of unprotected children sorely restrained any steps to fulfill their needs. Social programs persist as social agents rather than as independent angels of a Godly plan for Heaven on Earth.

Social Work and the Institution

Rothman's (1971) classic, *The Discovery of the Asylum*, summarizes the unfortunate history of programs for the insane, the criminal and the indigent through the nineteenth century in the United States. It repeats the story of the orphan trains and placing out: agents of society that despite individual good intentions fail to provide "standards of moral treatment" (ibid., p. 269). Indeed, moral treatment and its synonyms of asylum, order, safety, concern, care, and rehabilitation are often the soothing fictions of social welfare programs for people in need.

The early nineteenth-century institutions for people in need were reforms intended to "relieve overcrowding in the local almshouses and jails and provided more specialized and rational treatment...for inmates," including delinquent youth, the blind and physically hand-icapped, the physically ill and the seriously mentally ill (Lieby 1978, p. 49). The specialization, justified by the emerging status that science conferred, was probably wise if in fact the ability existed to address particular problems. However, then as now, rational treatment was a fiction, a term of commendation for serious attempts to address a problem more than the actual application of successful treatment derived from rigorous empirical investigation. The rational in the case of the asylum and corrections was a term of hope that referred to the promise of the institution: "to create a total environment that would furnish wholesome circumstances for change…[doing] the job that the existing community – the family, the neighborhood, economy, or polity – was not doing" (Rothman ibid., p. 56). This profoundly religious, utopian and even otherworldly vision only lasted as long as it was perceived to be both inexpensive and effective. In practice, the often ineffective search of the institution for cure, rehabilitation and socialization languished along with the social will to provide long-lasting substitutes for failed families and communities. Custodial care often declined into frank abuse, neglect, and regimentation.

> The American experiment with institutionalization was not a prolonged success. By the 1850's almost every type of asylum was losing its special qualities, and by the 1870's few traces remained of the original designs. In a majority of mental hospitals, the careful balance of moral treatment gave way to custodial care; in almost every penitentiary the unique arrangements of the Auburn and Pennsylvania plans disappeared before wardens' preoccupation with peace and security. Almshouses, never very attractive places to begin with, became even more disorderly, while houses of refuge frequently came to resemble poorly run state prisons. (ibid., p. 237)

Moreover, the science of philanthropy often went past any pretense of rational management, coming to rest on programs to fulfill the assumptions of eugenics and Darwinian sorting.

> It followed that the "mother state" should care for its "weaker children" in sequestered colonies where they would be comfortable and well provided for but unable to reproduce their kind… It seemed that science offered a real possibility that experts might distinguish the congenital criminal and the hereditary pauper, the hereditary lunatic and idiot, from those who could be rehabilitated, and that authorities might provide appropriate institutional care for each kind. Thus biology entered into a line of thought that was formerly dominated by religion and political economy, and custodial institutions were envisioned as a form of prevention. (Leiby, p. 110)

Subsequent efforts to improve conditions for dependent people also looked to noninstitutional, "homelike" placements and even occasional attempts to provide relief in people's homes. However, as suggested by the orphan train experience, placing out in one form or another after a short period of enthusiasm deteriorated to the same levels of neglect as institutional care. Moreover, decentralized programs were often less amenable to oversight and public scrutiny than care in large institutions. Still and all, the inadequacy of the programs for dependent populations—institutions or outplacements—probably reflected general unconcern more than any inherent financial inability of the contemporary economy to sustain people who could not provide for themselves.

Grob, an eminent historian of mental illness in the United States, argues that

> By the middle of the twentieth century, mental hospitals were widely regarded as the institutional remnants of an earlier social order – outdated institutions that disregarded the rights of sick and dependent persons by isolating and subjecting them to cruel abuse. The result was a renewed interest in other alternatives to institutional care... The rejection of the idea of mental hospital care proved to be a development of the utmost social significance. It affected not only nearly 450.00 patients in public mental hospitals in 1940 but families, psychiatrists and other mental health professionals, legislators, public officials and the general public. (Grob 1983, p. 5)

Yet the reforms, institutional and then community placements, were constrained by the principle of social efficiency. Solutions needed to be relatively inexpensive and compatible with social customs, implying a pervasive rejection of prolonged service that was better than abusive warehousing. While deinstitutionalizing the mental patient was a demonstrably plausible alternative to the failures of the mental hospital (Stein and Test 1980), American society never allocated sufficient funds to provide adequate community care. At the same time, the mental hospitals and their community alternatives drew staff—social workers as well as others—who abided their missions and their operations. Social workers and other staff became the tame managers of social priorities; the novelties of thought and program that they embraced replicated popular presiding assumptions.

Charity Organization Societies

During the approximately fifty years from the late 1870s and through the Progressive Era, two social work approaches to need contended with each other. The Charity Organization Societies focusing on home visits, differential diagnosis, and individual behavioral change anticipated the social clinic. In contrast, the iconic settlement houses at least initially sought systemic change. In practice, both converged around dominant social values offering little material support, largely recreational social services and infrequent challenges to reigning priorities and social preferences. Rather than material and political support, both approaches promoted soothing fictions of social reform largely based on personal relationships between the enlightened and gracious on the one hand and the unschooled and needy on the other. Not surprisingly, both were ineffective and not least because of their commitment to American romanticism of individual agency, paternalism, and the volunteer impulse rather than to social change.

Mary Richmond's *Social Diagnosis* (1917) laid out the core principles for the charity organization societies. The cause of individual need could be diagnosed on scientific grounds by a trained cadre of largely voluntary home visitors who would then apply the appropriate remedies. The obvious assumption was that need usually emerged from individual deficits of character that expressed itself in unemployment, behavioral problems, criminality, addiction, laziness, promiscuity, and other problems. The central aim of the charity organization societies was to avoid pauperism—the habitual reliance on public or private charity—and to achieve self-sufficiency, that is, independence from hand-outs.

> American social work, like its English counterpart, was an integral part of the liberal's answer to life under a system of free enterprise. Both began as an attempt to temper the cold wind of capitalism to the shorn lamb of a proletariat whose existence was both a rebuke and a threat to the more fortunate classes, and although in both countries social work changed as the framework of the existing social philosophy, the mark of the mint still remained. (Woodroofe 1971, pp. 92–93)

The solutions depended largely on counseling the assumed miscreant through a process of interviewing, home visiting, and investigation. Some charity organization societies engaged in more practical efforts. "The Buffalo society, for example, very early added to its work the maintenance of employment bureau, woodyards, laundries, work rooms, special schools, wayfarerers' lodges, loan societies, penny banks, fuel societies, creches, district nursing, sick diet kitchens and an accidental hospital and many other societies followed suit" (Woodroofe ibid., p. 96). Yet in an otherwise carefully documented book, Woodroofe does not document this claim nor prove that it was more than superficial and episodic if even that. Apparently only "a determined few" within the societies advocated for more material service. However, even these few were still committed to the "social worker's trained skill to use individual, group and community resources to help men and women to lead happier lives" (ibid., p. 97). Most charity societies and their workers were largely attentive to personal epiphany and self-help. Yet even the rosiest gloss on charity society activities cannot avoid the obvious conclusion that their efforts were grossly inadequate responses to need.

Mencher's (1967) summary of the philanthropic and religious impulse of the charity organization societies goes to the heart of their limitations and social blindness.

> Miss Richmond complained of the displacement of the volunteer by the professional worker. The professional symbolized the emphasis on scientific expertise and the decline of personal philanthropy. Whether there was ever any reality to Miss Richmond's romantic illusion about class relationships in America, the working people at the end of the nineteenth century were certainly not willing to accept paternalistic help. (ibid., p. 258)

The professional social worker was little different than the volunteer. Usually drawn from more comfortable social strata than the teeming multitudes but with an affection for scientific symbolism that conferred authority, the efforts of the trained social worker were just as ineffective as the volunteer. Neither one possessed or pursued even rudimentary knowledge capable of identifying the causes and solutions to social and individual problems. Social work practice then as now is typically marginal to contemporary political discussions but dominated by reigning orthodoxy, a consensus that paradoxically includes those to be helped.

Richmond's individual and clinical strategy was marginal to the political conflicts of the time that engaged more with the systemic problems of industrialization, urbanization, inequality, and immigration. The issues on the political table competed against the free market and limited government for greater public expenditures in health, education, income support, and the regulation of business. The goal of self-sufficiency was impossible then as it is now. Yet, Richmond's frank paternalism was apparently rejected by many in need but not by the dominant and influential classes of wealth. The Charity Organization Society was a programmatic failure but a political and social success. The narrative of social work as trained personnel applying scientifically effective interventions to social problems was the soothing fiction of a very unequal society with deep structural flaws.

Settlement Houses

In contrast with charity organization societies, the settlement house movement seemed to operate off of the premise that systemic failures created material and social deficits beyond the individual's capacity to address. However, the settlement house solution was as paternalistic and futile as home visiting and counseling and similarly lacked sufficient resources to meet the most basic material needs of food, clothing, shelter, education, and training. The settlements also failed to engage in the political conflicts over the social and economic inequalities that created systemic failures.

By the early twentieth century, there were more than 400 settlement houses in over 30 states with most located in large cities (https://social-welfare.library.vcu.edu/settlement-houses/settlement-houses/;   Karger 1984, p. vi). The description of settlement house services by Woods and Kennedy (1990), originally published in 1922, seems generally accurate or at least confirmed by a number of prominent sources (Lasch-Quinn

1993; Carson 1990; Trolander 1975; Pacey 1950; Barbuto 1999; Karger 1984; Fabricant and Fisher 2002; and even, for the most part, Addams 1998 [1923]): clubs for children; recreational programs; summer camps in the city and countryside; educational programs such as kindergartens, libraries, classes in grammar, history, sociology, and many other academic areas presumably taught by volunteer university faculty; training in a number of crafts with shop work for boys and needlework and domestic service for girls and other areas for both with the intention of encouraging more advanced vocational preparation; art exhibits along with training in arts and crafts such as weaving, basketry, pottery, wood carving and others. "The club and class scheme" dominated service provision at the settlements; however, its contributions to the society and most importantly for recipients are undocumented. Moreover, Woods and Kennedy and the literature itself provide few estimates, except in rare case studies, of the endurance, the depth or the outcomes of the services. Their description of settlement house advocacy in behalf of housing, factory, and health reform, the support of labor unions, and other political actions to benefit poorer groups seems largely restricted to Jane Addams at Hull House in Chicago and perhaps a few others. It was not broadly characteristic of settlement house priorities or activities.

The more common role of the settlements in addressing issues of labor, with Jane Addams in mind, was targeted to "prevent industrial conflicts by reaching sources of difficulty" (Woods and Kennedy ibid., p. 172). Quite to the point of clarifying the role of the settlements, a preference for social relations that depreciated the value of conflict minimized risks to the settlements—after all, their funding and many of their important volunteers were provided by industrial and commercial elites—but also limited their value and credibility in representing the interests of the poor and needy. No settlement house sought either election to their boards from residents of their areas or in any formal way asked for the sanction of service populations for settlement activities. There is little that is more paternalistic and condescending than telling the needy what they need. The propagation of goodness seems often to be a convenient substitute for addressing the material deficits of the poor.

Lacking detailed descriptions that address the degree to which the settlements satisfied prevailing needs, Woods and Kennedy compose a sentimental collective that pays tribute to the charitable impulses of wealthier classes, in particular their sympathy toward poorer, often immigrant populations. As symbols of philanthropy, they perpetuate the soothing fictions of small town self-help, the New Yorker magazine's charming fiction of the urban village but without its defining irony. The fact that the settlements also screened applicants for jobs further defines their role as adjunctive to the market rather than in opposition as an advocate for reform.

The Social Gospel, a Protestant movement that targeted social problems as systemic failures, was a major inspiration for the settlement houses. However, as Mencher argues, mainline religious opinion "continued to view reform as a personal rather than a social matter" (ibid., p. 259). A few settlement houses, notably Jane Addams' Hull House in Chicago and the Henry Street Settlement House in New York City, were politically active and still resonate as historical exemplars of social advocacy. Yet the so-called radical tradition in social work was notably unsuccessful. The more typical settlement house performed as a community center, providing recreation, athletics, arts and craft activities and some assistance for immigrants, mostly language classes, rather than social advocacy. In fact, many settlements offered casework and group work that were safely attendant to personal deviancy and belied their mission of social reform. "This type of program abbreviated the settlement's former commitment to altering the social structure to accommodate the individual. Instead, it stressed the need to alter the individual to fit the environment" (Lasch-Quinn 1993, p. 153). Personal risk in pursuit of social ideals has been a popular theme in social work rhetoric—heroic opposition to injustice in the nation's exceptional destiny. Yet social work practice itself has offered little more than the soothing fiction that the American system is fundamentally sound requiring only that the helping hand of service be extended to the few who either cannot or will not adapt to its virtues.

The hortatory intensity of the Social Gospel was insufficient to move the settlement houses to oppose deeply seated but unfortunate American preferences, notably for racial discrimination:

...The cherished creed of responsiveness to one's neighbors [the Social Gospel] and the view differentiating blacks from white immigrants prohibited the settlement movement from confronting the issue [of racial discrimination] directly. The mainstream workers provided tremendous leadership concerning the influx of huge numbers of European immigrants into the country, but faltered when it came to blacks. When the movement witnessed a major transformation during and after World War I, it underwent continual self-evaluation. The replacement of white immigrants by blacks in many settlement house environs presented a chance for a reorientation of the movement. True responsiveness to the community might have given the movement a new lease on life.

Instead, the movement's failure to adapt its plans for drastic community change to blacks hastened the migration of social service and civil rights activities into other organizations dedicated only to aspects of the integrated, ambitious settlement work programs. (ibid., p. 152)

The settlement house failure to address racial injustice was typical of its timidity in pushing against popular social preferences that contradicted its self-professed commitment to liberal democracy. "The National Federation of Settlements did not officially repudiate segregated settlements until the 1950's" (Trolander's Introduction to Woods and Kennedy 1990, p. xix).

While settlement house workers may have been "in the vanguard of Progressive Era reformers," judging by the programs of the settlements themselves, they were not in the vanguard of Progressive Era achievements (Barbuto 1999, p. vii). Karger's case study of the Minneapolis settlement house (1984) seems more faithful to the general record, such as it is, to consider the settlement movement and much of the progressive impulse of the time as a form of benign social control.

Throughout the progressive era the reformers were fearful of social upheaval....To the reformers, American cities were "swarming" and "seething" with the pernicious threat of the "dangerous classes."... Within the unstable political and social climate of early twentieth century America, the need for social control was thought to be of primary significance. Without social control there could be no social stability. For the progressive mind concerned with efficiency, rationality, stability, and social order, social control was the necessary ingredient in the social engineer of the period. (Karger, p. 281)

Importantly, the consilience between the progressive reformers and the industrial and social elites was not through conspiracy but through culture, "a commonality of values and a similar Weltanshauung" (ibid., 282). The shared values of social work leadership, elites and prevailing social values created programs of more ceremonial value than substantive.

Social control for the settlements meant the teaching and propagating of middle class values. If, in the meantime, it was humbling and paternal to the immigrant classes, that would have been a small price to pay for the benefit accrued by assimilation. (Karger, p. 284)

Yet it seems that no one in the settlements asked the swarming masses for their opinion about the trade-off between paternalism and assimilation. Unfortunately, even with regard to assimilation, the settlements seem to have played a marginal role. In any case, it is not at all apparent that settlement house programs and the insights and efforts of staff and board members had any effect on controlling the masses. Industrialization that produced jobs and good wages along with broadened political participation and labor unions probably offered much more than thin social services by way of taming the savage breast of revolution. Social work as ever seems dominated by its symbolism in affirming popular values rather than by contributing substantially to the resolution of social problems.

Mencher (1967) dilutes the Romantic strain in the settlement movement, preferring to characterize it as imbued by "the practical and the scientific" (ibid., p. 258). Yet the notion of localism running through the basic notion of neighborhood helping and reliance on local initiatives proved inadequate to handle the enormous problems created by economic failure and social isolation. The settlement houses for all their good intentions seemed out of touch with those they would help. Their notions of good government—"taking thought for its bookkeeping, safeguarding its finances, and enhancing its administrative efficiency"—made "but a sorry appeal among the tenements" (Woods and Kennedy op. cit., p. 227). The political machines despite the issues of corruption delivered more material benefits to poor people than the interminable preaching and thin, desultory provisions of social workers.

Jane Addams, the most prominent settlement house worker, also perpetrated the most telling delusion of the settlement house ideology.

> It is constantly said that because the masses have never had social advantages they do not want them, that they are heavy and dull, and that it will take political or philanthropic machinery to change them. This divides a city into rich and poor; into the favored, who express their sense of the social obligations by gifts of money, and into the unfavored, who express it by clamoring for a "share" – both of them actuated by a vague sense of justice. This division of the city would be more justifiable, however, if the people who thus isolate themselves on certain streets and use their social ability for each other gained enough thereby and added sufficient to the sum total of social progress to justify the withholding of the pleasures and results of the progress from so many people who ought to have them. (Addams as quoted by Mencher op. cit., p. 260)

Addams saw the settlements and her role as arbitrator between contending factions, especially between commercial ownership and organized labor (Addams 1998 [1923], p. 228). She advocated the unity of the population: "settlement workers are bound to regard the entire life of their city as organic, to make an effort to unity it, and to protect against its overdifferentiation" (ibid., p. 261). The reality was quite different. Citizens were deeply divided between wealth and ownership on the one hand and the poor and the worker on the other. Addams, among the most willing among the settlement workers to advocate justice temporized its content in pursuing a fantasy of solidarity that was largely irrelevant to existing problems. Compared to the labor movement and the policy positions of the urban political machines, the settlements had little to offer the very people that they claimed to care for. Contrary to Fabricant and Fisher's loyal hope for social work, there is little evidence that the settlements were ever able "to promote social solidarity and thereby help address the crisis of the community" (Fabricant and Fisher 2002, p. 239). The role of settlement workers "…to see the needs of their neighborhoods as a whole, to furnish data for legislation, and use their influence to secure it" was rarely if ever a vital service (ibid.). Indeed, Margolin (1997) might well argue that in light of their self-appointed mission—the "cover of kindness"—the primary role of the settlements worked out to be surveillance of the poor by keeping an eye on swarming and seething Americans for signs of rebellion.

It is a measure of America's core values at the time, that Addams' "acclaim and adulation" before World War I—at least according to Elshtain (2002, pp. 244–245)—was probably predicated on her temporizing goals of solidarity rather than advocacy. The heroic elevation of Addams symbolized the romanticism of American values—the curious conjunction between organic solidarity and extreme individualism. The settlements were the capitulation to those values at a time when conflicts between important forces offered more vital alternatives and greater promise.

Trolander's (1975) portrait of settlement house activities during the 1930s—the height of social need in the United States—gets past sentimentality. A few politically active settlements, usually in New York and Chicago that accepted the call to improve neighborhood conditions as their prime objective and pushed for the Social Security Act, aligned themselves with the labor unions, and organized groups of the unemployed for social and political changes. However, they were hardly typical of the 202 settlement houses—the core of the movement—that faced the Great Depression. "Many settlements were never really involved in social action. While most were eager to cooperate with private relief-giving efforts, some never went beyond this stage." They fulfilled settlement obligations by programs of "clubs and classes" (ibid., p. 149) with even less attention to social reform than during the Progressive Era.

Trolander's multitude of explanations for the decline of the settlement movement reduce to one: The settlements acceded to the safety of social preferences through the vehicle of funding. Without funding, they could not exist. Funding came from wealthier populations. Social activism in support of greater economic and social change threatened their finances and thus their existence. Most settlements did not take the gamble. Those that did were in less precarious situations that sustained their activism. Dominant social preferences prevailed even to the point of engendering what Leuchtenburg (1963) judged to be a very inadequate Social Security Act—the pinnacle achievement of the New Deal—even within the economic capacities of the time.

The Social Clinic in Social Work

Social work can be defined as an occupation in perpetual pursuit of professional standing. Its adoption of psychotherapy as its core intervention repeats its service history but with one large difference. The social clinic provided the field with a broader mandate to serve a much larger population than the poorest and neediest American citizens and increased the field's purview of social problems amenable to treatment. In addition to the impoverished and those with obvious and deep deficits in function, the social clinic laid claims to all mental and emotional problems along with social problems that are engendered by presumably deviant motivations including laziness, promiscuity, drug and alcohol addiction and a variety of criminal offenses. By 2002, social workers, comprising more than 60% of mental health professionals, provided more psychotherapy than psychiatrists and clinical psychologists combined (Gibelman 2004, p. 43).

Social work's development followed a mandate of popular values. It rarely challenged that mandate or the propriety of the reigning national ethos. Episodic social criticisms coming from social workers were muted under the employment weight of the field that was concentrated in social clinics obedient to dominant preferences. Those preferences defined a role for social work to correct the individual rather than address systemic failures. Its attempts to correct deviance were typically channeled through the social clinic, that is, talk therapy. Finally, the interventions of social work—typically clinical, much less commonly supportive or caring, and sometimes involving mediation that referred to liaison and resource mobilization—were near-uniformly unsuccessful. Psychotherapy is ineffective while resources are inadequate for supportive care limiting the possibilities for addressing need except by referral to other customarily resource-strapped agencies.

The field's history belies its heroic myth, namely that fearless avatars of justice competed for the good of all. To the contrary, the field had little choice but to accept the social values that defined its purposes and funded its services. Opposition would have been futile even while the field's acquiescence has been quick and graceless with little negotiation over the conditions of surrender. In short, social work was neither unfaithful nor angelic (as Specht and Courtney 1994 would have it) but staffed out with the rather humdrum range of citizens seeking a somewhat professional calling and some degree of social status. Social work seems to have realized Tocqueville's fears of democracy as elevating populist sloganeering to professional standing above the Enlightenment's hope for a science of human behavior.

Commissioned by the National Conference of Charities and Corrections, the 1915 Flexner report early on challenged social work's ambition to mature from a volunteer enterprise to become a profession. He laid out six criteria of a profession: intellectual operations deriving their core knowledge from science and learning focused on practical and definable ends, amenable to educationally communicable technique, tending to self-organization, and altruistic in motivation, that is, "responsive to public interest" (ibid., p. 156). A number of deficiencies in social work isolated it from professional standing. Its essential role was in mediating access to other professions rather than applying its unique knowledge. "The very variety of the situations he encounters compels him to be not a professional agent so much as the mediator invoking this or that professional agency" (ibid., p. 160). Social work "appears not so much a definite field as an aspect of work in many fields.... [It is] not so much a separate profession, as an endeavor to supplement certain existing professions pending their completed development" (ibid., p. 161). Further, Flexner claimed that its diffuse aims impeded training. While he judged that the material of social work "comes obviously from, science and learning, from economic, ethic, religion and medicine," it had still not become thoroughly professional in character and scientific in method (ibid., p. 164). He certainly did not think much of the field's appreciation for its uncertainties.

Social work has suffered to some extent from one of the vices associated with journalism, excessive facility in speech and in action.... For if social work is not definite enough to be called a profession, the social worker will at least be less cock-sure than the professional man he calls in. (ibid., p. 163)

In summary, Flexner argued that the field lacked true scientific information, a sharply defined role, autonomy and an appropriate mood to be a profession. Yet Flexner's meaning of scientific knowledge seems often synonymous with respected knowledge, e.g., the clergy and law, more than with professions based on the sciences themselves, e.g., medicine and engineering. In this light, social work appeared to have options in pursuing professional status. It could seek an objectively coherent practice expertise or it could choose a softer test for the value of its interventions. On the one hand, clinical rationality required definitive tests of its interventions and on the other hand only the criteria of social satisfaction mattered. In choosing first Freudian psychoanalysis and then the psychotherapies, social work followed the clergy's epistemologies of faith and revelation (along with the ecclesiastical test of social acceptance). It hedged the bet with the demulsifying fictions of the social sciences and the jargon of best practice, evidence-based practice, and then the concession of evidence-informed practice.

Arguably the best of the histories of social work's early development from 1880 to 1930, Lubove's *The Professional Altruist* (1967) portrays the consistency of psychotherapy with the field's earlier development, particularly the charity organization societies' use of case diagnosis, individual treatment, and home visiting. By the 1920s, "the emergence of a therapeutically oriented casework as [its] nuclear image and skill" broke little new ground in social work as a call on professional standing (p. 220).

Casework rooted in a psychiatric explanation of human behavior was a key, presumably, to a knowledge base and helping technique more "scientific" and hence more professional than "social diagnosis" or social reform which exaggerated environmental and rational factors in behavior and its control. (ibid., p. 221)

> Social work's emergence as a profession resulted not only in a devaluation of voluntarism but in a chronic tension between public and private welfare. In minimizing the desirability of relief in favor of character rehabilitation and close personal supervision of the poor, the charity organization movement discredited public assistance. Charity organization leaders convinced themselves and countless Americans that public outdoor assistance was incompatible with efficient, scientific philanthropy because it pauperized the recipients…[A]ccepted by the poor as a right, public relief disrupted the social and economic order by reducing all incentive to work. (ibid., p. 52)

Yet Mary Richmond's (1917) process of social diagnosis was impossible to achieve and remains so. Except in very unusual circumstances, methods for rationally identifying social cause cannot be applied in a humane society; moreover, the definitive methods of randomized controlled trials are technically impossible to apply to live social situations outside of the laboratory except in small scale, limited demonstrations. They would also be prohibitively expensive even if the legal, cultural, political, and moral questions could be addressed. The social sciences were attempts to develop a compromise with rationality in exploring social reality. Yet the triumph of psychotherapy in social work represented the rejection of even the semblance of objective coherence in favor of the a priori romanticism of the suite of psychotherapies.

Following Lubove, social work practice materialized embedded social values that gave rise first to the charity organization movement and then inspired the kindred assumptions of psychotherapy and the social clinic. Psychotherapy offered special knowledge to achieve "social adjustment," a term of art that implied that the techniques of personal treatment would effectively handle a variety of deviant behaviors including psychiatric problems, addiction, and criminality. By adopting psychotherapy as its core knowledge and skill

> Social workers undoubtedly acquired a more sophisticated awareness of the subtleties and ambiguities of personality, but in the process they undermined their capacity to promote institutional change and deal effectively with problems of mass deprivation in an urban society. (ibid., p. 117)

Lubove is surely accurate in describing the natural compatibility of psychotherapy with casework and thus the dominance of the field by the social clinic. Yet he probably makes a number of mistakes of emphasis, first in interpretation by exaggerating the field's autonomy from dominant social attitudes but then too by mischaracterizing both the power and success of psychiatry (e.g., psychotherapy) as well as alternative roles in systemic reform. He and the field itself also employ science as a term of commendation—being reasonable and sensible—more than as a collection of methods of rationality adjusted by the different disciplines that define the terms of objective reality.

As ever, social work practice depended on funding. Even the wealthiest of its enthusiasts have never been capable of sustaining even a small portion of social need. Thus, social work was obliged to defer to dominant values in defining its goals and developing interventions to achieve them. Then as now, the American ethos has been conservative and romantic with an extreme insistence at its core on personal agency and therefore personal responsibility. In promoting psychotherapy, social work also accepted another pillar of the romanticism that rejected objective coherence in favor of the truth of the inner life, that is, subjectivity (Epstein 2017). In spite of a paradoxical image as liberal, the social clinic is an organic social creation of the essential conservative tenets of American culture and society, insisting through its practice that the forms of rational induction implicit to psychotherapy are capable of encouraging the individual to adjust their dysfunctional behaviors. In contrast, to insist on systemic failure as the genesis of personal failure and then to organize affected citizens socially and politically around this theme would alienate the field from its sources of support. It is not a stretch to see social work as the first and quintessential postmodern profession and not least because of its delusional claims on scientific practice.

Lubove also misreads the alignment of social workers during the early formative period of the field with reform movements as well as their success. Most social workers and social service programs—as above, the asylums, settlement houses and fostering provisions for children—followed socially obedient paths. Only a few reflected either in practice or opinion even the moderate reform attitudes of Addams.

Few publicly supported democratic socialism let alone an activist and radical path such as communism. More to the problem of historical accuracy, Lubove does not document his assumptions of program accuracy and the power of a variety of interventions—an impossible task given the sparse record, the absence of credible program evaluations, and its many departures from systematic description; after all, he was an historian trapped by the gross incompleteness of the existing record. Lubove's affection for reform, the capacities of social work, and the correctness of its mission did not last long past the 1960s when he became an enthusiast for President Reagan and antagonistic to the claims of the poor.[3]

Concerning the social clinic generally, the ceremonial role becomes the naturally ascendant explanation without evidence of clinical prowess. Neither social work nor Lubove ever seriously questioned the effectiveness of psychotherapy. The field's assessment of its value followed the imperatives of social acceptability and organizational benefit more than clinical effectiveness. The persistence of social work as with the clergy and theology apparently depends on the popularity of a ceremonial role.

The Social Clinic, Social Work and the Bribe to Indolence

The pattern of activism for reform among service agencies quickly adapting to social imperatives that undercut its momentum is replicated repeatedly throughout the history of social work and social welfare in the United States. It is not surprising in an open society with few coercive influences over the formation of popular tastes that society

---

[3]I was enrolled in Roy Lubove's history of social work course in 1966 and stayed in touch with him and a number of his colleagues until the late 1980s. His political views became even more strident than those of the neoconservatives whom he supported. He also had a judgment of academic social workers in particular as uninformed, unintelligent and closed to objective argumentation. I do not disagree with this judgment that still seems largely accurate. He was in many ways a man of his beloved nineteenth century, born too late to participate in and too early to appreciate the nation's reenactment of it in the 1996 welfare reforms.

will usually reach a consensus on most important issues. Following the embedded romanticism of American social choices, the social clinic emphasizing individual responsibility for change has long been social work's principal incarnation. Serious social change with its eye on systemic reforms and the provision of supportive and surrogate services have been aspirations of few social workers and quite to the point only a small and ineffective proportion of citizens. The "bribe to indolence"—the classic trade-off between funding for services and activism for reform—is the soft touch of accommodation to the social will (Smith 2019 [1776]). Without regard to the circumstances of the external world, self-invention and its extension as the transformative power of the human will are romantic myths. These soothing fictions highlight the justice of success and of the penalties for failing to exert one's will and thus sustain policy minimalism rather than political rebellion.

The field deceives itself that service recipients have ever been its clients. This sleight of mind underscores the rejection in practice of the force of systemic failures in creating the needs of service recipients. To the contrary, the interventions of the social clinic that have always dominated social work in one form or another—grossly inadequate substitutes for common social institutions and psychotherapy that places the onus on the individual for change—are low-cost substitutes for substantial services and redistributive policies to address America's social and economic inequalities. The voice of social work that wished to address those inequalities has always been weak, marginal, and ineffective. At the same time, there is hardly any evidence that social work services and notably the social clinic at its core have ever been successful in addressing the mental, emotional, or moral deficits of those it claims to serve. All that is left is the beleaguered conformity of an ever aspiring weak occupation with popular values performing a pantomime of ineffective talking cures in denial of the material claims of those in need.

References

Addams, J. (1998 [1923]). *Twenty Years at Hull-House*. New York: Penguin Books.

Barbuto, D. M. (1999). *American Settlement Houses and Progressive Social Reform*. Phoenix, AZ: The Oryx Press.

Elshtain, J. B. (2002). *Jane Addams and the Dream of American Democracy*. New York, NY: Basic Books.

Carson, M. (1990). *Settlement Folk: Social Thought and the American Settlement Movement, 1885–1930*. Chicago: The University of Chicago Press.

Day, P. J. (2006). *A New History of Social Welfare* (5th ed.). Boston, MA: Pearson Education.

Epstein, W. M. (2017). *The Masses Are the Ruling Classes: Policy Romanticism, Democratic Populism, and Social Welfare*. New York, NY: Oxford University Press.

Fabricant, M. B., & Fisher, R. (2002). *Settlement Houses Under Siege*. New York, NY: Columbia University.

Gibelman, M. (2004). *What Social Workers Do* (2nd ed.). Washington, DC: NASW Press.

Grob, G. N. (1983). *Mental Illness and American Society 1875–1940*. Princeton, NJ: Princeton University Press.

Holt, M. I. (1992). *The Orphan Trains: Placing Out in America*. Lincoln and London: University of Nebraska Press.

Karger, H. J. (1984). *The Sentinels of Order: A Case Study of Social Control and the Minneapolis Settlement House Movement, 1897–1950*. University of Illinois at Urbana-Champaign, ProQuest Dissertations Publishing.

Lasch-Quinn, E. (1993). *Black Neighbors: Race and the Limits of Reform in the American Settlement House Movement, 1890–1945*. Chapel Hill: University of North Carolina Press.

Leiby, J. (1978). *A History of Social Welfare and Social Work in the United States*. New York: Columbia University Press.

Leuchtenburg, W. E. (1963). *Franklin D. Roosevelt and the New Deal: 1932–1940*. New York: Harper and Row.

Margolin, L. (1997). *Under the Cover of Kindness: The Invention of Social Work*. Charlottesville, NC: University Press of Virginia.

Mencher, S. (1967). *Poor Law to Poverty Program: Economic Security Policy in Britain and the United States*. Pittsburgh: University of Pittsburgh Press.

NASW Center for Workforce Studies. (2010). *2009 Compensation and Benefits Study: Summary of Key Compensation Findings*. Washington, DC: NASW.

O'Connor, A. (2001a). *Poverty Knowledge: Social Science, Social Policy, and the Poor in the Twentieth-Century U.S. History*. Princeton, NJ: Princeton University Press.

O'Connor, S. (2001b). *Orphan Trains: The Story of Charles Loring Brace and the Children He Saved and Failed*. Boston, MA: Houghton Mifflin.

Pacey, L. M. (1950). *Readings in the Development of Settlement Work*. Freeport, NY: Books for Libraries Press.

Richmond, M. (1917). *Social Diagnosis*. New York: Russell Sage Foundation.

Rothman, D. J. (1971). *The Discovery of the Asylum: Social Order and Disorder in the New Republic*. Boston and Toronto, Canada: Little, Brown.

Smith, A. (2019 [1776]). *An Inquiry into the Nature and Causes of the Wealth of Nations*. Amazon Digital Services.

Specht, H., & Courtney, M. (1994). *Unfaithful Angels: How Social Work Has Abandoned Its Mission*. New York, NY: The Free Press.

Stein, L. I., & Test, M. A. (1980). Alternative to Mental Hospital Treatment. I. Conceptual Model, Treatment Program, and Clinical Evaluation. *Archives of General Psychiatry, 37,* 409–412.

Trolander, J. A. (1975). *Settlement House and the Great Depression*. Detroit, MI: Wayne State University Press.

Warren, A. (1996). *Orphan Train Rider: One Boy's True Story*. Boston, MA: Houghton Mifflin.

Woodroofe, K. (1971 [1962]). *From Charity to Social Work in England and the United States*. Toronto: University of Toronto Press.

Woods, R. A., & Kennedy, A. J. (1990). *The Settlement Horizon*. New Brunswick, NJ: Transaction Publishers.

7

Contemporary Social Work and the Social Clinic

Social work has been courting professional standing for more than one hundred years. Despite a near-constant plea since Abraham Flexner's 1915 report to develop special knowledge, social work has never done so. Rather than the scientific practice of philanthropy, charity or caring, the field has expressed an obedience to policy minimalism by the choice of talk therapy of one sort or another as its base of practice knowledge. Ancillary to their dominant clinical role, social workers have often administered and staffed the deficient surrogate services that care for people unable to care for themselves. They have supervised the impaired in large barren congregate institutions and more recently provided similar oversight in small decentralized "fostering" settings that are equally barren but even less protected. Social workers have always been prominent in the provision of child foster care and other forms of protective services. In addition, the field has a minor presence in health care, schooling, and others. Talk therapy is employed in many of the practice settings in addition to the social clinic itself. Yet the clinical skills have not been successful in any of the field's practice settings.

The social clinic lost impetus during the Great Depression when the frank needs for material support overwhelmed a view of the poor as

© The Author(s) 2019
W. M. Epstein, *Psychotherapy and the Social Clinic in the United States*,
https://doi.org/10.1007/978-3-030-32750-7_7

undeserving of assistance and fears that relief would create dependency. Yet the voice of social work throughout the Great Depression was weak and largely restricted to the remnants of the settlement house movement. By and large, social work was silent, staffing out inadequate private social agencies and abiding by the dominant ethos of the time that attributed individual failure to individual faults. The pressure of social work for far more assistance than the Roosevelt administration offered was weak and unrepresentative of both the field and the nation (Trattner 1999, p. 286). The standard histories provide little evidence that the field itself, despite the ineffectual efforts of a few social workers—"an environmentalist voice crying in a wilderness of individualism"—transcended small town Republicanism before World War II (Woodroofe 1962, p. 129). It is haunting that the social clinic's dominance of social work practice took place after the devastations of economy and war when a truly sentient and caring society would have learned lessons of modesty concerning the individual's capacity for self-invention. The resilience of the romantic in American social welfare and society remains awesome, constant but unexplained except to point out that it is so.

Social work histories that draw distinctions between charity organization society's home visits and psychotherapy in the social clinic are too taken with what appears to be the break between religion and then psychological theory as a base of social work practice (Trattner 1999; Woodroofe 1962; Lubove 1967; Mencher 1967; Leiby 1978; and others). Yet, what had long been religious explanations of deviance—godless sin and the willfulness of sinners—became sanitized and updated through the scientisms of psychological theory. Psychotherapy offered a more modern version of old-timey preaching but both assumed that the locus for change lay in the individual not the society and both employed exhortation as the principal strategy to change unwanted, deviant and socially improper behaviors. The high points of each approach—the revivals, church meetings, and sermons on the one hand, individual psychotherapy sessions on the other—build to the cathartic climax of personal responsibility, enjoining the penitent to seek salvation by amending their sinful ways or the deviant to seek perfection by adapting their dysfunctional behavior to appropriate social norms. In this way, respect for religion blended with an awe of science to produce overlapping strategies of social welfare that reinforced social values. Psychotherapeutic theory had little advantage over religion in explaining "facets of human behavior hitherto ignored as irrelevant or dismissed as irrational" (Woodroofe ibid., p. 130). Its relative advantage was in style and appeal to a more rationalistic society, that is, an ethos appropriating the terms of science but not its substance. That neither strategy has ever had much of a demonstrable production function in material relief or social treatment says much about their robustness as ceremonies of cultural affirmation. The "technical and scientific elitism" (Lubove ibid., p. 84) of the social clinic emerged from the same well-spring of romanticism that produced the popular doctrines of American religion.

As ever, some social workers—along with a small minority of citizens—were active in pursuing substantial social reforms. Yet their identification as social workers often referred to their degrees but did not represent the preferences and roles of agency programs in which they were employed or the field itself. By the 1960s, the social clinic dominated social work practice abetting an increasing disengagement from the problems of poverty, lower paid groups, and the material needs of Americans.

Social work's clinical practice involves individual and group psychotherapeutic treatments performed by practitioners singly, in partnerships or under the supervision of psychiatrists and others. In addition, clinical social work services are often administered through school systems with the hope of correcting students' behavior and their families' functioning, in community settings for patients with chronic mental conditions (addressed in Chapter 9), in agencies devoted to family discord, through the child foster care system and others. The principal strategy of the social clinic in social work is to address social problems as if they were mental and emotional problems rather than deficits of material provision and of inadequate participation in basic social institutions. There is little evidence that psychotherapy provided by a social worker is distinguishable from psychotherapy provided psychiatrists, psychologists, counselors, or any of the other occupations of talk therapy; Smith et al.'s (1980) findings that the level of training has little effect on clinical outcomes have been repeated over the years. There is even some evidence that training in psychotherapy does not matter at all (Strupp and Hadley 1979).

Presumably, social work's unique perspective is based on the interaction between the individual and the environment. Yet theories of human behavior remain embattled over the relative contributions of internal motivation and external conditions. Social work's "person in environment" is more cant than professional canon—a jargon of empowerment, including "the strengths perspective," and the babble of psychotherapy. And without either the social and political power to change the environment, the material resources to provide caring surrogates for environmental deficits, or demonstrations that its clinical role is effective, social work has long bent in ritualized deference to social values of parsimony. Displacing the grand delusion of opposition and reform, the field has been reduced to talk therapy, information and referral, surveillance of the needy and administrative tasks.

The Social Work Therapist in the Social Clinic

Thyer's (2015) bibliography identifies an "astonishing" 740 randomized controlled trials published between 1949 and 2013 that were authored by at least one social worker *or that the services provided were performed by professional social workers* (emphasis added, pp. 753, 756). It did not contain a critical review of the research but still concluded with a prudent caution concerning their credibility. Most although not all of the studies appear to evaluate clinical practice.

> Many are, to be frank, methodologically quite weak, with small sample sizes yielding underpowered studies. Some investigations used outcomes of unknown validity, did not follow-up on the long-term maintenance of any apparent improvements, and so on. Also, some arrived at negative conclusions, finding no differences following intervention and others determined that social work services seemed to produce iatrogenic results, for example, harm. Many positive studies may lack external validity, in that the favorable results do not hold up well when the tested

intervention is applied to more diverse or complex client groups than those in the initial study, or when the social workers are less well trained or supervised than those in the published report. (ibid., p. 757)

Thyer also pointed to the possibility of file draw problems, that is, the preference to publish and submit for publication positive findings. In this regard, he might well have pointed to experimental evidence that social work journals and perhaps journals that cover the social clinic generally favor research that sustains the appearance of successful social work practice (Epstein 2006). The pitfalls in the best research give substance to Thyer's doubts. There is little to endorse clinical social work practice.

Swenson's essay defining clinical social work for the 19th edition of the Encyclopedia of Social Work (1995) covers the jargon of the field but ignores the issue of effectiveness. Grant (2013) in the most recent edition of the Encyclopedia of Social Work gives very brief attention to the desirability of outcome research to test clinical interventions, only that "accountability requires the clinical social worker to have some knowledge and competence in the use of evidence-based interventions" (p. 322). The encyclopedia entry minimizes the value of scientifically grounded "evidence based practice." Grant prefers to seat clinical social work within the romantic theories of postmodernism—"constructivism, solution-focused, existentialism, radical theory, and critical realist philosophy [that] frame the newer developments in clinical practice…" (ibid., p. 318)—attributing to clinical social work the heroic role of liberator of the oppressed. The potency of therapy is generally assumed in the manner of many descriptions and analyses of clinical social work (Gonzalez and Gelman 2015). Apparently, noble intent and a commitment to justice, equality and goodness are adequate justifications for practice.

Evidence-based practice with constant attention to rigorously tested outcomes of the social clinic seeks to substitute a more scientific authority for the intuitions of the experienced practitioner (Heineman 1982) as a basis for clinical social work. Drisko (2014) refers the evidence-based practitioner to the Cochrane Library for evidence of best practices and evidence-based treatments. However, the Cochrane archives of clinical trials provide no guarantee of quality but only some assurance that it contains the best of the research, that is, studies that incorporate randomized designs. Yet a randomized design, while a necessary condition of credible clinical research, is not nearly sufficient. As with previous studies discussed in earlier chapters, the Cochrane holdings and the larger literature that test clinical outcomes house a monotony of bias and otherwise impaired studies. There is little if any scientifically sustainable evidence of the ability of clinical social work to achieve cure, prevention or rehabilitation of emotional and mental problems or to demonstrate the value of its "person in environment" assumptions.

Drisko's and Grady's (2012) comprehensive text on clinical social work relies largely on material from the Cochrane Collaboration but also through their own systematic searches of the literature to sustain the effectiveness of clinical social work. They illustrate the value of the social clinic in social work with six case studies—a gay man with depression, a man with panic attacks, a 12-year old with "reactive attachment disorder," parents of a man with schizophrenia, a teenager with a drinking problem, and a homeless woman with borderline personality disorder. In each case, the practitioner is referred back to the most credible psychotherapy literature. The goal is to identify then apply the best practices in each area. Yet best practice may not be good at all. Drisko and Grady typically point to the invalidating deficiencies of the outcome research even while they recommend specific psychotherapeutic treatments of questionable value. Still, their own research logic and the evidence they put forward point to a more plausible alternative conclusion: The best research fails to sustain the value of clinical social work through scientifically credible evidence of successful treatment.

Drisko and Grady's case example in which parents of a schizophrenic child are referred to a support group epitomizes the problems of clinical social work's literature and the field itself. The Cochrane Collaboration came up short. Drisko and Grady learn of an untested program by searching the Web site of the National Alliance of the Mentally Ill. Thus, they were able to identify only one untested program after decades of similar efforts.

There is very little outcome research on these groups. Given the lack of alternative interventions, the social worker views this program as fitting the evidence based practice decision model's requirement to locate the best available research. No alternatives with stronger research support were located. The program fits with the couple's needs and interests quite well. (Drisko and Grady ibid., p. 207)

In other words, best practice is often as suspect as customary practice which appears to be routinely ineffective. It is noteworthy that the field of social work has paid little attention to a basic program for a population—the seriously mentally ill—who should be at the center of clinical social work's attention.

After an exhaustive review of the best of the outcome research, Amato et al. (2011) concluded that "adding any psychosocial support to standard maintenance treatments do not add additional benefits" in treating opioid addiction (p. 2). It is worth noting in this regard that the value of standard maintenance treatment, e.g., methadone, is questionable. Yet the base of research cited in Amato et al. is so impaired, often by enormous attrition and loss of data, that the possibility of routine harm persists. Yet Amato et al. are unusual in publishing negative findings.

Most frequently, the reviews of the outcome literature of clinical social work reinforce each other with consistent findings of effective treatment. Nonetheless, the absence of credible evidence of effective treatment—a debased body of primary research—undercuts the core interventions that define clinical social work. Byrne and Egan's (2018) review proceeded without any critical analysis but found, across a variety of studies, that improved "mentalizations skills" are a common factor in the successful treatment of bipolar disorder. Bender et al.'s (2011) meta-analysis of 15 randomized studies claims that individual and family-based treatments are moderately successful in reducing adolescent marijuana use. Marijuana use was self-reported in some of the studies. Attrition was large but ignored in the analyses of a number of studies. Follow-up was uncertain. The amount of abuse appeared to be slight—"experimental"—in some studies. Only a few studies compared treatment to a non-treatment control.[1]

McPherson's (2012) review of 8 randomized controlled trials concludes that narrative exposure therapy reduces post-traumatic stress disorder in survivors of mass violence. The studies however are seriously undercut by their small samples and lack of blinding. On the basis of a meta-analysis of 14 randomized studies, Lundahl et al. (2008) conclude that "process-based forgiveness interventions increase hope and positive emotions and relief from negative emotions, cognitions and behaviors" (p. 465). The study ignored attrition, intention to treat, blinding and other potential sources of bias.

Similarly, porous meta-analyses and systematic reviews reached similarly positive conclusions: Psychosocial interventions for women help women with AIDS/HIV (Hernandez and Macgowan 2015); young people in outpatient treatment for nonopioid drug use benefit from cognitive behavioral therapies (Lindstrom et al. 2016); a variety of psychosocial interventions reduce late-life depression in long-term care facilities (Yoon et al. 2015). And on and on with hollow, misleading claims that clinical social work can treat the effects of sexual abuse in children (Parker and Turner 2014), mental health problems in people with intellectual disabilities (Gustafsson et al. 2009), depression (Gellis and Kenaley 2008), alcohol abuse (Thomas and Corcoran 2001), and the range of mental, social, and emotional problems.

---

[1]The review articles and the primary research in this section were located by searching two prominent journals that cover clinical social work: the Clinical Social Work Journal and Research on Social Work Practice. The former is dedicated to Clinical Social Work and the latter has the highest impact score among research journals listed in the Web of Science's social work category that is edited under social work auspices. Undoubtedly, there is superior outcome research concerning the social clinic that is authored by social workers but published in psychology journals and others. However, Thyer's (2015) bibliography does not distinguish between authorship and provision nor does it identify the social worker's position among the authors (i.e., primary author, secondary author, or simply one of many). Thus, the field produced only about twelve studies per year that incorporated an experimental design; many of these were inadequate as Thyer acknowledges while the importance of the social worker in conducting the research (their position among the authors), if in fact they were authors, is not clear. As discussed in earlier chapters, the clinical research that this body of work represents is poor and fails to sustain the value of the social clinic. The current work in this chapter probably represents the best of social work's research that is published within the field itself and often by social workers.

The summary research is impaired by a tolerance for the serious pitfalls of the base of primary outcome studies. Perhaps the overriding defect that baits the many research distortions emerges from the fact that hardly any of the primary studies or summaries are conducted by truly independent researchers. Almost all of the authors are therapists themselves or work under the auspices of those with professional stakes in sustaining the effectiveness of psychotherapy and clinical social work. Morrow-Howell et al. (1998) and Kim et al. (2018) exemplify the serious inadequacies that undercut even the best tests of clinical social work's effectiveness identified in the field's leading research journal.[2]

Morrow-Howell et al. (1998) evaluated Link-Plus, an enhanced telephone service attached to a suicide prevention hotline. Link-Plus was a free clinical social work service intended to prevent suicide among "the elderly at increased risk of suicide by virtue of depression, social isolation and unmet needs" (p. 28). The program assesses need through phone interviews with social workers then arranges necessary services from the existing network of mental, physical, and social care programs. The social worker provided continuing supportive therapy through phone calls with the elderly and when necessary the elderly person's family. The Link-Plus social worker maintained contact with recipients for a mean of eight months during which the social worker made a mean of 30 calls to the recipient and a mean of 24 calls to service providers.

Referrals to the hotline received standard crisis intervention services until the risk of suicide was considered low. At that time, participants were randomized either to Link-Plus care or to a four-month waitlist control. In all 80 participants were randomized, 19 of whom dropped

---

[2]Only six randomized evaluations of social work interventions emerged from a twenty-year search of Research on Social Work Practice. All six dealt with clinical interventions. One was authored and situated in Hong Kong (Lo et al. 2015). One did not incorporate a nontreatment control (Meezan and O'Keefe 1998). Another seemed trivial (Gellis et al. 2008). A fourth, Wolf and Abell (2003), was the only randomized study identified in this chapter that employed a placebo control; it will be addressed in Chapter 8 along with other research that evaluates mindfulness as a clinical technique.

out by not completing the evaluation protocol; 30 remained in the Link-Plus group and 31 in the control.

The major outcome measure was depressive symptomatology but measures of social need, service satisfaction, and others were also solicited from the service recipients and in one case service providers. All the information was collected by research assistants who "had not specific knowledge of the [participants'] treatment plans or progress." However, "they also solicited the [participants'] perspectives on the effectiveness of Link-Plus" and thus were not blind to group assignment (ibid., p. 35).

In the end, the treatment group reported only occasional and small improvements over the control group. Depressive symptoms and in-person contacts improved marginally in the Link-Plus group. Measures of needs, socialization, and loneliness did not differentiate the two groups. In contrast and not surprisingly provider assessments of the benefits to the elderly of their services indicated much greater improvement. They estimated that depression symptomatology was greatly improved in 42% of recipients and unmet needs greatly improved in 52% of recipients.

Yet even these small and occasional reported benefits by recipients need to be discounted by a number of likely biases. First, there were no objective measures of the recipients' conditions while the objectivity of the self-assessments of progress and need was probably compromised. The recipients received free care delivered by people with whom they had presumably established at least friendly and respectful relations and thus their assessments may reflect some degree of gratitude. Secondly, the assessors were not blind to the group assignments of those they were interviewing. Third, the evaluation took place under demonstration conditions rather than in routine practice. Staff may have been unusually motivated in both Link-Plus program and in agencies to which participants were referred. Finally, by the time of assignment, that is after customary hotline service when all of the participants had reached a point of low suicide risk, the research sample was not particularly needy either socially or psychologically thus reducing the likelihood of any improvement.

It appears then, that the benefits of Link-Plus are marginal and likely the result of report bias more than clinical intervention. The control group did not deteriorate and the experimental group did not gain much. Furthermore, since the initial callers to the hotline were not randomized to a nonservice group, it is impossible to assess the degree to which initial gains are the result of hotline service or simply natural remission. Recalling the earlier discussion of psychotherapy, it is doubtful that any treatment of the social clinic has been successful in relieving depression or preventing depression.

Still and all, many of the elderly are quite unhappy. They have great needs for recreation and opportunities to stay socially connected notably as they become older, unoccupied, and single. Social support and communal participation are two areas of traditional social work that have been crowded out by the social clinic and the American tolerance of social neglect.

Kim et al. (2018) evaluated the effectiveness of solution-focused brief therapy in treating "substance abuse and trauma related problems" (p. 1). Solution-focused brief therapy, usually provided in 6–10 sessions "views problems as fixable and change as viable by concentrating on the achievement of small, concrete behavioral goals" (p. 455). Thus, it concentrates attention on "solution building rather than problem solving…, desired future rather than past problems…, increasing current useful behavior…, small changes that can lead to larger changes…" and "assumes solution behaviors already exist in clients,…" as well as other assumptions and points of intervention (p. 454). Participants "were parents who have had their children removed from their custody and [placed] into foster care by child welfare service, have been referred by child welfare services for substance use treatment, and have a case plan goals of family reunification" (ibid., p. 3).

Sixty-four participants were randomized to either solution-focused treatment or treatment as usual. All outcomes were assessed by the self-report of participants. Data were collected before treatment began and again at the end of treatment or three months after treatment began, whichever occurred first. In the end, only small differences without apparent clinical importance favored the group receiving solution-focused brief therapy (about nine percentage points better than the treatment as usual group). While both groups improved somewhat over time, the study did not employ a nontreatment control that obviates attributing the improvements to the interventions rather than to some form of natural remission or the seasonality of the problems.

The authors acknowledge several limitations of their study: small sample sizes, nonrandom assignment of clinicians, a lack of data describing the treatment as usual services, and the fact that many of the participants were receiving other (unidentified) services during the study. By themselves, the acknowledged limitations severely hamper the credibility of the research. Yet other problems with the research are more serious threats to its credibility. The authors are obviously advocates of the interventions they are evaluating and thus lack impartiality which may explain the additional limitations that they did not mention. While attrition was considerable in both groups, no intention to treat analysis was conducted. Making the customary assumption that attrition represents failure and thus carrying forward the initial scores of those who dropped out would likely have wiped out any statistically significant finding in the study. Moreover, the samples are probably not representative of those with similar problems; the study groups contain motivated participants who want their children returned and are voluntarily seeking treatment for substance abuse. Yet the research loses even a tenuous claim on credibility by the use of self-reported data concerning substance abuse. It is beyond the limits of gullibility to accept a substance abuser's assessment of use. The research employed neither urine nor hair tests.

Kim et al. (2018) failed to protect against demonstration effects of unusual therapist motivation; the research ignored attrition, failing to employ intention to treat analyses; it did not incorporate a non-treatment control; it could not describe the nature of the treatment-as-usual control; and its data were all self-reported by participants with substance abuse problems, the principal reason for treatment and the principal outcome that was measured. Even so, reported outcomes were small in the few instances they occurred. The authors' conclusions that their study constitutes "an important contribution" (p. 459) and "significantly adds to the substance use and trauma literature by examining an innovative approach to engaging and treating parents in the child welfare system" (p. 460) are simply unfounded, even ludicrous. Rather, the study perpetuates the convenient myths of minimalism: that the cheap, short-term treatments of clinical social work are viable treatments for serious personal and social problems. The assumptions of solution-focused brief therapy and more generally the strengths perspective of social work reinforce the romantic fictions of the nation: People have within themselves the sufficient conditions of their reformation and redemption. The romantic assumptions of personal agency displace the importance of generous social supports.

Morrow-Howell et al. (1998) and Kim et al. (2018) are among the very strongest evaluations of clinical social work published during the past twenty years in the most highly regarded research journal within social work. Nevertheless, they are trivial both as practice and as theory. They are deficient as science. The clinical record of social work outcomes in traditional practice areas of foster children, schools, and family reunification is similarly disappointing—a multitude of poorly conducted studies that fail to support the field's claims of effective practice—but that perpetuate the soothing fictions of social welfare in America.

References

Amato, L., Minozzi, S., Davoli, M., & Vecchi, S. (2011). Psychosocial Combined with Agonist Maintenance Treatments Versus Agonist Maintenance Treatments Alone for Treatment of Opioid Dependence. *Cochrane Database of Systematic Reviews,* 1–93. http://dx.doi.org/10.1002/14651858.CD004147.pub4.

Bender, K., Tripodi, S. J., Sarteschi, C., & Vaughn, M. G. (2011). A Meta Analysis of Interventions to Reduce Adolescent Cannabis Use. *Research on Social Work Practice, 21*(2), 153–164. https://doi.org/10.1177/1049731510380226.

Byrne, G., & Egan, J. (2018). A Review of the Effectiveness and Mechanisms of Change for Three Psychological Interventions for Borderline Personality Disorders. *Clinical Social Work Journal,* 1–13. http://dx.doi.org/10.1007/s10615-018-0652-y.

Drisko, J. (2014). Research Evidence and Social Work Practice: The Place of Evidence Based Practice. *Clinical Social Work Journal, 42*(2), 123–133.

Drisko, J. W., & Grady, M. D. (2012). *Evidence-Based Practice in Clinical Social Work*. New York, NY: Springer.

Epstein, W. M. (2006). *Psychotherapy as Religion: The Civil Divine in America*. Reno, NV: University of Nevada Press.

Flexner, A. (1915). Is Social Work a Profession? *Research on Social Work Practice, 11*, 152–165. https://doi.org/10.1177/104973150101100202.

Gellis, Z. D., & Kenaley, B. (2008). Problem-Solving Therapy for Depression in Adults: A Systematic Review. *Research on Social Work Practice, 18*, 117–131. https://doi.org/10.1177/1049731507301277.

Gellis, Z. D., McGinty, J., Tierney, L., Jordan, C., Burton, J., & Misener, E. (2008). Randomized Controlled Trial of Problem-Solving Therapy for Minor Depression in Home Care. *Research on Social Work Practice, 18*, 596–606. https://doi.org/10.1177/1049731507309821.

Gonzalez, M. J., & Gelman, C. R. (2015). Clinical Social Work Practice in the Twenty-First Century: A Changing Landscape. *Clinical Social Work Journal, 43*, 257–262. https://doi.org/10.1007/s10615-015-0550-5.

Grant, D. (2013). Clinical Social Work. In *Encyclopedia of Social Work*. New York: Oxford University Press.

Gustafsson, C., Ojenagen, A., Hansson, L., Sandlund, M., Nystrom, M., Glad, J., et al. (2009). Effects of Psychosocial Interventions for People with Intellectual Disabilities and Mental Health Problems. *Research on Social Work Practice, 19*, 281–290. https://doi.org/10.1177/1049731508329403.

Heineman, M. B. (1982). The Obsolete Scientific Imperative in Social Work. *Social Service Review, 63*(3), 175–185.

Hernandez, J. P., & Macgowan, M. J. (2015). Psychosocial Interventions for Women with HIV/AIDS: A Critical Review. *Research on Social Work Practice, 25*(1), 103–116.

Kim, J. S., Brook, J., & Akin, B. A. (2018). Solution-Focused Brief Therapy with Substance-Using Individuals: A Randomized Controlled Trial Study. *Research on Social Work Practice, 28*(4), 452–462. https://doi.org/10.1177/1049731516650517.

Leiby, J. (1978). *A History of Social Welfare and Social Work in the United States*. New York: Columbia University Press.

Lindstrom, M., Filges, T., & Jorgensen, A. (2016). Brief Strategic Family Therapy for Young People in Treatment for Drug Use. *Research on Social Work Practice, 25*(1), 61–80.

Lo, H. H., Ng, S., & Chan, C. L. (2015). Evaluating Compassion-Mindfulness Therapy for Recurrent Anxiety and Depression: A Randomized Control Trial. *Research on Social Work Practice, 25,* 715–725. https://doi.org/10.1177/1049731514537686.

Lubove, R. (1967). *The Professional Altrusit.* Cambridge, MA: Harvard University Press.

Lundahl, B. W., et al. (2008). Process-Based Forgiveness Interventions: A Meta-Analytic Review. *Research on Social Work Practice, 18*(5), 465–478.

McPherson, J. (2012). Does Narrative Exposure Therapy Reduce PTSD in Survivors of Mass Violence? *Research on Social Work Practice, 21,* 153–164. https://doi.org/10.1177/1049731511414147.

Meezan, W., & O'Keefe, M. (1998). Evaluating the Effectiveness of Multifamily Group Therapy in Child Abuse and Neglect. *Research on Social Work Practice, 8,* 330–353. https://doi.org/10.1177/104973159800800306.

Mencher, S. (1967). *Poor Law to Poverty Program: Economic Security Policy in Britain and the United States.* Pittsburgh: University of Pittsburgh Press.

Morrow-Howell, N., Becker-Kemppainen, S., & Judy, L. (1998). Evaluating an Intervention for the Elderly at Increased Risk of Suicide. *Research on Social Work Practice, 8*(1), 28–46.

Parker, B., & Turner, W. (2014). Psychoanalytic/Psychodynamic Psychotherapy for Sexually Abused Children and Adolescents: A Systematic Review. *Research on Social Work Practice, 24,* 389–399. https://doi.org/10.1177/1049731514525477.

Smith, M. L., Glass, G. V., & Miller, T. I. (1980). *The Benefits of Psychotherapy.* Baltimore, MD: Johns Hopkins University Press.

Strupp, H. H., & Hadley, S. W. (1979). Specific vs. Nonspecific Factors in Psychotherapy: A Controlled Study of Outcome. *Archives of General Psychiatry, 36,* 1125–1136. http://dx.doi.org/10.1001/archpsyc.1979.01780100095009.

Swenson, C. R. (1995). Clinical Social Work. In R. L. Edwards (Ed. in Chief), *Encyclopedia of Social Work* (19th ed., pp. 502–513). Washington, DC: NASW Press.

Thomas, C., & Corcoran, J. (2001). Empirically Based Marital and Family Interventions for Alcohol Abuse: A Review. *Research on Social Work Practice, 11,* 549–575. https://doi.org/10.1177/104973150101100502.

Thyer, B. A. (2015). A Bibliography of Randomized Controlled Experiments in Social Work (1949–2013): Solvitur Ambulando. *Research on Social Work Practice, 25,* 753–793. https://doi.org/10.1177/1049731515599174.

Trattner, W. I. (1999). *From Poor Law to Welfare State: A History of Social Welfare in America* (6th ed.). New York, NY: The Free Press.

Wolf, D. B., & Abell, N. (2003). Examining the Effects of Meditation Techniques on Psychosocial Functioning. *Research on Social Work Practice, 13*, 27–42. https://doi.org/10.1177/104973102237471.

Woodroofe, K. (1971 [1962]). *From Charity to Social Work in England and the United States.* Toronto: University of Toronto Press.

Yoon, S., et al. (2015). Effective Treatments of Late-Life Depression in Long-Term Care Facilities: A Systematic Review. *Research on Social Work Practice, 28*(2), 116–130.

8

Clinical Social Work in Child Foster Care, Family Preservation, and the Schools

Clinical social work is also practiced in areas of the field outside of the clinic itself. Regrettably, the record repeats itself in child foster care, family preservation services, and applications in schools.

Child Foster Care, Family Preservation, and Family Reunification

Although certainly not the most popular area of practice among social work students and practitioners, child foster care is the signature social service of social work, an obligation that it often attends to through clinical interventions. Many foster children come into care with serious behavior problems. They are often placed with foster parents who also have serious emotional problems and even more often are largely motivated by the stipends rather than a humane commitment to fostering children without parents. It is a sign of the poor quality of care itself that so few evaluations of the physical and emotional environment of placements or of outcomes have been conducted. When they do exist, low quality undercuts the credibility of their conclusions.

© The Author(s) 2019

W. M. Epstein, *Psychotherapy and the Social Clinic in the United States*,
https://doi.org/10.1007/978-3-030-32750-7_8

Stipends for foster care (a state average of approximately $8500 per year plus a small amount of extra subsidy in some states) are customarily below the poverty line for single individuals and below estimates for costs of child support (DeVooght et al. 2012). Many foster parents take a large profit for themselves out of the stipends and spend little on the children for food, clothing, shelter, and other necessities. There is little evidence to refute the suspicion that poor children who were neglected and abused by their birth parents are still poor and neglected in foster care and often abused as well. The scarcity of quality evaluative research (Goldhaber-Fiebert et al. 2011) parallels the neglect of the children in care.[1]

One of the clearest indictments of foster care is the incapacity of foster children to handle life after they age out of the system—substantial difficulties with "independent living and self-sufficiency" (Scannapieco et al. 2007, p. 425; Kushel et al. 2007). The defense of the system that many foster children come into care too damaged to respond to any intervention rings as a hollow excuse for the deficiencies of the program. Many of these presumably failed cases have spent most of their youth in foster care bouncing from one inadequate placement to another. Scannapieco et al. (2007) detail the problems well however their solutions—youth-focused practice, better communication, and satisfying unmet material and emotional needs, presumably through permanent connections with responsible adults—if taken seriously entail resources that have never been provided and clinical interventions that remain uncertain and probably ineffective. Indeed, their list of "practice principles for child welfare workers" concentrates on process and personal interactions with the youths but minimizes the difficulty of providing material resources including financial supports, jobs, supplementary education, training, medical and mental health services, and others.

Perceptions of the inadequacies of foster care encourage the growing hope that parenting skills training will prevent many foster care

---

[1] The recurrent scandals of savagery by foster parents are customarily covered by journalists better than by the social work literature. There is little money allocated for the oversight of foster care while the private moneys seem to produce tepid reports. As examples, see Pecora et al. (2006) and much of the other subsidized research by the Casey Foundation.

placements. In a randomized controlled trial of 700 foster and kinship parents, Chamberlain et al. (2008) tested a program "to reduce children's problem behaviors by strengthening foster parents' skills" (p. 17). "The experimental group received a 16-week course of training, supervision, and support in behavioral management methods" (p. 19). The control group received the customary services of the child welfare department. The study reported benefits for training, particularly among children with greater behavior problems. However, the few statistically significant benefits were very modest (about 10 percentage points) and of dubious relevance; 38% of those invited to participate refused; no attrition was reported during treatment; there was no follow-up to test the sustainability of effects; all data were self-reported by the foster parents. In the end, the study produced little beyond skepticism that skills training for foster parents has the ability to repair the behavior problems of foster children. It does however reinforce the popularity of these programs, reducing the possibility of more substantial and material attention to the serious deficits of foster children and the conditions under which they live. Still, superficial interventions such as "family finding to engage relatives with foster children" and "natural mentoring" remain popular but ineffective or unsupported (Vandivere et al. 2017; Thompson and Greeson 2017).

Therapeutic foster care is a more intense form of foster care that concentrates clinical interventions, applying a psychotherapeutic logic to treat particularly troubled youth, that is, "children most at risk of poor developmental outcomes" (Frederico et al. 2016). It is intended as a diversion program both to minimize the costs of extremely expensive group residential care, including incarceration, and to improve outcomes for the youth. Hahn et al.'s (2005) review of the few evaluations of therapeutic foster care that exist recaps the general findings about clinical social work.

Two studies of therapeutic foster care for children with severe emotional disturbance yield inconsistent results; evidence to date is inconclusive. Three studies of therapeutic foster care for adolescents with chronic delinquency…indicated that this intervention can reduce subsequent violence in this population. (Hahn ibid., p. 72)

However, those three studies are seriously impaired. One of them (Chamberlain 1990) evaluated a sample of only 16 youths and employed a matched comparison group in community residential care. It is not clear whether the positive outcomes resulted from a convenient comparison group of severe risk, the maturation of the experimental group, or other factors apart from the therapy itself. The second study (Chamberlain and Reid 1994) did not employ any control group leaving doubts that the positive outcomes—fewer arrests after treatment than one year before treatment—were the result of therapeutic foster care rather than maturation, the loss of data, or other factors. However, "during the program, aggressive behavior problems reported by foster parents increased among girls," a finding reported in other studies (Hahn et al. ibid., p. 79). The third study (Chamberlain and Reid 1998) employed a randomized design and reported that therapeutic foster care lowered the *self-reported* incidence of violence such as aggravated assault, sexual assault, and gang fights. The authors consider the self-reported data to be more accurate than official referrals, again a choice between bad and worse that does not improve the reliability of the research. In any event, the outcomes, such as they are, could be attributed to the harms of care that control groups received as much as to the therapeutic foster care or to simply reporting bias. Most notable, all three studies were conducted by the same principal investigator who was apparently committed to the value of the intervention.

In a separate retrospective study of "enhanced foster care," Kessler et al. (2008) reported that alumni of private foster care had better emotional and physical health 1–13 years after leaving care than children in public programs. However, the study did not incorporate a randomized design to secure comparability between the samples and attrition was large. Moreover, it is not clear whether the large outcome differences between groups were due to the benefits of the private programs, the characteristics of the samples, the quality of the foster parents, or the abusive conditions of the control group rather than the benefits of enhanced care, that is, the skills of staff and clinical interventions.

The absence of evaluations of therapeutic foster care, let alone high-quality assessments, is generally true across child welfare. The common fare is hopeful but not definitive—statements by humane researchers that some novel but inexpensive form of care will improve outcomes. Unfortunately, the common fare gets by with nonrandomized, uncontrolled research relying on unreliable data and open to numerous sources of bias (Frederico et al. 2016; Madigan et al. 2017). The evaluative research of child welfare programs remains more like advocacy research—factional studies—than credible evaluation.

Pecora et al.'s (2006) attempt to assess the outcomes of foster care is limited by a retrospective design. It summarizes the educational and employment achievements of foster care alumni, but it cannot estimate the contribution of foster care itself to those outcomes. It is simply a statement of inequality. Yet their comments about research in foster care and the system itself seem accurate. Due to many problems of design, comparability, measurement, and neutrality as well as law and ethics, "It is difficult to demonstrate that what happens for foster children is the result of being in foster care, and not merely something which happens as a consequence of pre-determined characteristics of those entering the foster care system" (ibid., pp. 143, 462). Yet even accepting the influence of "predetermined characteristics," the simple issue of decency and equality intrudes—what needy children without resources or family merit simply as citizens of a wealthy nation. What they currently receive seems more like punishment and abuse than therapy or care. Predetermination reverberates as the hollow excuse for the inertia of failed minimalism. The effects of foster care may be less germane and secondary to the conditions of foster care as an appropriate social concern—a point of decency and equality rather than efficiency and effectiveness.

The goal of intensive family preservation programs, emphasized in a federal set-aside for foster care, is closely aligned with foster care. The programs provide short-term (perhaps six months) intensive services, notably including counseling and psychotherapy but also referrals for more material support as well as medical and mental health care, to families often in crisis and at risk of out-of-home placement of a child. To the extent that families at risk of breaking apart or otherwise having their children removed can be held together, the foster care rolls will be minimized along with the public costs of care. Moreover, it is generally felt and probably true that children fare better with their own parents, assuming that they are not frankly abusive or neglectful, than in foster care. This conclusion, given the low quality of foster care placements, is only the better of two evils and a rebuke to the refusal of a very wealthy society to protect and nourish its children.

Two of the most recent meta-analyses summarizing the outcomes of intensive family preservation programs agree with each other (Dagenais et al. 2004; Channa et al. 2012); the programs do not reduce placement although they have a modest positive effect on family functioning. Channa et al. (2012) were more thorough in detailing the weakness of the base of research than Dagenais et al. (2004). However, only three of the Channa et al.'s studies reported on family functioning.

A number of the Dagenais et al.'s findings raise questions about the quality of the underlying research as well as the effects of intensive family preservation programs. "Studies that were not published showed more negative effects…than journal publications…or book chapters/reports…. Negative effects were also found in randomized controlled trials…, whereas positive effects were found in quasi-experimental studies with a nonmatched control group" (ibid., p. 1475). The negative effects in the stronger studies were marginal while the positive effects in the studies with weak designs were moderate. Placement rates are obviously easier to measure than family function and less amenable to bias. In short, the more credible studies found smaller effects. Yet even this important qualification understates the failure of intensive family preservation as well as the fundamental problems of the research itself.

Channa et al. only considered basic study design in rating the quality of the research. They ignored issues of attrition, intention to treat, blinding, and others and failed to apply any standard quality of research instrument such as the Cochrane risk-of-bias tool. The three studies that Channa et al. cite to conclude that intensive family preservation improved family functioning do not in one instance and cannot in all instances sustain that conclusion. Meezan and McCroskey (1996) were concerned with family functioning, not placement although they reported no difference in placement between their experimental groups and the customary service control. Initially, both groups reported that they did not have "significant problems with family function in any of the six overall areas" that were measured (ibid., p. 19). In contrast, caseworkers considered the members of both groups to exhibit serious problems in family functioning. After one year and in comparison with controls, intensive service recipients reported modest improvements in only two of six areas of family functioning: living conditions and family conditions with the latter significant only at $p = .09$; however, neither condition seems to be an appropriate measure of family *functioning*. "By the close of service, the [case]workers saw statistically significant improvements in four areas of family functioning" (ibid., p. 19). In other words, the researchers accepted the caseworkers' evaluations of their own efforts. All of the ratings were made by caseworkers and service recipients; no independent, objective assessments were made. Attrition was considerable, 19% by the end of service, 37% by the one-year follow-up. The intention to treat procedure is not explained, and follow-up data are not reported. More to the point, it is not clear that the caseload met the criteria of need—imminent risk of placement—for intensive family preservation services. The study provided no data tables and seemed to selectively present information that best fit its intentions; it was published in a marginal journal.

The two other studies cited by Channa et al. relative to family functioning—Feldman (1991) and Lewis (2005)—are replications in ambiguity. All of the measures in Lewis's (2005) randomized experiment were drawn from the parents of the families; there were no objective assessments. In contrast with the control families, the intensive services provided to the experimental group may have created a special bond between the workers and the families receiving intensive services that induced exaggerated reports of improved family functioning. Still, family functioning reportedly improved in only two of three measured areas and failed in the third, "parent effectiveness/parent–child relationships," which would seem to be the core of family functioning. The changes in the other two areas while statistically significant appear to be modest at best rather than "a strong positive effect," and their clinical and practical significance is not at all clear (Lewis ibid., p. 505). The experimental intervention also provided concrete services, notably with finances and community support, but the study makes no estimate of degree to which the concrete services rather than counseling contributed to outcomes. The follow-up period was only three months, but the study touts the enduring benefits of the intervention. Finally, Lewis (2005) provides scant evidence that the families were at imminent risk of disruption.

Feldman (1991), the third of Channa et al.'s cited tests of intensive family preservation programs in improving family functioning, was not published in a peer-reviewed journal but appeared in an edited volume. Relative to family functioning, families that received intensive family preservation services "did not generally improve to a greater degree than did control families" (p. 63). It is not clear how Channa et al. merged this study with the other two to arrive at their positive finding about the ability of intensive services to improve family functioning. Feldman found that the differences in placement rates, that is, family disruption rates, were modest but favored the intensive service group throughout the one year after the end of intensive services. During the year, placements rates converged and increased greatly from 7 to 46% in the intensive service group and from 15 to 58% in the control group. It is speculative whether the small differences were due to intensive services, to the differences between the groups (perhaps in the degree of need), to the suppression of placement by fiat in the experimental group, or to demonstration effects generally—in particular unsustainable and thus unique motivations of demonstration workers that cannot be transferred to the customary service setting. Workers in the experimental condition may have been motivated to do all in their power to prevent placement, even taking risks in this regard, or in other ways to artificially but briefly maintain families. The short-term benefits may suggest, as Feldman argues, that intensive services should be continued for a longer period. In contrast, the argument seems more plausible that the benefits were so small that far more intensive provisions concerning employment, education, childcare, housing, and others are necessary if imminent risk conditions are to be reduced and families are to be preserved.

Each of the three intensive family preservation studies that Channa et al. cite relative to family functioning is seriously impaired and thus fail as credible estimates of their findings. Among many other shortcomings, a fundamental lack of neutrality among the researchers may go far to explain the outcomes of essentially porous research. As a prominent example, Schuerman et al. (1994) conducted one of the most highly cited evaluations of intensive family preservation programs. It concluded that intensive family preservation was ineffective. On its face, the study displayed many of the most desirable features of good research: randomized design, large samples, multiple measures and multiple sites, follow-up, and others. However, like the intensive family preservation research generally, in practice the study undercut almost every other crucial feature of scientific credibility. Actually, the invalidating seriousness of its design imperfections was obvious early on, and the decision to continue the research raises questions about the intentions of the researchers: to provide unbiased, neutral findings or to support their preconceptions.

Schuerman et al. (1994) set out to assess the effects of the intensive family preservation program in Illinois that provided enriched, short-term casework services including counseling and psychotherapy in comparison with the customary services of the state's Department of Child and Family Services. The target population as in other studies of family preservation programs was families at imminent risk of disruption.

The evaluation produced no consistent, significant, or substantial benefits for the intensive family preservation program. The additional services did not preserve families. The authors found that there was

> little evidence that the [family preservation] program affects the risk of placement, subsequent maltreatment, or case closing and some evidence that the program may be related to short-term progress on case objectives. However, these results must be viewed in the context of considerable variation among sites and variations in outcomes that are due to characteristics of cases and the services provided to them. (Schuerman et al. 1994, p. 188)

Nonetheless, numerous failures in the design and conduct of the study undercut the credibility of all its conclusions. First, the subjects of the research were probably not representative of the intended population of those at imminent risk of placement. As the authors acknowledged, there are no accurate predictors of imminent risk. Second, randomization was ignored in more than 24% of cases—16% due to worker preference and the rest usually due to court orders. While these cases were not considered in findings, they probably reduced the level of imminent risk within the pool of remaining subjects. The authors were quite attentive to the possibility of creaming—the likelihood that the experiment enrolled subjects was unrepresentative of the target population.

Third, many measurement problems plagued the evaluation. The study used existing instruments to evaluate outcomes. But those instruments, as the authors stated, never achieved high or convincing reliabilities. The authors concede that "evaluations of family preservation will continue to make use of measures of uncertain reliability, validity, and sensitivity" (ibid., pp. 212–213). Fourth, procedures "to gather information [were] different for the experimental and control group" (ibid., p. 212). Workers in the private agencies provided information by filling out questionnaires; workers in the public agencies were interviewed. More serious, interviews with subjects were conducted by two different groups of interviewers. The interviewers who collected later data were more experienced and better trained. They were employed by the highly respected National Opinion Research Center. The early interviewers employed by the study were judged to be inadequate, apparently too affected by the subjects' living conditions to provide credible interviews. As a consequence, the data may have been reflected differences in interviewer characteristics rather than the live situations of subjects.

Fourth, treatment integrity—the assurance that services were delivered as intended—could not be assured. The evaluation failed to corroborate the actual receipt of services. Many subjects who were referred to agencies by caseworkers may not have shown up for their appointments, the agencies may not have provided what the referring caseworker assumed, or the agency of the initial referral may have sent the subject on to other agencies.

Fifth, neither subjects nor raters were blind to the assignment of subjects to family preservation services or customary services. Without blinding, expectancy biases, reporter biases, or others may easily affect the accuracy or subject responses.

Sixth, the basic measure of outcomes—placement—may have been sensitive to worker motivation more than the conditions of the subjects.

Workers in the family preservation program were obviously motivated to reduce placements. They may have taken risks of judgment or in other ways sought to suppress the behaviors that would naturally lead to the appropriate decision to separate maltreated children from their parents. Control group workers knowing that they were being scrutinized for placement decisions may have been similarly motivated. The research did not evaluate the appropriateness of worker decisions either to place the children or to maintain the families.

Finally, the evaluation was conducted under demonstration circumstances that by themselves undercut the representativeness of its findings and defies replication in customary situations for which it is intended. The motivations of workers and evaluators along with novel sensitivities among other participants (notably the participating public and private social service agencies) are likely to be different than under normal operating conditions. Yet the workers hired for demonstrations are probably more skilled and dedicated than the workers who would be employed in replications of the service.

The authors enumerated a number of the research limitations that were created by faults in its design. However, they remained sufficiently confident in their findings to reach extended conclusions about family preservation programs and child welfare in general.

The expansion of the purview of the child welfare system that has occurred in the last few decades should be stopped and reversed. This requires that lines be carefully drawn between our aspirations and what can be reasonably expected... The state cannot accept responsibility for the optimal development of all children. Nor should it even endeavor to assure the "well-being" of all children, given the impossibility of achieving that goal, even if well-being could be adequately defined and measured.... Emotional harms can, of course, have serious effects on the child on his or her development, and the state should encourage the development of services to help parents better relate to their children. But these services should be voluntary, outside the abuse and neglect response system. (ibid., p. 245)

Nothing in the authors' evaluation of intensive family preservation in Illinois leads to this conclusion. It simply confesses their basic assumptions about child welfare and the desirability of a minimal role for government in social welfare. Yet the design problems and their severity were obvious early in the research—it could not address its basic task of evaluating the family preservation program. Nonetheless, the authors refused to abort the research.

Schuerman et al. (1994) may be among the best tests of intensive family preservation, but such deficient research impeaches the broader enterprise of program evaluation and indicts the neutrality of the community of scholars from which it emerges. The authors held prestigious positions at the University of Chicago and enjoyed great respect and success within the field of social work. Yet their success at competing for research grants resonates back to their obedience to cultural preferences for minimal expenditures on social welfare. The orientation of the researcher in weak fields such as clinical social work may be the best predictor of the research findings.

Still and all, family preservation programs cannot succeed. Short-term intensive services including clinical social work are insufficient to address deep material deficits in families and long-standing emotional and behavioral problems. Only the public sector accepting the strong mandate of a population desiring greater social and economic parity has the resources to provide the caring supports of education, employment, day care, housing, and others that are necessary to protect the nurturing family. That mandate does not exist in the United States.[2]

There are caring alternatives to foster care and its jury-rigged programs of family reunification and preservation. However, they are very expensive. Boys Town provides unusually generous homelike environments to troubled youth. Taking housing costs into consideration, each of its cottage beds may cost more than $100,000 per year that amounts to more than ten times the annual cost of a child in foster care. Boys

---

[2]For a more detailed analysis of the Illinois evaluation, see Epstein, W. M. (1997). "Social Science, Child Welfare, and Family Preservation: A Failure of Rationality in Public Policy." *Children and Youth Services Review*, 19(1&2): 41–60.

Town justifies its services as therapeutic contributions to social adjustment, emotional health, and school performance. However, there are no credible studies that sustain these claims. More important, these outcomes should not be the critical criteria to evaluate services for children without parents. Rather, the basic social obligation embraces greater equality in social provisions rather than pursues specific outcomes of emotional or social adaptation. It is implicit in the logic of greater equality that its realization generally justifies differences in outcomes— the common precept that a fair game requires an even playing field. Yet simply as an issue of common decency, a just society will provide a generous and caring homelike environment to children without resources or family. The foster care program in the United States is a brazen statement that American society refuses to do so.

Boys Town adapts to American parsimony and does not characterize itself in terms of greater equality but rather casts itself as a clinical intervention that employs the "teaching family model" although without a staff of psychotherapists. Nonetheless, the model is an expression of learning theory—punishments and rewards, mentoring, self-exploration, and personal agency that underpin most of modern psychotherapy. However, unlike the typical foster care home (either personal or congregate), it provides a truly homelike environment; the children have personal spaces, clothes, toys, a relatively special long-term and intimate relationship with emotionally mature parent surrogates, and access to physicians, dentists, and other specialists. Boys Town in Las Vegas, Nevada, operates as a residential treatment center that aims to meet its goals usually within 12–18 months at which time the child is returned to their parents, to another fostering situation, or ages out of care.[3]

The overwhelming majority of foster children need such a program, not for a few months but rather for the entirety of their youth. The public's refusal to provide long-term expensive care and Boys Town's

---

[3]Boys Town closed its Las Vegas cottage program that served 30 children at any time. The state of Nevada refused to provide the necessary resources for more than 90 days while the Boys Town teaching family model requires longer support.

inability to compensate with private donations reduces the program to medium length residential treatment and also restricts its caseload to those whom the program judges can adjust to its requirements. Since there are no randomized trials of similar care, there are no credible estimates of its superiority to customary care. This creates a situation in which a program justifying itself in clinical terms on grounds of empirical evidence does not in reality have that evidence.

Yet the program's profound value rests with the quality of the environment it provides to children as a point of decency and justice. However, the advocacy of greater equality runs political risks even when provided for children. Social welfare programs have long made the safe decision to subordinate advocacy to service and their organizational health. Nonetheless, Boys Town is the epitome of high-quality childcare outside of the family: a demonstration that decent congregate care is feasible and desirable, at least from the child's perspective. American foster care and clinical social work are patently inadequate substitutes.

Moreover, the common language of behaviorism that dominates congregate care for children—rewards and punishments in maintaining control—might yield to more emotionally enriched choices that emphasize the child's human legacy rather than their animal descent. The provision of decent circumstances realized as greater equality for poor children without parents probably precedes the ability to engineer specific behavioral outcomes; indeed, it may be the crucial ingredient in successful socialization.

The Social Work Therapist in the Schools

The schools play a central role second only to the family in socializing children, first through classroom education but also through a variety of activities that contribute to the psychological and social maturation of citizens. Clinical social work, the dominant form of social work practice in schools, is designed to enhance these functions through psychosocial interventions with disturbed children and their families (Franklin 2016, p. 427).

The best known and most widely used model is the traditional clinical model, which focuses on individual students with social and emotional problems that interfere with their potential to learn. The model's primary base is psychoanalytic and ego psychology. The model's major assumption is that the individual child or the family is experiencing difficult times or dysfunction. (Allen-Meares 2013, p. 4)

The literature of school social work that evaluates practice is even weaker than the clinical literature itself. If anything at all, it documents a consistent failure to correct targeted behaviors in the children or their families. Among the best of the outcome research but still an impaired effort evaluates Communities in Schools (CIS), a private, nonprofit national program housed in participating public school systems to address school dropouts. Clinical interventions dominate its service strategy. In pursuit of lessening dropouts, CIS provides school-wide services for all students regardless of their risk that include assembly presentations, motivational speakers, and health fairs. Its individual services provided through clinical social work case management include "one-on-one academic tutoring, linkages to legal or medical resources, or substance abuse and anger management counseling" as well as professional mental health services, college and career preparation, family counseling, and life skills training. Behavioral health services (i.e., psychotherapy of one sort or another) covering almost 250 hours for some students in higher-performing schools were the most intense service that CIS provided. The services were typically provided through "community partnerships" with local organizations and volunteers. The CIS *Spring 2014 National Impact Report* states that the program "reached 1.3 million students in 375 school districts through 2250 schools at every level." It goes on to state that in 2012–2013, "41,758 volunteers worked with affiliates across the country...[providing] more than 1.4 hours of service..., an estimated value of $31,127,467" (p. 5).[4]

In the current fashion of private charities, CIS hired a for-profit, private contract research firm to evaluate its effectiveness. Their

---

[4]For a detailed analysis of CIS and the evaluation, see Epstein (2017, Chapter 6).

multivolume study included a quasi-experiment that compared CIS schools to a matched group of nonparticipating schools as well as three small randomized experiments in three cities. On the basis of these studies, CIS boasts that "independent research demonstrates that Communities in Schools is one of the very few organizations proven to keep students in school and the only one to document that it increases graduation rates. The study also shows that a higher percentage of students served by Communities in Schools reach proficiency in 4th grade and 8th grade reading and math" (Communities in Schools of Nevada, n.d.).

The research compared 30 schools that faithfully implemented CIS and 17 schools that partially implemented the model with matched nonparticipating schools. Relative to their matched schools, those that faithfully implemented the model improved 3.6% and those that partially implemented the model improved only 1.5%.

In reality, the research could sustain none of these conclusions or others. For one, the comparison schools were in fact different than those that participated and notably because they did not opt into CIS to begin with and were probably not as motivated as participating schools. Propensity score matching could not adjust for motivation. The reports also lacked important information about the reliability of the data; the services themselves were not systematically evaluated to assure their quality and their delivery. The data on retention and graduation, collected only as enrollments, did not include transfers. The more credible but costlier procedure would have been to follow each enrolled student. Moreover, the math and reading tests may have reflected test preparation rather than actual achievement.

Austin, Texas, was the most successful of the randomized experiments. Over the two years of the experiment, outcomes were consistently small, often not statistically significant, and sometimes favored the control group. Slight differences in attendance (2.3%), dropouts (1.1%), and grade points (1.9%) favored the CIS sample. There were no differences in math scores and in completed credits, but the reading scores favored the controls. Disciplinary referrals declined for both groups, but much more for controls (75%) than CIS students (59%).

Yet even the partial, small, and various findings of the Austin experiment are not credible. Randomization is a necessary but certainly not a sufficient condition of scientific credibility. Yet even if measured accurately, the Austin results might well be explained by a variety of research biases that emerged from the study's substantial pitfalls. As in the quasi-experiment, reliability was not checked, student behaviors were reported by staff, attrition was substantial, intention to treat analyses was not performed, and the experiment was conducted without consideration of the unusual motives, efforts, and expertise of demonstration staff. Moreover, the samples in both types of studies were probably unrepresentative of the population of concern—many parents and students refused to participate. The final samples may have contained the most motivated students and supportive parents. Thus, a sample of relatively motivated students who do not improve meaningfully after receipt of CIS services suggests both the failure of CIS and the inability of clinical social work to improve outcomes. The evaluative literature of clinical social work in schools does not threaten this conclusion.

Coren et al. (2016) conducted a meta-analysis of all programs—domestic and international—attempting to reintegrate "street-connected children and young people" into mainline social institutions, notably schools, and to reduce their harmful behaviors. They concluded on the basis of 13 minimally qualified studies that there was "no consistently significant benefit for focused therapeutic interventions compared with standard services such as drop-in centres (sic), case management and other comparable interventions" (n.p.). Moreover, they judged the quality of the research to be poor while "no studies measured the primary outcome of reintegration and none reported on adverse effects" (ibid., n.p.).

The Response to Intervention (RTI) program and the similar Positive Behavior Supports program (PBIS) in K-12 schools are designed to handle both academic and behavioral problems. PBIS in the form of school-wide positive behavior support has been adopted by more than 5000 schools (Flannery et al. 2009). Both programs claim to only provide "research based" interventions that "have strong empirical support from the behaviorist literature" (Kelly 2014, n.p. citing Kelly, Berzin et al. 2010).

Providing the lead article on school social work for the most recent Encyclopedia of Social Work (2005), Kelly (2014) offers presumably the most credible research that endorses the effectiveness of both programs. Yet the cited literature cannot sustain the claim that the two programs enjoy a "significant and sizeable literature supporting their effectiveness" (p. 8). Kelly et al. (2010) and Kelly, Frey et al. (2010) rest this claim on the National School Social Work Survey. However, the survey does not address the outcomes of clinical interventions to change undesirable student behaviors. It largely addresses the different activities of school social workers.

The randomized trial by Horner et al. (2009) does not in fact credibly support "the use of PBIS…to positively impact student behavior" (p. 6). The crucial measure of student behavior in the research counts "office discipline referrals." However, the research did not collect the necessary data to report on this outcome (p. 140). Towvim et al. (2012) report a series of nonexperimental case studies of PBIS implementation. They are journalism at best, a bit of contracted support for the National Center for Mental Health Promotion and Youth Violence Prevention. Flannery et al. (2009) report on another survey, this one polling program administrators of school-wide positive behavior support; it provides no objective evaluation of the program. Hale et al. (2010) are simply a discussion of "critical issues" in RTI providing research findings of typically weak studies concerning its effectiveness and only addresses learning disabilities not emotional and behavioral problems. Reynolds and Shaywitz (2009) are far truer to the literature than Kelly (2014) in summarizing the problems of the RTI and PBIS: "the apparent lack of student-based data to guide the most effective choice of approaches to, and specific components of intervention" (p. 44). There is no credible research that supports the ability of either RTI or PBIS to address the concerns of clinical social work in the schools. Even under optimal conditions, a few hours of counseling are insufficient to address serious emotional and behavioral problems of children.

According to the Encyclopedia of Social Work, "one of the most promising areas of intervention for Solution-Focused Brief Therapy (SFBT) is with children, adolescents, and teachers in school settings" (Franklin and Belciug 2015, n.p.). SFBT has been applied to behavioral and emotional problems as well as academic performance, social skills, and dropout prevention. It is based on the assumptions of the strengths perspective "that it is important to build on resources and motivations of clients because they know their problems the best and are capable of generating solutions to solve their own problems" (Kim and Franklin 2009, p. 464 following Saleebey 1996). SFBT is usually completed within four months.

> At the core of SFBT is the collaborative relationship between the client and the helper, with focus on letting clients discover their own solutions. SFBT also makes use of solution-talk and co-construction of meaning in the conversations between people, which is a major therapeutic mechanism for change.... This means that social workers practicing SFBT listen carefully and position questions and dialogue that challenges the client to identify present competencies and new behaviors that can be enacted in the future, and that have the potential to accomplish desired goals.... (ibid., n.p.)

However, the extensive research that Franklin and Belciug (2015) cite in support of SFBT—much of it authored by Franklin—is at best ambiguous and provides little if any evidence of effectiveness.

The review by Kim and Franklin (2009) identified just seven studies of SFBT that met their minimal inclusion criteria, only one of which incorporated a randomized design. Presumably the best of these seven studies, the randomized study by Froeschle et al. (2007), employed SFBT to prevent drug use among eighth-grade students who reported that very few were using illicit drugs. The study found "large" differences in reported drug use and thus concluded that SFBT was successful in prevention. However, attrition reached 25% in both control and experimental groups; no intention to treat analysis was performed. "For ethical reasons," parents were informed about the group assignment of their children thus preventing participant blinding (ibid., p. 502). Drug use was self-reported which should by itself invalidate the research. Moreover, school performance measured by grade point average, the only objective data in the research, was equivalent between the groups. Neither hair tests nor urinalysis were performed.

The recent study by Bond et al. (2013) reviewed the most methodologically credible and relevant studies that evaluated SFBT with children and families. However, these 38 studies only contained ten that employed randomized designs. Of these ten only two conducted follow-up evaluations, only one of which maintained improvements of the experimental group. Moreover, one of the ten employed a sample of only two. An additional five of the remaining nine showed no gains for the BSFT group compared with the control. Of the remaining four randomized studies, one experienced 60% attrition in the control. Two of the final four provided mixed outcomes. The last two randomized studies reported positive findings; one was conducted in Korea and the other in Romania. The credibility of these two studies by Shin (2009) and by Violeta and Dafinoiu (2009)—the best of the best reviewed by Bond et al.—is undercut by additional serious problems in addition to small samples and a lack of follow-up.

However, contrary to Bond et al. (2013), Violeta and Dafinoiu (2009) do not consider their study to be randomized but rather a "non-randomized pilot study" (p. 185). The control group was matched by "gender, age and the number of absences before beginning counseling" (p. 189). The objective of the intervention was to reduce truancy. The success with the experimental group was small (reduced from 13 to 5%) but statistically significant. The absence of randomization prevents attributing the results to the therapy rather than characteristics of the experimental group or simply unidentified and chance factors.

The last man standing, Shin (2009) employed SFBT to treat youth on probation for assault and theft in Korea. The experimental group showed great improvement over the control in aggressiveness, social adaptation, and goal attainment while aggressiveness in the control group apparently increased.

> Most of the participants achieved their expected level of change. Such a result appears to be attributable to the fact that they opened up while participating in the program, sharing their personal stories and experiences of failure, interchanging feedbacks (sic), and consequently realizing why they must change. (Shin, p. 283)

However, all of the data were self-reported by the youth. No objective measures were taken of the youths' behaviors during probation. The samples were questionably representative of Korean youth on probation and probably not representative of American youth convicted of crimes. There were no controls for expectancy biases, and the researcher may have provided the therapy and supervised the self-reports (the description of procedures is incomplete). There was no attrition which is not surprising during probation although the scrutiny and threats of probation may affect self-reports. Shin does not question the increased reported assault in the control group which is surprising for youth being supervised by a probation officer.

The wonderment lies in SFBT's persistence in spite of its ineffectiveness. While it offers little hope of improving the emotional conditions or academic achievements of school children, it endorses two important social values. In the first instance, it promises substantial outcomes at minimal cost. A few chats with a psychotherapist and often in groups are far less expensive than providing all children with the social and family conditions that encourage social, emotional, and intellectual growth.

Second, and probably more important than even cost, the strengths perspective at the core of SFBT is an expression of American romanticism both of which insist on personal agency rather than social reliance to resolve personal problems. By assuming that people with problems have the inner strength to resolve them, SFBT denies the role that systemic failures and deprivations—in this case the absence of supportive, nurturing families—play in creating personal problems and thus minimizes the legitimacy of claims on public resources. Character dominates social conditions as explanations of wayward behavior. Indeed, social work itself and not simply its clinical expressions perch on self-help, repeating the popular conservative mantra of "a hand up not a hand out." The strengths perspective is just one among the field's many soothing fictions that accompany the interminable sloganeering of clinical treatment.

Clinical Social Work Considered

Clinical social work fails to credibly demonstrate the ability to achieve its goals. Yet it remains popular, offering relatively inexpensive interventions that are compatible with social mores as solutions to serious emotional and social problems. In every aspect of its practice, clinical social work repeats the experience of clinical psychology, routinely failing to cure, prevent, or rehabilitate. It persists as ceremony reinforcing America's romantic values that exaggerate the power of personal agency and denigrate attention to the nation's many systemic failures. Cultural loyalty is apparently sufficient to account for durability.

Clinical social work rests its claims to effectiveness largely on the seriously impaired psychotherapy literature. The field's own efforts at clinical research are even weaker. Notwithstanding the century-old ambition for professional standing on grounds of specialized scientific information and decades emphasizing research in doctoral education (Berzoff and Drisko 2015), clinical social work and social work itself have failed to develop a scientifically credible practice or a suitable theory of intervention and social need. Even a definition of the social work clinic expanded beyond psychotherapy to include the core techniques of social casework—contracting, case management, and psychosocial analysis—does not improve the outcomes of clinical practice.

The field depreciates the value of systematic knowledge and program evaluation in favor of a priori wisdom and self-certifying belief that recapitulate popular preferences. Every area of clinical social work acts as though the length of a bibliography constituted proof. Without objective and coherent evidence of effectiveness, the literature of clinical practice in social work and its extensive research efforts reduce to missals of treatment sacraments and catalogs of rituals.

Evidence-based practice in clinical social work still awaits the development of "empirically supported treatments" to get beyond the amorphous but comforting intuition that best practice is by itself effective practice. In tribute to style over substance—words over meaning—clinical social work has appropriated the language of evidence-based practice to generate soothing fictions that displace attention to enduring social and personal problems.

The soothing fictions of service have frequently been organized around presumptions that efficiency begets effectiveness—lower cost but equivalent or superior outcomes. At other times, programs with tested superiority but that cost more than existing services—Stein and Test's (1980) demonstration of feasible community care, Boys Town, and the story of the asylum in the United States, as examples—are inaugurated but deprived of sufficient funding and shortly revert to the deficiencies of customary practice. Successful but costly demonstrations of care are almost invariably replicated in skeletal form as if the magic of their success rested on spirit rather than material resources, enduring service and professional skill—e.g., the Harlem Children's Zone and the Quantum Program in Philadelphia.

The rewards and the demands for evidence of programmatic effectiveness and efficiency suborn research neutrality and the integrity of a community of scholars. Clinical research follows along with distorted evidence that endorses psychotherapeutic approaches to foster care, family preservation, and clinical social work practice generally. In the end, social efficiency—the demand for inexpensive social welfare programs compatible with social values—displaces the goal of effectiveness as well as the pursuit of greater equality.

Foster care and its variants remain inadequate substitutes for generous care that might truly protect the integrity of families and the socialization of individuals. The soothing fictions of clinical social work and the social clinical are best understood as political ideology. The popular amalgam of social liberalism and economic conservatism transforms neglect and greed into a sacred ritual of individual freedom that minimizes public responsibility for individuals and wider problems.

Social work's failure to achieve the requisite knowledge that defines a clinical profession may be explained in two ways. On the one hand, the field lacks the necessary research skills and its community of scholars lacks neutrality. On the other hand, clinical practice may simply be ineffective and the evidence, such as it is, of positive outcomes marks the biases, inaccuracies, and misstatements of a beholden guild. If persistence is the goal, then social work's intellectual and academic weaknesses are its strengths. Indeed, the modern history of social work acknowledges the force of social cohesion rather than the independence of intellect in a liberal democracy. Even in its academic garb, the field is tolerated for its mythic affirmation of cultural values rather than as a serious intellectual presence. Tocqueville's exaggerated fear that democracy would descend into mediocrity is invigorated by social work theory and practice.

Plausible alternatives to the social clinic are justified primarily in terms of greater equality, fairness, and justice yet also in the hope that harm will be repaired and prevented. Boys Town is an earnest example of this possibility. Unfortunately, it is very costly and just as earnestly the society refuses to support it.

There have been rare but trenchant criticisms of the quality of social work research covering its clinical role among others. Wootton (1959) conducted one of the most thorough reviews of psychotherapeutic interventions concluding first that the research was inadequate and secondly that the field itself was misguided. A good Fabian socialist, she preferred handling systemic deficiencies rather than the "very comfortable" turn of policy toward individual failure (p. 329). Segal's (1972) greater focus on clinical social work repeated Wootton's comments about the poor quality of the literature that often uncovered the harmful effects of psychotherapy. Fischer (1973) screened the outcome research of casework to identify the best of the research. Only eleven studies satisfied his minimal criteria of quality: any control group, treatment delivered by social workers, and research conducted in the United States. Not one of the eleven established the effectiveness of clinical social work. "In slightly under 50 percent [of the] studies clients receiving services in the experimental group were shown either to deteriorate to a greater degree than clients in the control group or to demonstrate improved functioning at a lesser rate than control subjects" (pp. 15–16). Yet the surprisingly negative findings may have been due less to research rigor than to the persistent tendency to reflect the spirit of the times, in this case the skepticism and hostility to authority of the 1960s; ten of the eleven studies were published after 1961. Wood (1978) provided more reason for skepticism in a similar but more inclusive review. Yet

even the research that reported effective outcomes was seriously undercut by procedural pitfalls (Epstein 1993).

The field seemed to take a lesson from negative findings. Subsequent
research, including by Fischer, was far more hopeful, complimentary,
and rewarding of social work efforts. Outcomes improved and science
was presumably served. Yet the actual quality of research methods—the
ability to protect against bias—hardly advanced except for the introduction of more sophisticated statistics and the greater prevalence of randomized trials, neither of which proved adequate to the task of assuring
credible findings. Clinicians and those with obvious interests in positive
findings conducted the research with predictable results that inflated
the success of social work interventions. Measurement tools were routinely suspect. Raters were not blinded. Placebo controls were rarely
employed, and follow-up measures were seldom taken. Samples were
not representative. Attrition was high. Evaluations were usually conducted in demonstration situations rather than in live practice.

After a few years of floundering attempts on the basis of an avalanche
of suspect research to redeem the effectiveness of social work practice
with behavior modification and then with the empathy, warmth, and
genuineness of practitioners, Fischer (1981) announced a scientific
revolution in the field. He achieved the conversion from agnosticism
to faith on the basis of "material presented at social work conferences,
from the literature and from less concrete sources of evidence such as
the new 'spirit' or 'world view' that seems to be emerging among many
social workers" (p. 199). The field followed apace with experiments and
reviews of the literature all discovering the prowess of clinical social
work and social work in general although with only an occasional and
weak note of caution (Reid and Hanrahan 1982; Thomlison 1984;
Sheldon 1986; Wakefield 1988a, b; Gorey 1996; Rosen et al. 1999).

> All but two or three of the twenty-two studies yielded findings that could
> on balance be regarded as positive...Also in contrast to the earlier exper-
> iments, no recent study that involved a comparison between treated and
> untreated groups failed to yield at least some evidence of the positive
> effects of social work intervention. (Reid and Hanrahan 1982, p. 331)

The outcome data reporting on programs to produce individual change, such as those for anxiety disorders, sexual problems, psychosis, obesity alcohol and drug problems, all attest to positive results obtained with behavioral therapy. (Thomlison 1984, p. 52)

With rare exceptions, none of the reviews and none of the research that they included are credible. This conclusion has been strengthened by the repetitive pitfalls of more recent research and reviews covered in these chapters. Yet the falsity of the research is coincidental, and not by accident, with the emergence of clinical social work and accompanied by the field's abandonment of typically needy populations, notably the poor and others requiring material supports. Indeed, clinical social work has long been displacing basic, material, and practical activities by social workers. Rather than public service to those in need, private clinical practice has become the beau ideal of the field and the goal of most social workers. Social work is complicit but as ever not creative in its destiny. The dominance of the social clinic occurs in a society enthralled by the privateering values of business and commerce that accept growing inequality as natural and just and eased along by the fiction of entrepreneurial self-invention.

Cloward and Epstein (1965) documented this shift through an historical analysis of more than sixty years of private social work agencies that is still relevant one half century after its publication. They pointed out that even after the enactment of broad but inadequate public programs addressing poverty,

There was, and still is, ample opportunity for private agencies to continue programs of financial assistance for many emergency situations, for supplementation of inadequate public assistance grants, and for other purposes. There was, and still is, ample opportunity for private agencies to concentrate their resources on problems experienced by the poor which are not dealt with adequately in public programs, especially in such spheres as medical care, homemaking, housing and employment. (p. 33)

Instead, private agencies and social work itself became dominated by the social clinic under the excuse of serving the whole community rather than only those who most needed support. Cloward and Epstein explain the abandonment of the poor in terms of the concern of "the social work profession for its own status, which has led it to seek a more prestigious clientele, and the feeling that the psychological technology of social work is more amenable to middle-class than to lower-class socialization" (ibid., abstract).

Yet Cloward and Epstein largely attribute the choice of clinical practice to the field itself rather than to the near inescapable forces that determine the decisions of social institutions. The freedom of individuals to attempt heroic defiance is rarely shared by organizations dependent on social support. The story of the social clinic is more an acknowledgment of irresistible social imperatives than a drama of individual choice.

Specht and Courtney's (1994) respected history of social work's "mission drift" into psychotherapy repeats the error of blaming the field itself for its adaptation to dominant values. However, they also repeat Cloward and Epstein's insistence that there are alternatives to clinical practice that stay true to its avowed mission to help the poor and historically successful. Unfortunately, the choice seems to exist only between clinical programs that fail and earlier roles that also failed but not because of bad choices by the field. Rather, both types failed because the society refused to allocate sufficient resources or priorities to the goals of socialization and greater equality.

Even while chastising the field, Holden et al.'s (2017) documentation of the eccentric new areas of clinical social work implicates the social preferences that sustain them. Indeed, the strangeness of the new practices is the fruits of enduring popular reliance on the miraculous, the fantastic, and the otherworldly for quick, painless, personal transformation. Psychotherapy and its infusion into the guided self-help industry fit nicely with the pervasive and dominant popular culture. Once again, social work is exploring new markets through which to achieve professional standing.

Holden and Barker scoured the Internet and other sources for areas of social work practice that press against the "fuzzy borders" of social work practice. *Should Social Workers Be Engaged in These Practices?* lists more than three hundred practices and their Web sites. Most appear to incorporate some form of psychotherapy or are at least phrased in a way to suggest a basis in psychotherapy. A sampling of this Very New Age in clinical social work hints at the ripening of professional aspiration into shameless self-promotion.

21st Century Relationship Psychic, Access Consciousness Energetic Facelifts, Accessing Universal Intelligence mentor, A Course in Miracles, Amma Therapy, Ancestor work, Archangel Light, Be Set Free Fast, Beyond the Inner Child Work: Parts Work, Body Talk System, Certified Emotion Code Practitioner, Certified Flower and Gem Essence Therapist, Certified Humanistic Sand Tray Therapist, Certified in BrainWorking (sic) Recursive Technique, Color Puncture, Crystal bowl healing, Depossession work, Elemental Divination, Extraction (removing localized spiritual intrusion), School for Shamans, Oracles, Priest/esses. Healers, Intuitives and Alchemists, Guidance from the angelic realm, Harner Shamanic Counseling, House Blessings, Induced After Death Communication, Inner Courage Therapy, Intuitive Channeler, MariEl (sic) Healing, Mind Frequency Shifting, Polarity Therapy, Psychic Psychotherapy, Psychotherapist and Animal Communicator, Qualified Therapeutic Touch Teacher, Spirit attachment work, Splanka Therapy, Thought Field Therapy, Trauma Conversion Therapy, Vipassana Therapists, White Time Healing, Womanrunes.

Most of these examples are based on unsubstantiated superstition, quasi-religious faith, spiritualism, voodoo science, and perhaps even alien abduction. Yet too, so is clinical social work and the social clinic itself. The debased science of clinical social work erases the distinction between the approved and the crackpot. Both lack the dignity of credible evaluation and, consequently, credible evidence of success. Holden and Barker confirm the tenuousness of social work's attachment to objective coherence and modern professionalism while subtly if not silently raising questions about the quality of academic preparation in the field. Citing others and reporting his own analyses, Stoesz et al. (2010) put the issue to rest: Academic social work is woefully deficient.

In the manner of most disciplines and professions, the intellectual life of social work and preparation for clinical practice are vested in the faculties of schools of social work. Never a particularly fertile terrain, schools of social work have aged into a contemporary desert of lazy incompetence that satisfies social expectations. The torpor of social work's intellectual life measured by journal reputation, the scholarly publication of journal editors and editorial boards—the gatekeepers of social work's specialized knowledge—school leadership, and the performance of its two principal professional organizations has been forcefully captured by Stoesz et al. (2010).

In the ten years from 1992 to 2001, the editors of five middling psychology journals (as measured by Journal Citation Reports) published almost seven times more journal articles and received eight times more citations than the editors of the top five social work journals published under a social work auspice (as per Journal Citation Reports). The scholarly productivity was similarly weak among the consulting editors, the gatekeepers to publication, of Social Work, the field's leading journal, and *JSWE*, the principal journal of social work pedagogy.

> Another way to capture the scholarly inexperience of consulting editors is to liken their productivity to standards for promotion to associate professor with tenure. Hypothetically, if a minimal standard were six publications in Social Sciences Citation Index journals, then 35.1% of consulting editors for *Social Work* and 61.8 percent of *JSWE* consulting editors would not likely have been promoted or tenured based on their scholarship. (Stoesz et al. 2010, p. 46)[5]
>
> More than one fourth of deans and directors of MSW programs had apparently published no journal articles [in Social Sciences Citation Index journals] over their entire careers. Almost 52 percent had published only two or fewer articles, 70 percent had five or fewer articles. (ibid., p. 90)

It is also worth keeping in mind that most articles have more than one author. This is an extraordinarily low level of scholarly output among academics who occupy positions of leadership.

---

[5] *Social Work* is the leading journal in the field, and *Journal of Social Work Education* (*JSWE*) is as its title suggests the principal journal of social work pedagogy in a disciple that claims internship education as its core.

Stoesz et al. (2010) go on to detail the enormous growth of social work programs at all levels, baccalaureate, masters, and doctorate— overall, 52% between 1985 and 2009. Yet student enrollment did not keep up with the growth of programs, thus exacerbating a competition for students and an inevitable decline in both qualifications for enrollment and graduation. In 2005, the Graduate Record Examination scores for social work students (896) were the second lowest in the nation; only physical education students had lower scores (894).

Apparently, social work opens a backdoor to clinical practice for students who are not academically competitive for entry into clinical psychology programs. Yet the quality of preparatory courses for practice may not matter much in light of the ineffectiveness of the social clinic generally. The point is one of symbolism not substance; self-invention has its prerogatives. More privileged and wealthier citizens with emotional problems see practitioners with Ph.D.s in clinical psychology; less privileged and poorer citizens get to speak with social workers with master's degrees.

Underfunded universities and colleges found a benefit in sustaining inexpensive social work programs that provided a tuition dividend they could apply to more favored programs. Social work salaries in the academy as well as in practice have declined. Social work courses have been increasingly taught by relatively untrained adjunct and part-time faculty. Stoesz et al. (2010) conclude that

> Social work education's adherence to a growth model is based on the assumption that social programs will require an infinitely elastic supply of professionals.... In replication of the industrial model of professional education, social work has chosen to stress uniformity over customization, and efficiency over competence.... Among the casualties of such arrogance has been the quality of social work education. (p. 69)

However, Stoesz, Karger, and Carrilio may err in describing the field's weak academic life as a "secret that cannot be kept indefinitely" (p. 77). He also makes the common error of emphasizing the responsibility of the field for its current condition. The recursive story of weak programs poorly preparing weak students to enter a public service market that provides only modest compensation hardly seems a situation that the field created by itself or can alter. Rather, the low status of the field mirrors the low status of the recipients of social work services. Its services are symbols of concern rather than the real thing—the soothing fictions of American charitability that sum up popular sentiments. Poorer and lower status Americans receive the same inferior quality clinical services that replicate their experience in the other institutions of the culture. The situation is not accidental; it is intended and deemed quite acceptable.

In fact, the poor quality of social work's academic and intellectual life never was hidden nor was it a threat to the field. It has always been known and accepted by the culture. The field simply obliges prevailing sentiments. Those sentiments are captured in work that epitomizes the dominant intellectual assumptions of practice and closely tracks the policy romanticism of American society. The style of social work is clothed in the talk of science, while proof and effectiveness are a fiction of practice.

Heineman (1981) argued that science was "obsolete," that is, irrelevant, for social work. Science was inevitably biased by a number of researcher intrusions and limitations of measurement while the assumptions of logical positivism were imperfect. Instead, she argued for less restrictive methods of research that equated the value of retrospective designs with prospective experimental designs. There was strong reason to consider empathy "as a valid instrument of observation" (p. 379) and practitioner wisdom as a valid measure of outcomes. Heineman argued for the primacy of problem-solving that was not restricted simply to operationalized standards of research but incorporated the political and social situations of the research. Thus, the resolution of the service "problem" became a negotiation among those involved in practice— patients, therapists, and the broader society—over standards of effectiveness as well as the measures of the outcomes themselves; objectivity was no longer a necessary requirement of measurement or meaning. This purposive equation of the objective standards, measures, and procedures of rational clinical research with the subjectivities of social preferences permitted clinical practice to certify its own value so long as it remained attentive to social imperatives. In appreciation of Orwell, the social clinic remained independent to affirm social values.

The published reaction to Heineman eloquently picked apart her position and reaffirmed the importance of scientific standards in clinical research. However, the criticism has had little influence on the field. Indeed, the critics themselves, have routinely violated the tenets of science in their own work. A corrupted form of research prevails that esteems ineffective murky oddities of the social clinic such as the strengths perspective and even spiritual practice (Derezotes 2006). Science in clinical practice becomes debased as "science talk" to bolster the professional status of social work and the social clinic (Blau 2017). The health of social work practice is the heart of Heineman's argument, and the problem to be resolved is professional standing based on social acceptance rather than service measured by the objective gains of recipients.

The controversy over Heineman's essay became a struggle between anti-science and distorted science—between those who simply reject empiricism in favor of implicit wisdom and those who wish to employ the forms of science to satisfy factional ambitions. As evidenced by the research, the community of scholars of the social clinic have routinely manufactured defective tests of practice while refusing to turn over sensitive research to independent evaluators. The talk of method has become the breastplate of bogus professionalism; the actual issue has always been sectarian precedence as though in a competition among religions.

Millenarian visions of clinical social work—personal transformation, social adaptation, and institutional change through a variety of talk therapies—are as futile and unrealistic as messianic belief in the rapture and the Second Coming. They have not inspired an effective practice of treatment. Yet they symbolize popular opposition to social policies of greater sharing and decency, deferring attention to the material inequalities of the here and now with a longing eye on the eternal bliss of self-actualization through clinical treatment. The field exists in a dream-state of its ambitions in which cultish true-belief certifies its imagined virtues and distorts both practice and the independence of its intellectual life. A superficial commitment to scientific practice along with the rejection of pragmatism signals the field's romantic core: personal agency as the operative assumption of the social work clinic, implicit belief in its rightness and effectiveness, and a sense of professional exceptionalism that echoes the society's sense of its chosenness. Clinical social work is professionalism hollowed out of measurable meaning and replaced by the long-standing, insistent, and popular preferences of American society, the true client of social work.

The deficiencies of clinical social work are a piece with the pretensions of social work itself as Abram's lamp of spontaneous insight radiating beams of enlightenment, social justice, fairness, and goodness to an attentive society (Abrams 1953). The reality of the field is quite different. There is little credible evidence that social work practice actually pursues let alone achieves any of its grand goals, notably including its clinical promises of successful treatment. In fact, the role as a paladin of the poor and the oppressed is rarely if ever sustained in its social mandate or enumerated in the job descriptions of social workers. Instead, clinical social work and the field generally have succumbed to the rewards for exuding the pietistic gas common to occupations without material purpose but that enjoy redemptive virtue parading the banner of popular values. The retreat into the ineffable, enveloping miasma of altruism, goodness, helping, and an enraptured martyrdom for suffering humanity masks social work's betrayal of the needs of poorer and lower status Americans. The sin of clinical social work and its exculpation both lie in the fact that it mirrors the American culture, neither able to go its own way nor willing to do so.

The prospect of greater equality and decent care in American social welfare has usually succumbed to the reality of American depravity, cruelty, and selfishness. The nation's barbaric abuses of many populations were not seriously challenged until the Civil War and then routinely ignored during American apartheid and continued afterward by a determinative consensus to do little about American inequality. The enormous capacity of the nation to address the deficits of its population was not only the inadvertent result of differential luck and development but often a product of the theft of labor and a ruthless disregard of human liberty and dignity. Social work and the social clinic are steps backward—soothing fictions that personal and social distress are easily repaired.

If Rothman were alive today, he might reconsider his faith in American social development that "since the Progressive era, we have been gradually escaping from institutional responses, and one can foresee the period when incarceration will be used still more rarely than it is today" (ibid., p. 293). The deinstitutionalized system of care for the seriously impaired has become as cruel and inadequate as the large hospitals, sanatoria, and poor houses that it replaced. More broadly, the material deficits of American citizens have been increasing even while national wealth increases. The failure is even more glaring with the realization that expectations for productive participation in both the market and the society have become increasingly demanding and complex. The social clinic including social work's preference for psychological cures is not the solution but a distraction and an impediment to finding one.

Clinical social work as well as the practices of community psychology, community psychiatry, and the discipline of corrections fabricates romantic escapes from the pains of reality, the soothing fictions that endorse the rightness, and inevitability of embedded social priorities. None of the clinical practices are free to create themselves or to plan their own programs without deference to dominant social dictates. Their genius lies in self-deception, not service.

References

Abrams, M. H. (1953). *The Mirror and the Lamp*. New York: Oxford University Press.

Allen-Meares, P. (2013, May 8, 2018). School Social Work. *Encyclopedia of Social Work*. http://dx.doi.org/10.1093/acrefore/9780199975839.013.351.

Berzoff, J., & Drisko, J. (2015). Preparing PhD-Level Clinical Social Work Practitioners for the 21st Century. *Journal of Teaching in Social Work, 35*, 82–100. https://doi.org/10.1080/08841233.2014.993107.

Blau, J. (2017). Science as a Strategy for Social Work. *Journal of Progressive Human Services, 28*, 73–90. https://doi.org/10.1080/10428232.2017.1310543.

Bond, C., Woods, K., Humphrey, N., Symes, W., & Green, L. (2013). Practitioner Review: The Effectiveness of Solution Focused Brief Therapy with Children and Families: A Systematic and Critical Evaluation of the

Literature from 1990–2010. *Journal of Child Psychology and Psychiatry, 54,* 707–723. https://doi.org/10.1111/jcpp.12058.

Chamberlain, P. (1990). Comparative Evaluation of Specialized Foster Care for Seriously Delinquent Youth: A First Step. *Community Alternatives International Journal of Family Care, 2,* 21–36.

Chamberlain, P., & Reid, J. B. (1994). Differences in Risk Factors and Adjustment for Male and Female Delinquents in Treatment Foster Care. *Journal of Child and Family Studies, 3,* 23–39. https://doi.org/10.1007/BF02233909.

Chamberlain, P., & Reid, J. B. (1998). Comparison of Two Community Alternatives to Incarceration for Chronic Juvenile Offenders. *Journal of Consulting and Clinical Psychology, 66,* 624–633. https://doi.org/10.1037/0022-006X.66.4.624.

Chamberlain, P., et al. (2008). Prevention of Behavior Problems for Children in Foster Care: Outcomes and Mediation Effects. *Prevention Science, 9*(1), 17–27.

Channa, M. W., et al. (2012). A Meta-Analysis of Intensive Family Preservation Programs: Placement Prevention and Improvement of Family Functioning. *Children and Youth Services Review, 34*(8), 1472–1479.

Cloward, R. A., & Epstein, I. (1965). *The Adjustment of Social Welfare to Social Change.* Available from ERIC.

Communities and Schools of Nevada. (n.d.). https://www.cisnevada.org/.

Coren, E., et al. (2016). Interventions for Promoting Reintegration and Reducing Harmful Behaviour and Lifestyles in Street-Connected Children and Young People. *Cochrane Database of Systematic Reviews, 1,* (Article number CD009823).

Dagenais, C., Begin, J., Bouchard, C., & Fortin, D. (2004). Impact of Intensive Family Support Programs: A Synthesis of Evaluation Studies. *Children and Youth Services Review, 26,* 249–263. https://doi.org/10.1016/j.childyouth.2004.01.015.

Derezotes, D. S. (2006). *Spiritually Oriented Social Work Practice.* Boston, MA: Pearson.

DeVooght, K., Fletcher, M., & Cooper, H. (2012). *Federal, State, and Local Spending to Address Child Abuse and Neglect in SFY 2012.* The Annie E. Casey Foundation. https://www.childtrends.org/wp-content/uploads/2014/09/SFY-2012-Report-for-Posting-July2015.pdf.

Epstein, W. M. (1993). *The Illusion of Psychotherapy.* New Brunswick, NJ: Transaction Publishers.

Epstein, W. M. (1997). Social Science, Child Welfare, and Family Preservation: A Failure of Rationality in Public Policy. *Children and Youth Services Review, 19,* 41–60.

Epstein, W. M. (2017). *The Masses Are the Ruling Classes: Policy Romanticism, Democratic Populism, and Social Welfare.* New York, NY: Oxford University Press.

Feldman, L. H. (1991). Evaluating the Impact of Intensive Family Preservation Services in New Jersey. In D. Biegel (Ed.), *Family Preservation Services: Research and Evaluation.* Newbury Park, CA: Sage.

Fischer, J. (1973). Is Casework Effective: A Review. *Social Work, 18*(1), 5–20.

Fischer, J. (1981). The Social Work Revolution. *Social Work, 26*(3), 199–207.

Flannery, K., Sugai, G., & Anderson, C. M. (2009). School-Wide Positive Behavior Support in High School. *Journal of Positive Behavior Intervention, 11,* 177–185. https://doi.org/10.1177/1098300708316257.

Franklin, C. (2016). *Social Work Essentials: Selections from the Encyclopedia of Social Work.* Washington, DC: NASW Press.

Franklin, C., & Belciug, C. (2015). Solution-Focused Brief Therapy in Schools. *Encyclopedia of Social Work.* https://doi.org/10.1093/acrefore/9780199975839.013.1040.

Frederico, M., Long, M., McNamara, P., McPherson, L., & Rose, R. (2016). Improving Outcomes for Children in Out-of-Home Care: The Role of Therapeutic Foster Care. *Child and Family Social Work, 22,* 1064–1074. https://doi.org/10.1111/cfs.12326.

Froeschle, J. G., Smith, R. L., & Ricard, R. (2007). The Efficacy of a Systematic Substance Abuse Program for Adolescent Females. *Professional School Counseling, 10.* http://dx.doi.org/10.1177/2156759X0701000507.

Goldhaber-Fiebert, J. D., Snowden, L. R., Wulczyn, F., Landsverk, J., & Horwitz, S. M. (2011). Economic Evaluation Research in the Context of Child Welfare Policy: A Structured Literature Review and Recommendations. *Child Abuse & Neglect: The International Journal, 35,* 722–740. https://doi.org/10.1016/j.chiabu.2011.05.012.

Gorey, K. M. (1996). Effectiveness of Social Work Intervention Research: Internal Versus External Evaluations. *National Association of Social Workers.* https://doi.org/10.1093/swr/20.2.119.

Greenberg, G. A., & Rosenheck, R. A. (2010). Correlates of Past Homelessness in the National Epidemiological Survey on Alcohol and Related Conditions.*Administration and Policy in Mental Health and Mental Health Services Research, 37*(4), 357–366.

Hahn, R. A., Bilukha, O., Lowy, J., Crosby, A., Fullilove, M. T., Liberman, A., et al. (2005). The Effectiveness of Therapeutic Foster Care for the Prevention of Violence. *American Journal of Preventative Medicine, 28,* 72–90. https://doi.org/10.1016/j.ampre.2004.10.007.

Hale, J., Alfonso, V., Berninger, V., Bracken, B., Christo, C., Clark, E., et al. (2010). Critical Issues in Response-to-Intervention, Comprehensive Evaluation, and Specific Learning Disabilities Identification and Intervention: An Expert White Paper Consensus. *Learning Disability Quarterly, 33,* 223–236. https://doi.org/10.1177/073194871003300310.

Heineman, M. (1981). The Obsolete Scientific Imperative in Social Work Research. *Social Service Review, 55,* 371–397. Retrieved from http://www.jstor.org.ezproxy.library.unlv.edu/stable/30011495.

Holden, G., et al. (2017). Self-Efficacy Regarding Social Work Competencies. *Research on Social Work Practice, 27*(5), 594–606.

Horner, R. H., et al. (2009). A Randomized, Wait-List Controlled Effectiveness Trial Assessing School-Wide Positive Behavior Support in Elementary Schools. *Journal of Positive Behavior Interventions, 11*(3), 133–144.

Kelly, M. S. (2014). Response to Intervention in Schools. *Encyclopedia of Social Work.* https://doi.org/10.1093/acrefore/9780199975839.013.1013.

Kelly, M. S., Frey, A. J., Alvarez, M., Cosner Berzin, S., Shaffer, G., & O'Brien, K. (2010). School Social Work Practice and Response to Intervention. *Children & Schools, 32,* 201–209. http://dx.doi.org/doi.org/10.2137/145960610792912602.

Kessler, R. C., Pecora, P. J., Williams, J., Hiripi, E., O'Brien, K., English, D., et al. (2008). Effects of Enhanced Foster Care on Long-Term Physical and Mental Health of Foster Care Alumni. *Archives of General Psychiatry, 65,* 625–633. https://doi.org/10.1001/archpsyc.65.6.625.

Kim, J. S., & Franklin, C. (2009). Solution-Focused Brief Therapy in Schools: A Review of the Outcome Literature. *Children and Youth Services Review, 31,* 464–470. http://dx.doi.org/doi.org/10.1016/j.childyouth.2008.10.002.

Kushel, M. B., Yen, I. H., Gee, L., & Courtney, M. E. (2007). Homelessness and Health Care Access After Emancipation: Results from the Midwest Evaluation of Adult Functioning of Former Foster Youth. *Archives of Pediatrics and Adolescent Medicine, 161,* 986–993. https://doi.org/10.1001/archpedi.161.10.986.

Lewis, R. E. (2005). The Effectiveness of Families First Services: An Experimental Study. *Children and Youth Services Review, 27,* 499–509. https://doi.org/10.1177/106342669700500204.

Madigan, S., Paton, K., & Mackett, N. (2017). The Springfield Project Service: Evaluation of a Solihull Approach Course for Foster Carers. *Adopting & Fostering, 41,* 254–267. https://doi.org/10.1177/0308575917719373.

Meezan, W., & McCroskey, J. (1996). Improving Family Functioning Through Family Preservation Services: Results of the Los Angeles Experiment. *Journal of Family Strengths, 1*(2), 1–21. Retrieved from http://digitalcommons.library.tmc.edu/jfs.

Mizrahi, T., & Davis, L. E., (2005). *Encyclopedia of Social Work* (20th ed.). Washington, DC: NASW Press.

Pecora, P. J., Kessler, R. C., O'Brien, K., White, C. R., Williams, J., Hiripi, E., et al. (2006). Educational and Employment Outcomes of Adults Formerly Placed in Foster Care: Results from the Northwest Foster Care Alumni Study. *Children and Youth Services Review, 28,* 1459–1481. https://doi.org/10.1177/030857590703100126.

Reid, W. J., & Hanrahan, P. (1982). Recent Evaluations of Social Work: Grounds for Optimism. *Social Work, 27*(4), 328–340.

Reynolds, C. R., & Shaywitz, S. E. (2009). Response to Intervention: Prevention and Remediation, Perhaps. Diagnosis, No. *Child Development Perspectives, 3,* 44–47. https://doi.org/10.1111/j.1750-8606.2008.00075.x.

Rosen, A., Proctor, E. K., Staudt, M. M. (1999). Social Work Research and the Quest for Effective Practice. *Social Work Research, 23*(1), 4–14.

Saleebey, D. (1996). The Strengths Perspective in *Social Work* Practice: Extensions and Cautions. *Social Work, 41,* 296–305. http://dx.doi.org/doi-org.ezproxy.library.unlv.edu/10.1093/sw/41.3.296.

Scannapieco, M., Connell-Carrick, K., & Painter, K. (2007). In Their Own Words: Challenges Facing Youth Aging Out of Foster Care. *Child and Adolescent Social Work Journal, 24,* 423–435. https://doi.org/10.1007/s10560-007-0093-x.

Schuerman, J. R., Rzepnicki, T. L., & Littell, J. H. (1994). *Putting Families First: An Experiment in Family Preservation.* New York: Aldine de Gruyter.

Segal, S. P. (1972). Research on Outcome of Social Work Therapeutic Interventions—Review of Literature. *Journal of Health and Social Behavior, 13*(1), 3–17.

Sheldon, B. (1986). Social Work Effectiveness Experiments—Review and Implications. *British Journal of Social Work, 16*(2), 223–242.

Shin, S. (2009). Effects of a Solution-Focused Program on the Reduction of Aggressiveness and the Improvement of Social Readjustment for Korean Probationers. *Journal of Social Service Research, 35,* 274–284. https://doi.org/10.1080/01488370902901079.

Specht, H., & Courtney, M. (1994). *Unfaithful Angels: How Social Work Has Abandoned Its Mission.* New York, NY: The Free Press.

Stein, L. I., & Test, M. A. (1980). Alternative to Mental Hospital Treatment. I. Conceptual Model, Treatment Program, and Clinical Evaluation. *Archives of General Psychiatry, 37,* 409–412.

Stoesz, D., Karger, H. J., & Carrilio, T. (2010). *A Dream Deferred: How Social Work Education Lost Its Way and What Can Be Done.* New Brunswick, NJ: Aldine Transaction.

Stokey Kelly, M., Cosner Berzin, S., Frey, A., Alvarez, M., Shaffer, G., & O'Brien, K. (2010). The State of School Social Work: Findings from the National School Social Work Survey. *School Mental Health, 2,* 132–141. https://doi.org/10.1007/s12310-010-9034-5.

Thomlison, R. J. (1984). Something Works—Evidence from Practice Effectiveness Studies. *Social Work, 29*(1), 51–56.

Thompson, A. E., & Greeson, J. K. (2017). Prosocial Activities and Natural Mentoring Among Youth at Risk of Aging Out of Foster Care. *Journal of the Society for Social Work and Research, 8,* 421–440. https://doi.org/10.1086/693119.

Towvim, L., et al. (2012). *Positive Behavioral Interventions and Supports.* National Center for Mental Health Promotion and Youth Violence Prevention. http://www.promoteprevent.org/sites/www.promoteprevent.org/files/resources/positive_behavioral_interventions_snapshots.pdf.

Vandivere, S., Malm, K. E., Allen, T. J., Williams, S., & McKlindon, A. (2017). A Randomized Controlled Trial of Family Finding: A Relative Search and Engagement Intervention for Youth Lingering in Foster Care. *Evaluation Review, 41,* 542–567. https://doi.org/10.1177/0193841X17689971.

Violeta, E., & Dafinoiu, I. (2009). Motivational/Solution-Focused Intervention for Reducing School Truancy Among Adolescents. *Journal of Cognitive & Behavioral Psychotherapies, 9,* 185–198.

Wakefield, J. C. (1988a, June). Psychotherapy, Distributive Justice, and Social Work. Part 1: Distributive Justice as a Conceptual Framework for Social Work. *Social Service Review, 62,* 187–210.

Wakefield, J. C. (1988b). Psychotherapy, Distributive Justice, and Social Work Part 2: Psychotherapy and the Pursuit of Justice. *Social Service Review,* *62*(3), 353–382.

Wood, K. M. (1978). Casework Effectiveness: New Look at Research Evidence. *Social Work, 23*(6), 437–458.

Wootton, B. (1959). *Social Science and Social Pathology.* London: George Allen and Unwin.

Part III

Other Practices of the Social Clinic

9

Community Psychological Practice and a Note on Rehabilitation in Corrections

What a curious muddle. Social work pursues professional standing by abandoning its traditional commitment to the poor and needy in favor of a psychotherapeutic clinical practice aimed at emotional comfort and attitude change. Political and social activism along with community practice, always minor themes in social work and rarely successful, have been obliterated by the dominance of clinical practice. In contrast, community psychology and community psychiatry—combined as community psychological practice—initially committed to an individual psychological approach to human dysfunction have adopted a professional strategy to become more like classical social work, emphasizing the provision of material and caring services to needy and marginal populations—notably schizophrenics and others with serious mental illnesses. Community psychology stresses community practice including political and social activism. From its founding at the Swampscott Conference in 1965, "Community psychologists were encouraged to be active participants in solving the general problems of society and to become 'social change agents, political activists, and participant conceptualizers'" (Rickel 1987, p. 511). Less ideologically driven and politically engaged than community psychology, community psychiatry

© The Author(s) 2019
W. M. Epstein, *Psychotherapy and the Social Clinic in the United States*,
https://doi.org/10.1007/978-3-030-32750-7_9

has largely abandoned the arena of services in favor of biological treatment—psychopharmacology—that by itself cannot succeed. While the forms of appropriate treatment have been developed, notably supportive community-based alternatives to hospitalization, by and large they have not been adequately funded.

There remains considerable overlap between social work and community psychology although not community psychiatry with its grounding in medicine. The liberationist rhetoric of social work and community psychology is almost identical. Both are freeing the human spirit, pursuing justice, and committed to marginalized groups. Both assume the interaction between person and environment, that is, the "ecological perspective" provides clinical services and claims evidence-based success for their interventions. Both place an emphasis, approaching the romantic transcendence of spiritualism, on the capacities of change agents (the therapist, the activist, the organizer, the intellectual) to motivate passive populations and resistant individuals (Dalton et al. 2001; Levine and Perkins 1997; Kagan et al. 2011; Nelson et al. 2014). Both have a tendency to substitute imagination and intuition for reality.

Yet social work and community psychological practice differ in a fundamental regard. Social work's defining role has emerged in the social clinic that despite the field's avowed ecological perspective assumes enormous personal agency—the ability of people to transform themselves. In contrast, community psychological practice assumes the overriding influence of the environment on human behavior rather than the determinative power of self-creating character and human will. While the disciplines of community psychological practice may have to a great extent abandoned psychotherapeutic interventions, talk therapies are yet routinely provided by the community mental health centers that employ psychologists and psychiatrists.

Thus, community psychological practice seeks to change the individual's environment through the direct provision of material and caring services that provide material supports (crucially housing) and surrogates for failed social institutions, notably the family, the peer group, and the community. Secondly, community psychology seeks to influence policy through political engagement, community organization, and programs of empowerment.

In spite of their noble liberationist hopes, the programs of all three fields consistently fail. Psychotherapy is ineffective and thus the social clinic is a functional dead-end. Community psychological practice fails but largely because funds are inadequate to sustain its programs, notably housing, and supportive care. The resistance to adequate funding—popular antagonism to higher taxes and the needy populations themselves—has not been surmounted by strategies of political activism. The organization of vulnerable, needy, and poorer people for political power—a form of localized self-help—is very unlikely to succeed. The list of similar attempts contains a greater number of heroic tragedies and tyrannies than successes. There is no successful discipline of political, social, or psychological liberation. Moreover, the provision of decent community care, notably for patients with chronic mental and emotional disorders but many others as well, is very expensive. The social clinic is much less expensive. Neglect is even cheaper.

Even though a planned change in human consciousness is about as likely as the Messiah's often-scheduled return, some of the programs of community psychological practice provide clues to successful interventions. The provision of care, that is, a new environment for a short period often results in modest benefits although they wear off quickly when the recipient is returned to the old situation. The provision of more intense care over a relatively long period and perhaps even with no limit seems likely to produce a dose effect. If the concern is with successful service, then the provision of care calibrated to need rather than fiscal parsimony is surely superior to the distorted bulletins of beholden researchers that superficial interventions have performed miracles.

Community Psychological Practice

Community psychological practice was largely initiated by federal legislation, the 1963 Community Mental Health Act that funded a multitude of community mental health centers and Medicaid that provided reimbursements for patient services. The centers were established primarily to facilitate the accommodation in the community of long staying mental hospital patients. Community living was assumed to be superior to long stays in the mental hospital. Successful adjustment to the community was predicated on the ability of psychotropic drugs to control psychotic behaviors and the provision of supportive services: case management, psychosocial rehabilitation including skills training, socialization services, some amount of clinical referrals, housing, employment when possible, and direct supervision when needed and others. The community mental health centers also had secondary functions to provide the broader community access and referrals to mental health services, public education about mental health, mental health services research, and prevention.

In a powerful demonstration, Stein and Test (1980) demonstrated the feasibility of community psychological practice. "Training in community living" that has become known as "assertive community treatment" provided an alternative to the mental hospital in Dane County (Madison) Wisconsin.

> The program was implemented by a retrained mental-hospital ward staff who were transplanted to the community. Staff coverage was available 24 hours a day, seven days a week. Patient programs were individually tailored and were based primarily on an assessment of the patient's coping-skill deficits and requirements for community living. Most treatment took place in vivo: in patients' homes, neighborhoods, and place of work. More specifically, staff members on-the-scene in patients' homes and neighborhoods taught and assisted them in daily living activities such as laundry, upkeep, shopping, cooking, restaurant use, grooming, budgeting, and use of transportation. In addition, patients were given sustained and intensive assistance in finding a job or sheltered workshop, and the staff then continued daily contact with patients and their supervisors or employers to help with on-the-job problem solving... Providing support to patients, patients' families, and community members was a key function of the staff. The program was "assertive"; if a patient did not show up for work, a staff member immediately went to the patient's home to help with any problem that was interfering. Each patient's medical status was carefully monitored and treated. Medication was routinely used for schizophrenic and manic-depressive patients. (Stein and Test, pp. 393–394)

The treatment phase of the demonstration program lasted for 14 months and was evaluated through a randomized design. Patients were followed for an additional 14 months after the end of treatment. All the patients had sought admission for inpatient care at a single hospital. They had accumulated a mean of five previous mental hospitalizations totaling a mean of 14.5 months. Only 17% of patients had no previous mental hospitalizations. Sixty-five patients were randomized to training in community living, the experimental condition, and sixty-five were randomized to a treatment as usual control. The control condition was unusual in providing a considerable range and intensity of inpatient and out-patient services, setting a high bar for the success of the experiment. After 28 months, attrition only reached about 16% in the experimental group and 15% in the control group. Still, an intention to treat analysis would presumably have slightly reduced the positive outcomes.

The outcomes were compelling. During the 14 months of training in community services, experimental patients compared with control patients accumulated significantly fewer hospital days. This reduction in hospitalization did not eventuate in more jail time or supervised living in the community. Training in community living patients were also substantially less unemployed and earned more than control patients. By the end of treatment, experimental patients compared with control patients showed fewer psychotic symptoms, were more compliant with their medications, and reported greater satisfaction with their lives and living situations. Outcomes measuring leisure time, social relationships and quality of environment showed few differences between the groups.

The experiment writes a brief for prolonged and intensive services. Fourteen months after terminating treatment all the experimental group gains evaporated, returning to the levels of the control group: less employment, more symptoms, less compliance with medication, and less satisfaction with life.

The authors' conclusions stay true to their data:

> With minimal use of the hospital, it was possible to treat in the community a [representative] group of patients who applied for admission at a state mental hospital. While most of the control subjects were admitted to the hospital and many were subsequently readmitted, almost all of

the experimental patients had a sustained community tenure for the year. Most important, the data indicated that their sustained community living was not gained at the expense of their quality of life, level of adjustment, self-esteem, or personal satisfaction with life. (ibid., p. 396)

A related cost-benefit analysis of the experiment (Weisbrod et al. 1980) concluded that training in community living cost approximated $800 more per patient than customary care although the authors also argued that it provided about $1200 more per patient in benefits. More speculative, an attempt to measure social costs concluded that the provision of training in community living imposed no greater burdens on families and the community than traditional services (Stein and Test 1980).

Nonetheless, a number of considerations constrain the applicability of the demonstration and perhaps even its meaning, converting the service notion of community care into a soothing fiction. The beneficial outcomes may have been due to the voluntary and substantial efforts of families and relatives. The patients enjoyed considerable attachment to families that wanted them to succeed outside of the hospital and wanted them at home. Thus, many patients had free housing to rely on. Furthermore, the research does not detail the amount of voluntary care that patients required and thus the cost analyses do not estimate the finances to provide crucial substitutes for voluntary care when it is not present. Secondly, it is not clear whether decisions over patient hospitalization reflected true patient needs rather than the staff's ambition to minimize the incidence of hospital care. Stein and Test (1980) acknowledge that their diagnoses and subsequently decisions over hospitalization "were based on clinical judgment rather than on research diagnostic criteria. [After initial diagnoses] further reliability estimates were not made" (p. 396). Furthermore, the experiment was conducted as a demonstration that employed a highly motivated staff working over a relatively short period of time. Similar levels of motivation may not be easily maintained under customary conditions and similarly well-trained personnel may not be common.[1]

---

[1]Kirk et al. (2013) provide a far bleaker interpretation of the training in community living experiment. They question its outcomes, design, and use of coercion. To the extent to which their

The issue of cost inhibits the replication of the experiment that was conducted in a relatively affluent, rural homogeneous community—"a nonindustrial, progressive community that was receptive to this type of study" (ibid., p. 396)—with low crime. The situation for most chronically mentally ill patients without wealth or adequate insurance coverage is quite different. They lack families and support networks. They are outcasts in dangerous urban centers rather than members of tightly knit and safe rural communities. There is a paucity of volunteers to offer the daily uncompensated care of the experiment. Publicly supported and charitable programs in most states are far less adequate than in Dane County. Thus, the replication of the success of training in community living would need to bear enormous additional costs, notably for housing and for the crucial supportive care that was provided by volunteers. Recall too that the additional costs of the experiment were modest only in comparison with the well-funded customary care of the control. The additional costs would be much greater and large in the customary situation of neglect.

In a word, the experiment seems to have been a success but community psychological practice has not been. Substitutes for hospitalization cannot exist when they are not funded. While homelessness is in part a problem of the economy, education, and employment, much of it results from neglecting the needs of the chronically mentally ill. The experiment provides credible evidence of the benefits of intensive care; however, it does not address the routine absence of housing, safety, and family support for the many with chronic and serious mental health problems.

The clubhouse model of community care and its predecessor the Fairweather Lodge provide many of the same services for the seriously mentally ill but additional ones as well (Beard et al. 1982). They share the same goals as training in community living that are perhaps best

---

analysis is correct, the problem of providing care for the chronically mentally ill is that much more problematic and the community of mental health practitioners and scholars that much more incapable of addressing their defining problems. Also see, Gomory (unpublished).

summed up as "maximum individual functioning" (Fairweather 1980, p. 89). The clubhouse model has existed since 1948 and by 2012 grew to 335 programs worldwide (Battin et al. 2016); although its literature is infused with the hyperbole of liberation, rehabilitation and empowerment, the clubhouse model is a practical approach to providing safety and greater equality of living conditions for seriously mentally ill patients. It encourages active participation but compensates for incapacity with a range of supportive services, optimally including housing. The clubhouses are managed by members and staff and rely on mutual support among members themselves. Services include case management for food, housing, and income support, transitional employment, supported education, personal dignity ("identity development"), socialization, participation in services including their management and citizenship, and others—in short, services that provide social equality to the extent possible (Jackson 2001). However, all clubhouses do not provide the full range of services.

> Clubhouses offer a range of activities and support, including social and recreational events, and aid in accessing education, employment and housing. These are carried out during what is called a "work-ordered day, usually a period of 8 hours per day, from Monday to Friday, which is intended, first, to develop members" empowerment in reason of their responsibility for maintaining the essential functions of the clubhouse... itself, and, second, to mirror the work patterns of society outside of the clubhouse. Members and staff collaborate in open forums to discuss issues of management and governance... (Battin et al. 2016, p. 305)

While the clubhouse tends to be justified in terms of therapeutic success, it is basically predicated on goals of greater equality and fairness—the presumed right of citizens to common freedoms (unless limited through legal processes) along with a safe and caring environment that nurtures their capacities. In consideration of the limitations and vulnerabilities of many patients with serious, chronic mental disabilities, the priority of comparable circumstances seems a more reasonable concession to reality and more humane than promises of rehabilitation. Yet the concession acknowledges a longtime burden of costs.

Clubhouses strive to help member participate in mainstream employment, education opportunities, community based housing, wellness, or health promotion activities, reduce hospitalizations or involvement with the criminal justice system, and improve social relationships, satisfaction, and quality of life. (McKay et al. 2018, p. 29)

The evidence of the clubhouse's is at best equivocal. The systematic review by Battin et al. (2016) only identified one randomized controlled trial—Yau et al. (2005)—among only 14 studies that met their minimal inclusion criteria. The single randomized study was conducted in China but failed to incorporate either a nontreatment control or a customary care control but rather compared clubhouse participants to a training in community living control. Employment was the only evaluative criteria; 74% of the control group was employed compared with 60% of the clubhouse. The other studies—longitudinal and quasi-experimental comparisons—provided consistently equivocal results relating to quality of life, employment, hospitalizations, symptomatology, and social functioning. In addition to questionably relevant controls, the base of research often could not assure fidelity—many of the studies may not have faithfully implemented clubhouse procedures and services. More important, the adequacy of services was not assured in any of the research. Battin et al. (2016) were only able to conclude that "other more reliable, more comparable studies are needed to reach evidence-based conclusions on the effectiveness of the clubhouse model" (p. 311).

The systematic review by McKay et al. (2018) evaluated the effects of the clubhouse on comprehensive criteria of psychosocial rehabilitation. It concluded that the clubhouse confers substantial benefits of rehabilitation in all areas: employment, psychosocial functioning, rehospitalization, quality of life, and others. However, its base of studies although larger than Battin et al. (2016) was similarly impaired. The authors acknowledge "methodological limitations in some studies" but the same limitations and others often apply to the twelve randomized studies they identified, presumably the most credible: impaired fidelity, lack of blinding, attrition, lack of reliability checks, uncertain accuracy in reporting outcomes, uncertain replicability, partial evaluations of the clubhouse model, neutrality of measures, and others. None of the research reached the sophistication of the evaluations of training in community living. None were definitive tests.

Furthermore, it is not clear that the clubhouses provided adequate living conditions, notably housing, relied on samples that had access to housing or were in other ways unrepresentative of the needy population. The evaluations focused on psychosocial rehabilitation and largely ignored issues of parity and greater equality. Nonetheless, the randomized controlled trials that employed training in community living as the control reported largely equivalent outcomes but not necessarily outcomes that were comparable to the Wisconsin experience or that reflected humane expectations.

Yet, the clubhouse is not suitable for all seriously mentally ill, many of whom avoid clubhouses, refuse to adjust to its demands, or simply find it uncongenial. Thus, clubhouse participants and the sample in the Dane County Wisconsin may be less debilitated and needy than the larger population of the seriously mentally ill who require more intensive care and supports than the clubhouse provides. Still, the clubhouse appears to be an attractive alternative to hospitalization. It is even more apparent that there is an enormous deficit of community supports, in particular, appropriate housing.

The promise of community psychological practice rested on two pillars: successful medication and sufficient caring services. Both have been problematic—uncertain or in short supply—and thus it is not surprising that training in community living has rarely been replicated. Yet under the soothing fiction of community care, many public mental hospitals were closed and public auspices refused to compensate by allocating sufficient funds for effective supportive care. As a result, many chronically mentally ill patients long abandoned by family have had no place to live but the streets, prisons, and deficient congregate homes in which they are drugged into plasticity. Moreover, many of the centers operating under the broad mandate to provide mental health service to the entire community diluted attention to the critically ill with talk therapy to the less troubled. This curious triage decision was compatible with professional preferences more than patient need.

Housing programs for deinstitutionalized mental patients—an obvious need for an obviously deserving people with limited ability to provide from themselves—have never been adequately funded. A federal survey of homelessness in 2017 counted more than 550,000 Americans living in emergency shelters, in transitional housing or in unsheltered arrangements (file:///C:/Users/epstein2/Downloads/HUD%202017%20Continuum%20of%20Care%20Homeless%20Assistance%20Programs%20Homeless%20Populations%20and%20Subpopulations.pdf 6/28/18). It estimated that about 112,000 (20%) of the homeless were severely mentally ill. Other estimates of the incidence of serious mental illness among the homeless range from 20 to 50% (Greenberg and Rosenheck 2010). Additional millions of the American poor at imminent risk of homelessness are living in precarious "doubled up" situations. The rates of addiction to alcohol and drugs among the homeless may approach 50% (Benston 2015).

Unrestricted housing programs—Housing First—paired with supportive care are customarily justified as cost-effective.

> Although positive research outcomes helped build national support for the Housing First model, it also gained legitimacy because researchers and policy makers framed chronic homelessness as an economic problem with a market-based solution [i.e. competition for public funding]. By defining the problem as an affliction among individuals with mental illness who are frequent and expensive users of public services, advocates spread the message that Housing First could address a public eyesore while saving communities money. (Benston 2015)

However, it is apparent that the supply of Housing First programs is insufficient. It is also not at all clear that the programs are routinely successful in permanently housing the homeless or reducing cost. Marginal cost reductions are likely to be far less than the commonly reported reduction in average costs. More to the point, the service outcomes of the programs themselves do not clearly sustain the value of either Housing First or its less well funded and more restrictive alternatives.

A systemic search for the best the evaluations of permanent housing programs for the seriously mentally ill is remarkable for its careful attention to the methodological quality of the base of research. Benston (2015) identified the most credible 14 evaluations of programs that promised permanent housing for the seriously mentally ill. Numerous study pitfalls undercut the credibility of all 14 studies; among other problems, none of the studies contained a no-treatment control; the programs were poorly described; fidelity of implementation was not assured; five lacked randomized controls; attrition was often high, over 30% and unadjusted by intention-to-treat procedures or handled poorly with data imputations of questionable value; data were often collected only from interviews with program participants without checking for accuracy; demonstration effects may have distorted outcomes; there were apparent selection biases in the samples; and most of the studies were not comparable with substantial differences in design and implementation.

There are no definitive studies of housing programs for the seriously mentally ill and the existing research is too disparate to arrive at any general conclusion except one. It is quite apparent that housing programs for the homeless with serious mental illness have failed. Far too few housing units have been funded to satisfy need and far too few services have been provided to the few mentally ill in supported housing to keep them there; retention rates in the programs were variable and none achieved high enough rates to claim prima facie success in housing or the reduction of psychiatric symptoms. The prisons persist as the most common alternative to hospitalization along with dangerous shelters and the common hellish conditions of congregate home care in which resident patients are often drugged into immobility. The streets are often preferable to the risks in shelters or housing. As with many programs for the poor and disabled in wealthy nations, the issue remains ethical rather than economic. Sufficient resources exist to provide a humane standard of living for people who cannot provide for themselves; the nation refuses to make the allocation.

The small-scale programs of community psychological practice have been routine failures, at best providing weak hints that more intensive provisions might be proportionately more effective. Community services to maintain children with serious psychological impairments in their homes have been poorly evaluated but seemingly ineffective

(Shepperd et al. 2009). Shepperd's meta-analysis identified only seven randomized studies that addressed the outcomes of community-based psychiatric services for children as an alternative to hospitalization. At four-month follow-up, there was little improvement among children in the experimental groups. On some measures, controls did better.

One of the seven randomized studies evaluated three different programs intended to maintain children with "serious mental disturbances" in their homes (Evans et al. 1997, 2003). The experiment took place in the Bronx of New York City, among a very poor Hispanic and black population likely to be living in notoriously impoverished neighborhoods with enormous rates of drug abuse and violence; only 12% of the children were "white or other." 279 children were randomized to one of three service models. "All three models were intensive, short-term interventions, lasting approximately 4 to 6 weeks and conducted in homes and other natural settings (e.g., schools)" (Evan et al. 2003). The Homebuilders model provided full-time counselors trained in the program who were assigned only two concurrent cases. The counselors sought to resolve the "immediate crisis, teaching caregivers communication and other relevant skills, helping families improve relationships and linking the child and families to needed services" (ibid., p. 93). The second model augmented the Homebuilder model with "a bilingual, bicultural family advocate who established a parent support group and provided individualized parent support and advocacy, $100 in discretionary money, and respite care for emergencies" (ibid., p. 93). The third model, Crisis Case Management "was a less labor intensive intervention that [unlike the other two interventions] did not offer clinical treatment services in the home" (ibid., p. 93). Crisis Case Management served as a treatment as usual control. Nontreatment controls were not employed. Evaluative data were collected before treatment, at the end of treatment and six months later.

There were hardly any systematic, statistically significant differences among the three groups. Approximately 80% of the children in each group were maintained in families without episodes of hospitalization. The children in all the models demonstrated few substantial improvements over time. Only occasional improvements reached statistical significance and they were of questionable clinical importance.

The few significant differences usually occurred between the customary care group and the two Homebuilders interventions. However, neither the Homebuilders model nor its enhanced version conferred much benefit over customary care; in fact, customary care was occasionally superior (e.g., internalizing scores). Apparently, enhanced clinical interventions and greater cultural sensitivity added little to customary care. Nevertheless, without a nontreatment comparison it is impossible to attribute any of the changes, small and episodic as they are, to the interventions rather than to natural remission and the seasonality of mental problems.

A number of problems impair the research itself. There were important differences among the randomized groups that may have influenced the outcomes: educational attainment, temper tantrums, substance abuse, "functional impairments," and dangerousness. It is doubtful that blinding was maintained. Post-discharge attrition reached thirty-three percent and missing data were provided through statistical imputation and thus the authors' contention that little if any deterioration effects took place at follow-up is suspect. If anything at all, the research suggests that intensive short-term crisis intervention may have little effect on serious childhood mental and emotional impairments. Homebuilders and similar temporary family preservation efforts routinely fail and not least because of the absence or inadequacy of superficial supports. Contrary to Staudt and Drake (2002), the key to success may depend on attention to the material roots of family distress rather than on the choice of clinical orientation. Sustained, intense improvements in the material conditions of poorer people's lives may show proportionate improvements in the behavior of their children. Yet the weakness of the clinical research itself remains an impediment to identifying truly effective programs.

Mentoring is a recurring theme in community psychological practice especially for troubled youths and those at risk of developing problems. The effulgent glow of an upstanding member of the community shining on the needy youth or the nascent miscreant is intended to have restorative, transformative, and blossoming effects like springtime sun on cherry trees. In an analysis of a nonexperimental national longitudinal study, Timpe and Lunkenheimer (2015) estimate that "total lifetime benefits to having a male *natural* mentor was approximately $190,000 for all fatherless youth and $458,000 for African American fatherless youth" (p. 12, emphasis added). However, evaluations of the Big Brothers Big Sisters do not sustain the positive value of mentoring programs and probably because they do not provide *natural* mentors who replicate the relationships of caring parents to children in need.

Big Brothers Big Sisters (BBBS) is the prototype of mentoring programs, pairing youths from single-parent households with adult role models. The experimental design randomized youths between the ages of 10 and 16 to BBBS services ("the treatment group") or to a waitlist control in eight of the largest of BBBS's more than 500 local agencies—"only agencies with relatively large caseloads and waiting lists were considered" (ibid., p. 406). A variety of measures were taken before randomization and eighteen months afterward. All the outcome data were drawn from interviews with the children and their parents; additional descriptive information was provided by case managers.

> The volunteer and youth meet two to four times per month for at least one year, with a typical meeting lasting three to four hours. BBBS is not a program targeted at ameliorating specific problems, but rather at providing a youth with an adult friend. The friendship forged with a youth by the Big Brother of Big Sister creates the framework through which the mentor can support and aid the youth. (ibid., p. 405)

In addition, BBBS carefully screened both the volunteer mentors and the youths to assure that both desired the relationship and that the mentors did not pose any risk or would be incapable of developing the appropriate relationships. Presumably too, the youths were screened to weed out those with problems that would obviate a mentoring relationship with nonprofessional volunteers. The relationships were closely monitored. During the experiment, the mentors actually spent considerably more time with the youths than the prescribed minimum: 70% met at least three times per month; 45% met at least once per week; meetings lasted on average 3.6 hours.

The authors' general conclusions are provided against a backdrop of skepticism.

The past decade has seen widespread enthusiasm for mentoring as a way to address the needs and problems of youths but no firm evidence that mentoring programs produce results. In this article we provide solid evidence that BBBS has many positive and socially important effects on the lives of its young participants. (ibid., p. 403)

The research goes on the detail the statistically significant benefits for the BBBS treatment group: less use of alcohol and illegal drugs, a bit lower incidence of hitting, slightly better grades, slightly better family relations, and fewer skipped times that a day of school was skipped. It also details many outcomes that did not differ between the two groups: weekly hours spent in cultural activities, attendance at cultural events, global self-worth, social acceptance, self-confidence, parental communication, parental anger, and alienation.

However, the actual positive outcomes were typically small and exaggerated by the authors while serious design problems undercut the applicability and credibility of the findings. The authors report that the treatment group youths were "45.8% less likely to start using illegal drugs…." The actual incidence of drug use in the control group was only about 11% creating a net benefit of only about 5%. It is true that "for every 100 minority boys [in the control group] who start using illegal drugs, only 33 similar minority boys who have a Big Brother will start using drugs" (ibid., p. 413). But very few in the control group experimented with illegal drugs or alcohol and the benefit in absolute numbers given the size of the samples was less than 20. Moreover, to put the comparison in these terms falsely suggests that the treatment sample is comparable to the general population of minority boys between 10 and 16. The sly claim of comparability with problem youth crosses the line of research probity by proposing that this largely recreational program of pleasant sociability has an important relationship to handling serious youth problems of alienation and addiction.

The sample itself is unlikely to be representative of troubled youth. First, 109 of the 554 (22%) treatment group youths were unable to be matched. Presumably these were the most difficult and troubled youths whose absence in treatment sample of matched youths created a sample of the relatively untroubled and predisposes the research to positive outcomes. Even so, the few small positive outcomes were often significant only at the convenient level of 0.1.[2]

In addition, the outcomes were judged by the matched youths and their parents who after voluntarily spending considerable time with presumably agreeable and informed mentors may well have exaggerated their reports in gratitude for the relationships. The research reports no objective and independent assessment of the youths' needs. In addition, BBBS mentoring was sought out by parents and youths desiring the service. These attentive parents are not typical of the troubled parents of troubled youth. Thus, a motivated group of questionably needy youths with an attentive parent received relatively intensive mentoring services for 18 months from qualified adults that resulted in few and questionable positive outcomes.

Mentoring is a soothing fiction akin to religious conversion that stresses personal responsibility, low costs, and social compatibility but underplays the pernicious effects of inequality. With a few hours of volunteer mentoring wayward youths and those at forks in the road of maturity are given the opportunity of personalized encouragement to follow the one true path of cultural obedience. Mentoring fails as treatment but succeeds as myth.

BBBS was evaluated by Grossman and Tierney (1998) who were employed by Public/Private Ventures, a contract research operation that was a component of the Foundation Center before it disbanded in 2012. Public/Private Ventures was typically contracted by social services in the private sector and by charitable foundations to evaluate favored programs. The great Renaissance artists sacrificed truth for beauty in the portraits of their patrons. Contract researchers sacrifice truth for employment in pleasing their clients. Beauty better justifies the concession.

It could be argued that the BBBS experiment failed to test the effects of intensive mentoring on troubled youth. However, other evaluations of mentoring programs and similar superficial programs of peer support

---

[2]The data in the study's tables often conflict with the data in write-ups, a point of sloppiness or deceit that raises additional questions about the credibility of the research.

reinforce conclusions of routine ineffectiveness (Lipman et al. 2018; Larose et al. 2018; Heller et al. 1991).

Similar problems undercut the most credible evaluations of community psychological practice but reinforce the conclusion that superficial responses to serious deprivations are anodynes, at best, for systemic pain. The meta-analysis by Turner et al. (2018) report small benefits for psychotic patients of social skills training compared with a variety of comparison groups. Much of the base of research was compromised and at risk of bias. Social skills training did not show any superiority at six-month follow-up. Social skills training replicates the experience of supported living, education, and employment programs. As isolated efforts, they confer little advantage over controls but they are valuable in support of more thoroughgoing interventions such as clubhouses and community skills training programs.

Knight and Alarie (2017) conducted a retrospective review of patient charts to conclude that day treatment for moderately depressed geriatric patients was valuable. There was no control group. The outcome of a meta-analysis of two studies concluded that cognitive behavioral therapy fails to reduced auditory hallucinations in patients with chronic schizophrenia (Kennedy and Xyrichis 2017). However, the patients were not in crisis but in remission and the authors acknowledge that they had "little data to reliably assess how distressed participants actually were" (ibid., p. 131). Apparently, the therapist's multicultural competence has little effect on therapeutic outcomes (Tao et al. 2015); moreover, the base of research in this meta-analysis was impaired by publication biases, data reliability, and other defects.

Stewart et al.'s (2017) retrospective case study of a "community mental health initiative on outcomes for offenders with a serious mental disorder" did not employ randomized control groups and relied on administrative data. Differences between groups were small but statistically significant; however, without randomization it is impossible to attribute the outcomes to the intervention rather than to attributes of the samples.

Barton's (1999) systematic review concludes that "the essential direct service elements of psychosocial rehabilitation – skills training, family education, and vocational services – are supported by substantial empirical evidence of improved clinical and economic outcomes" (ibid., p. 532). As in many other summary reviews, Barton's base of research is seriously impaired. Smith et al. (1996) lacked a comparison group and studied a screened amenable sample. Marder et al. (1996) were demonstrated mixed results for social skills training in comparison with group therapy for psychotic patients; however, the patients were already stabilized in community settings and the advantages of skills training were only apparent when combined with drug treatment. The clinical and practical value of the learned skills is not demonstrated in Eckman et al. (1992). Moller and Murphy (1997) claim that their intervention—The Three R's Rehabilitation Program—lower rehospitalization rates for seriously mentally ill patients and saved an immense amount of money. The controls were not randomly assigned from the same group of patients. Treated patients were self-referred and apparently highly motivated. The comparison group was not similarly motivated. Moreover, it was not apparent whether the researchers decided on rehospitalization. Additionally, the program provided an intensity of services to the patients in the community but most importantly, the patients seemed to have considerable voluntary supports. Similar to other summaries of the outcome literature in community psychological practice, Barton (1999) fails to rigorously evaluate the base of research in the review, accepting conveniently weak research as definitive. If anything at all, the Barton review suggests marginal and mixed benefits for psychosocial inventions but contingent on the circumstances of coincidental support.

Similar problems deeply undercut other reviews of community psychological practice and their base of studies: as examples, Repper and Carter (2011) on peer support; Bryan and Arkowitz (2015) on peer administered psychosocial interventions; Pistrang et al. (2008) on mutual help groups; and Painter (2012) on evidence-based practices in community mental health. There are few if any definitive tests of practice and meager recognition of the problem.

In short, the small, poorly funded programs in community psychological practice seem largely ineffective, often trivial and poorly researched. Indeed, aside from the carefully documented comprehensive community programs for chronic psychiatric patients such as training in community living, the literature seems more protective of professional efforts than true to the obligations of scientific research. Some of the research can be reinterpreted to suggest that supportive efforts might become helpful if adequately funded for a sufficient amount of time in combination with comprehensive programs that seek greater equality for the seriously mentally ill. However, even this conclusion is tentative without randomized controlled comparisons followed over time and evaluated by neutral judges applying reliable measures. However, the field is professionally insular resisting independent evaluation and scrutiny (e.g., Cook and Shaddish 1982).

Liberation, empowerment, political intervention, community organization, and even efforts at mass mobilization infuse the literature of community psychological practice with a bouquet of hope, dedication, and farsighted altruism. A large portion of the field seems to assume that there is great latent support for the wisdom and humanity of providing a nurturing environment for the chronically mentally ill. Thus, the principal task of community psychological practice is to demonstrate the effectiveness and cost/efficiency of its programs. This literature has achieved by debasing the logic of scientific proof. However, the demand for "transformative change" that persists particularly in the textbooks and literature of community psychology is not paired with strategies to achieve it. The typical transformation concerns the patient, the therapist, the agency, and the immediate service community. In spite of an avowed sensitivity to the ecological perspective, community mental health and community psychological practice avoid confronting the encrusted meanness of the society itself. There are successful interventions to address the needs of the seriously debilitated mental patient notably through supportive housing and allied community services. They are not funded, a decision reached democratically throughout the world's most open nation. The failure to provide appropriate care is obvious on the streets, in the jails, and in the recurrent scandals of congregate homes that serve as alternatives to mental hospitals.

Indeed, community action for social change, that is, planned efforts to effect systemic changes typically fail and notably because the intended beneficiaries are late on the long line queueing for public sympathy.[3] The empowerment of the powerless has not been realized in an effective planned practice—it remains a ceremony of opposition (Epstein 2013). The pious volubility and sloganeering of community psychology are perhaps a tip-off that it is more soothing fiction than service. Another science of everything—the "embodied social ecological model" (Tebes 2016)—rivals in obliviousness social work's conceit that it treats the whole individual. They are the faux wisdom that obscures ineffective practice and its accommodations with society as it is.

There are voices that recognize the problems of community psychological practice. Hartmann et al. (2018) argue that

> Community psychology abandoned the clinic and disengaged from movements for community mental health to escape clinical convention and pursue growing aspirations as an independent field of context-oriented, community-engaged, and values-driven research and action. In doing so, however, community psychology positioned itself on the sidelines of influential contemporary movements that promote potentially harmful, reductionist biomedical narratives in mental health. We advocate for a return to the clinic – the seat of institutional power in mental health – using critical clinic-based inquiry to open sites for clinical-community dialogue…" (p. 62)

The point of their clinical-community dialogue was to "investigate transformative change locally and nationally" (ibid.). Thus, the failure

---

[3]Nelson et al.'s (2014) *Community Psychology and Community Mental Health: Towards Transformative Change* is a fine example of the genre. To demonstrate the success of mass mobilization, Levine and Perkins (1997) point to school desegregation but fail to acknowledge the resegregation of the public school system, the rise of public funding for private education, and increasingly homogeneous living patterns. Dalton et al. (2001) are confident community organization and empowerment are successful and ignore the most glaring obstacle to their success: Poor neighborhoods and communities—the objects of community organization and empowerment efforts—lack the resources or political strength to address their problems. Community organization as outreach—agricultural extension workers, public health nurses—has demonstrated some success. However, if the goal is political and social change through mass mobilization, it has been a consistent failure in the United States and internationally. Kagan et al. (2011) build an argument for "critical" community psychology—the authors' injunction to "Think!"—that attributes to weak research and professional agency the glow of scientific coherence while assuming that political decision making was grounded in the rational.

to change social attitudes as advocates and organizers—an accurate assessment of the field—was to be redressed by the reengagement and control of clinical practice. For one, it is unlikely that public funding agencies would put community practice in the hands of rebels. For another, even if they gained control, the record of insurrections in the United States suggests that they are unlikely to succeed.

In contrast, Becker (2015), a psychiatrist, is quite clear about the "nowhere" of contemporary community psychological practice.

> Motivated by economics, states moved increasing numbers of patients from hospitals into communities that were unprepared to care for them. The developing community psychiatry programs struggled to keep patients from becoming homeless and rehospitalized. Before harmful federal funding shortfalls for the new community programs could be corrected, Reagan's New Federalism terminated social-community psychiatry funding.... The survival of community-based services, research, and training became tenuous. Soon homelessness and arrest and incarceration replaced hospitalizations and community services.... Without federally funded community and social psychiatry activities, drugs became the most economical, medically indicated, and humane responses to serious mental illnesses. (ibid., p. 1098)

The shortfalls of community care are embedded in the inadequacy of public funding, a reflection of popular American priorities.

> Society has subjected psychiatry's patients to a sad social experiment that no Ethical Review Committee would allow medical investigators to pursue. These unacceptable experimental options – use of jails, medical errors, false claims for therapies, denials of health care access, and demoralizing conditions for the profession and its patients – are prevalent conditions today. Society chose and will choose the conditions affecting psychiatry. (ibid., p. 1099)

These choices have not yielded to empowerment practice, liberation strategies, or other professional rebellions against enduring American preferences. While biomedical interventions, i.e., psychoactive drugs, have been an understandable fallback position in the absence of services, they come along with many of their own deficits, not least, an enormous rate of failure along with unpleasant and harmful side effects.

Research concerning the effectiveness of psychopharmacology for serious mental conditions provides grounds for considerable skepticism. The eminent Archives of General Psychiatry in 2006 published a study by Lieber (2006) that tested the effectiveness of two generations of anti-psychotic drugs to treat schizophrenia. They reported only one substantial finding: 74% of 1432 patients who received at least one dose "discontinued the study medication before 18 months" (p. 1209). The intention-to-treat logic, a hallmark of scientific clinical research, interprets attrition failure. Against the backdrop of enormous attrition "indicating substantial limitations in the effectiveness of the drugs," the small differential rates of effectiveness among the drugs are clinically meaningless (p. 17).

In a two-part essay reviewing prominent books that discuss the state of biomedical psychiatry, Marcia Angell, a former editor of the New England Journal of Medicine, concludes that pills for the treatment of mental and emotional problems are routinely ineffective and often dangerous. The range of pills for depression are about as effective as placebos, that is, not effective at all. Angell (2011b) also finds the argument plausible that psychotropic drugs to handle schizophrenia and other serious mental conditions have actually increased their seriousness without effectively treating them.

> Antipsychotics cause side effects that resemble Parkinson's disease, because of the depletion of dopamine (which is also depleted in Parkinson's disease). As side effects emerge, they are often treated by other drugs, and many patients end up on a cocktail of psychoactive drugs prescribed for a cocktail of diagnoses. The episodes of mania caused by antidepressants may lead to a new diagnosis of "bipolar disorder" and treatment with a "mood stabilizer," such as Depakote (an anticonvulsant) plus one of the newer antipsychotic drugs. And so on. (Angell 2011a, p. 22)

Yet despite routine ineffectiveness and consistent harms, psychotropic medications are immensely popular. Angell explains this curiosity by lax federal oversight, the undue influence of the pharmaceutical industry and "the way psychiatry is now practiced – the frenzy of diagnosis, the overuse of drugs with sometimes devastating side effects, and widespread conflicts of interests" (Angell 2011b, p. 22). However, these three factors would not prevail without popular support. However, the use of psychiatric drugs that presumably facilitate participation in care became prevalent as the sole alternatives to unavailable community services (Becker and Greig 2010). The American people have refused to allocate sufficient funding for the care of seriously impaired citizens and notably those who must rely on public subsidies. The pills are the soothing fictions of treatment and social concern.[4]

Community psychological practice has not distinguished itself with program success despite evidence that some of its programs if better funded and expanded might meet some of its goals. It stumbles on a lack of resources for material care for the chronic mental health patient. Hundreds of thousands of the mentally ill live on the streets and in shelters. Many others become psychologically disabled and at risk of serious mental and physical disability by the absence of reliable housing, poor living conditions, dangerous streets, failing schools, and other persistent inequalities of American society. Community psychological practice is a soothing fiction more than a reality.

It is clear that we now do know how to tackle many of the problems faced by those who are mentally ill and homeless.... Now, we fail because we

---

[4]Much of the research concerning the effectiveness of psychopharmacology is ambiguous and misleading. As Angell noted, the Federal Drug Administration must certify a medication as safe and effective before it can be sold. However, certification requires only two demonstrations of effectiveness among what could be a much larger number of randomized controlled trials. Not surprisingly, positive findings are widely publicized; negative findings are kept in file drawers. Rush et al. (2006) offer an example of the common gaming of research in psychiatry—the complicity of government, industry, and professional practice sustained by popular belief. The experiment explores whether switching antidepressants is effective after the first drug fails. Patients with a nonpsychotic major depressive disorder who failed to respond to Citalopram were randomized to one of four groups to receive one of four different antidepressant medications. Remission rates were between 18 and 25% and the authors declare success. However, the research did not include a placebo control and thus the outcomes can be attributed to natural remission, in this case, the seasonality of depression. There was no credible finding that the remission was due to the new drugs. The authors of the study list extensive commercial ties to the pharmaceutical industry. The research was published in the New England Journal of Medicine.

won't, not because we can't, address these issues. (Goldfinger 2006 in Gillig and McQuistion, p. 166)

Community psychological practice and the social clinic are not situations of well-meaning people making unavoidable mistakes but rather fulfillments of the persistent social motives to stint on resources for needy populations, in this case for the seriously mentally ill but more generally for poorer citizens and those in need. They substitute for programs such as training in community living, the clubhouses, and others that hold promise for effective care although at considerable cost. As a substitute for effective care, the social clinic has been sanctioned by use and broad consent. As homelessness increased and became obvious, many made the assumption that the American public would be horrified to witness the mentally impaired, children, and the infirm living rough. Instead, the abandoned have been blithely accepted as kinetic street sculptures.

A Note on Rehabilitation in Corrections

A scientific discipline builds to definitive tests of theory, in this case, applications of theory to corrections and more broadly the objective value of the social clinic to rehabilitation of offenders. Presumably but only this, the program's success indicates the theory's value. Departures from decisive tests measure the distance of a field from true science. Definitive tests of rehabilitation programs must include representative samples, randomization into control and experimental groups including placebos when appropriate, as well as reliable and valid measures along with protections against bias, notably researcher bias. The tests need to be replicated and the researchers should be neutral. There are no definitive tests of rehabilitation services in the field of corrections.

The most consistent finding in the corrections literature is that incarceration and deterrence programs such as Scared Straight and boot camps are associated with increased offenses (recidivism) while supervision (probation and parole) has only very small effects on recidivism (Lipsey and Cullen 2007 and many others). For decades, even centuries, the hope has been to find alternative approaches to corrections that reduce rates of reoffense. The rehabilitation of offenders through psychological interventions—the social clinic approach to deviance—has become popular for a few reasons. It is socially efficient—less expensive than prison and it conforms to contemporary styles of social service in its emphasis on personal responsibility and choice. Enhancing their social efficiency, psychological approaches to rehabilitation are reportedly effective, at times enormously so. Successful rehabilitation through psychological interventions may also reduce the necessity of considering more complex and expensive approaches that entail the provision of social supports and alternative environments that reduce inequality. However, without credible evidence of effectiveness rehabilitation becomes a soothing fiction, a diversion from more profound, disruptive, and costly alternatives.

Rehabilitation of criminal behavior through psychological interventions has been developed and promoted through the social sciences, notably criminal justice, and clinical psychology.[5] It conforms closely with the social assumptions of the American ethos including its preference for the rational style. The process of science dictates that the causes of criminality are researched and defined, presumably through rigorous scientific analysis; interventions are designed to interfere with those causes; outcomes are evaluated and perhaps replicated (La Bonta and Andrews 2015 is a prime example).

The process of psychologizing criminal behavior assumes that attitude change precedes behavior change. Thus, interventions are designed through one form of behavioral learning theory or another—customarily a process combining rational induction with reinforcement—to reward

---

[5]The literature concerning the effectiveness of clinical rehabilitation programs in reducing criminal recidivism is too vast be summarized in a few pages. It deserves a multi-volume treatment. The present effort to characterize the credibility of the research attempts a few tentative conclusions concerning the credibility of the evidence and its broader implications for social policy. As in previous chapters, this discussion relies on the best meta-analyses and the most credible primary research. The current process is necessarily less intense than previous discussions and fewer examples are provided. Still, a curious challenge to the research is not easily dispelled. The consistently but by no means universally reported positive effects on recidivism may be better explained by nonclinical factors associated with treatment than by treatment itself.

prosocial choices and discourage the continuation of antisocial behavior. In addition to keeping people out of prison, a humane achievement in itself, the motives to discover and institute successful programs of rehabilitation are considerable. Innovators of successful social programs that save money and conform with institutionalized values gain prestige and material awards. They also become emblems of American virtue and evidence of its exceptionalism.

The field's conclusions of effectiveness are derived from meta-analyses of the primary evaluations of individual programs and systematic reviews of the meta-analyses themselves. Even when they fail to find credible benefits for the applications of the social clinic to corrections they stay loyal to the possibility of success, they do not stretch their speculations to consider the usefulness of broader social reforms.

In an immensely influential meta-analysis, Andrews et al. (1990) sustained their risk-need-responsivity model of rehabilitation. The largely psychotherapeutic model targets "changing antisocial attitudes, feelings, and peer associations; promoting familial affection in combination with enhanced parental monitoring and supervision; promoting identification with anticriminal role models; increasing self-control and self-management skills; replacing the skills of lying, stealing and aggression with other more prosocial skills, reducing chemical dependencies..." among others. In short, the model seeks to modify "contingencies within the home, school, and work by way of an increased density of reward for noncriminal activity..." (p. 375). The interventions themselves include "modeling, graduated practice, rehearsal, role playing, reinforcement, resource provision, and detailed verbal guidance and explanations (making suggestions, giving reasons, cognitive restructuring)" (ibid.).

The Andrews et al.'s (1990) findings sustained the effectiveness of their model that Lipsey and Cullen interpreted as a 60% reduction in recidivism. Appropriate services were effective in all settings—incarceration, community, and supervision. As of June 2018, Andrews et al. were cited 844 times. They concluded that appropriate services—targeting the needs of higher risk cases with relevant services—had a strong effect on reducing recidivism among adults and juveniles. Thus, Andrews et al. concluded that "there is reasonably solid clinical and research basis for the political reaffirmation of rehabilitation" (ibid., p. 384). As an extension, the disruptions of deep social reform to prevent criminality were proportionately less important.

Lipsey and Cullen's (2007) often-cited systematic review of correctional meta-analyses sustained Andrews et al. with additional research although more narrowly. Parole and probation (supervision) were associated with slightly reduced recidivism; intermediate sanctions with mixed but often notable increases in recidivism; and confinement with consistently higher recidivism. Rehabilitation treatment itself—usually clinical-type intervention—was associated with a modest 18% mean reduction in recidivism. In considering specific treatment types, the heart of their analysis, they reported an immense variation. However, social clinic interventions, usually employing a form of psychotherapy along with other unspecified conditions, were often associated with dramatic decreases in recidivism between 45 and 60%. Not surprisingly, positive effects were consistently much larger for juveniles than adults.

Lipsey and Cullen (2007) pointed to the immense variation, a "substantial heterogeneity" (p. 307), among the meta-analyses and even more among the much larger number of primary studies they summarized. Heterogeneity poses a problem for the logic of meta-analysis questioning the propriety of combining individual studies that differ in critical elements rather than imposing the enormous burden of handling them separately. In any event, addressing rehabilitation

> Within any broad sample of studies, one finds many near-zero and even negative effect sizes at one end of the effect size distribution, whereas the other end extends to impressively large effects representing reductions in recidivism of 50% and higher.... Much of it is related to substantive characteristics of the treatments and the offender samples to which they are applied. The most important challenge for contemporary rehabilitation research is to identify the factors that most influence the likelihood of positive treatment effects. (ibid., p. 306)

Thus, the research has still not identified the essence of treatment, whether it was actually based on psychotherapy or other, coincidental non-psychological elements. Moreover, their calculations assumed an average recidivism rate of 50% in the control groups. The assumption was employed to "make the magnitude of the recidivism rate more interpretable" (p. 300) but may magnify the importance of reported gains if in fact the actual control group recidivism was lower than 50%. Rather than only estimating the percentage change in recidivism compared against an assumed and apparently capricious standard of 50%, reporting the actual recidivism rates in treated and control groups would better describe the gains or losses of treatment especially in light of generally modest effect sizes. Additionally, measurements such as the phi statistic—the common statistic of the summaries, basically a two by two table—truncate data.

Employing similar methods, other systematic reviews of meta-analyses, and other large reviews of primary data at times sustained the effectiveness of clinical rehabilitation of offenders, sometimes did not, and sometimes were equivocal. Weisburd et al. (2017) found substantial positive effects for a range of interventions including rehabilitation programs that employ cognitive behavioral therapy. The meta-analysis by Morgan et al. (2012), largely concerning the noncriminal effects of psychiatric care, identified three studies that reported on changes in recidivism, only one of which was successful, two reported higher recidivism in the treated groups. The meta-analysis by Grietens et al. (2003) concluded that residential treatment for juvenile offenders reduced recidivism only modestly, by 9%. Wilson's (2014) meta-analysis assessing effects of clinical interventions on recidivism for those with antisocial personality disorder was not supportive of treatment; all three of the randomized controlled trials failed to report statistically significant differences in outcomes between treated and untreated groups.

The meta-analysis by Whitehead and Lab (90) renewed the controversial proposition that juvenile correctional treatment is routinely ineffective. They claimed that even their "lenient" standard for effective treatment "fails to support claims of efficacy by most interventions" (p. 291). It is not at all clear that the responses to the Whitehead and Lab meta-analysis by Lipsey and Cullen (2007) among others settled the issue or retrieved the value of rehabilitation (Lab and Whitehead 1990).[6]

---

[6]For a more detailed discussion of the controversy, see Epstein (1993).

A number of considerations impair the credibility of the summary reviews. They typically accept with few reservations the findings of their base of individual research studies thus acknowledging the absence of definitive tests. Otherwise, the reviews would only discuss evidence that is scientifically credible. Thus, the summaries draw useful, not dispositive, inferences from impaired research. In this way, they state only a consensus reached on the basis of partial, conflicting and often incommensurate evidence rather than a credible scientific conclusion. At best they should be tentative and focused on serious pitfalls in the research.

Additional design and measurement problems in the primary base of research and the reviews impede a clear assessment of clinical treatment for criminal behavior, that is, the effectiveness of rehabilitation for offenders. The studies often lack randomized controls or any controls at all. This is acknowledged in the summaries. However, the comparisons of high quality and lower quality studies rely only on randomization as the criterion of quality ignoring many other important design protections against faulty conclusions. Samples are not commensurate across studies. Thus, lumping together studies of residential community treatment as one example obscures enormous differences in what is provided by the different programs. Moreover, outcomes of studies of serious offenses are often conflated with studies of minor offenses.

The comparability of treatment is not assured but inappropriately assumed in many of the comparisons. Evaluative standards of success seem both capricious and perhaps self-serving. Moreover, the simplistic categorization of types of treatments may create false outcomes. Research is rarely replicated and initial reports of success may be due to demonstration effects that cannot be transferred, as one example, Cullen et al.'s (2018) "bad news" that the effects of Project Hope were not repeated. Furthermore, reported results are often trivial (e.g., Alexander and Parsons 1973).

There is a recurring disingenuousness in reports of rehabilitation programs. The Community Treatment Program, conducted by the California Youth Authority from 1961 until 1974, was an experiment in diversion from prison. It was intended initially to test whether intensive community treatment, often containing psychotherapies of one sort or another, would lower recidivism. The second phase of the experiment tested whether short stays in residential care for the more resistant youths would lower recidivism. Youths were randomized to the experiment or to the customary services of the California Youth Authority. The outcomes of the first phase showed small gains for community care. Yet Palmer (1974) claimed that during the second phase of the experiment delinquent behaviors of the more troublesome youths were substantially reduced through residential care.

However, numerous deficiencies in the research undercut the findings. The actual receipt of services was not measured well and control subjects may have received many of the same services as experimental subjects. By way of minimizing recidivism, home detention was often substituted for actually revoking probation. Relying on direct project information rather than the published research reports of the California Youth Authority, Lerman (1975, 1984), the program's principal critic, concluded that the Community Treatment Program acted as detention program far more than as a treatment program. In short, the experimental youths, detained in community substitutes for prison, were not free to commit crimes. Thus changes in recidivism measured only changes in the way that the delinquent youth were handled by the program rather than changes in actual criminal acts.

The same problem of reinstituting highly restrictive conditions in community and residential programs for juvenile offenders may often account for their lower reported recidivism. This is false support for diversion strategies. The systematic reviews and much of the primary research itself fail to consider this problem: Call it prison or call it community care, children under lock and key are unlikely to commit crimes.

Even recidivism as a measure of outcomes seems problematic not least because officially documented offenses undercount the true amount of crime and different jurisdictions may report and handle crimes differently (Elliott and Voss 1968). Coding errors may occur in transferring recidivism data from public records—Kirigin et al. (1982) documented a 20% error rate in this regard. Definitions of recidivism, that is what the different studies measure as recidivism, change from study to study—arrests, adjudications, serious crimes, all crimes, the severity of sentences, and deviant but not criminal behaviors (Gendreau and Leipciger 1978; Gendreau 1980; Griswold 1978; Andersen and Skardhamar 2017). The periods over which it is measured—by the end of treatment, six months after, one year afterward or many years afterward—vary from study to study while some research relies on self-reports to document offenses. Thus, the choice of recidivism measures may pose serious challenges to the credibility and utility of rehabilitation research.

Nonetheless, recidivism in the correctional literature in contrast with most of social clinical research is probably a more reliable and objective measure of outcomes unless there is frank bias in data collection—processes to identify recidivism that differ between treated groups and comparisons. Even more problematic, neither the summaries nor the primary research discuss at appropriate length the measures of recidivism they employ. Few studies even bother with reliability checks.

Yet in spite of numerous design flaws that impugn the credibility of the research, the huge number of studies employing a somewhat reliable measure of outcome (recidivism) suggests that some programs may in fact be valuable, particularly for juveniles. However, their success may have less to do with the psychological elements in correctional treatment and more to do with the degree to which the clinical elements are associated with important material supports, long-term surrogates for failed social institutions, notably the family and community and program characteristics such as the mix of juveniles in residential care. Success that is often attributed to psychological treatments, in particular, cognitive behavioral therapy, in fact, may be due to factors other than psychotherapy. The currently popular risk-need-responsivity model of treatment at the heart of clinical approaches to rehabilitation may itself depend on the provision of long-term supportive care designed as surrogates for the absence of common social institutions—families, communities, and appropriate peer groups. Furthermore, the apparent superiority of rehabilitation programs may be due more to the harms of imprisonment than the actual benefits of community treatment. Until rehabilitation programs are compared with a nontreatment control (perhaps, and with some modification, release with warning as a sentence or the decision not to place out of the home or to supervise), the value of ostensible benefits will remain unclear.

Much of the primary literature, some reporting success and some at least partial failure, begin to suggest the necessity of sustained care rather than short-term clinical interventions. For one, Kirigin et al. (1982) tested the teaching-family treatment approach that defines many group homes for juvenile offenders as well as others such as Boys Town. In a nonrandom design, 13 teaching-family homes were compared with nine "conventional residential programs in Kansas" (p. 3). Youths in the teaching-family group homes committed statistically fewer crimes during their stay in the program than youths in comparison with programs. However, the benefits of lower rates of criminal activity during teaching-family treatment were not sustained during the year after leaving the program. The authors' initial observation about juvenile corrections is affirmed by their own experiment: "Juvenile crime is a serious problem for which no treatment approach has been found to be reliably effective" (Kirigin et al. 1982, p. 1).

Nevertheless, the reported reduction of criminal activity along with other social and personal improvements while residing in a kind, supportive, emotionally, and materially enriched environment suggests that more than one year is required—the value of long-term residential care rather than short-term residential treatment. In fact, the clinical component may only be incidental to provisions that copy the critical substance of common social institutions, notably the family. That is, good foster parenting may be enriched by clinical advice but not dependent on its simplistic truisms. It may not have been the conditions of behavioral therapy that lowered criminal activity during residence but the nonclinical conditions of decent care. Without the surrogate provisions, the clinical component would most likely have failed. The point is that the research did not test the value of the social clinic. Yet this dose effect is difficult to achieve without considerable expense. Moreover, the superiority of the teaching-family group homes over the comparison group homes may have been due at least in part to more successfully reinstituting the conditions of detention in the manner of California's Community Treatment Program.

Chamberlain and Reid (1998) sustain the idea that long-term replication of decent families rather than clinic intervention is necessary to reduce juvenile recidivism. Adolescent boys with histories of chronic and serious crime were randomized to either multidimensional treatment foster care or to traditional community care. One year after the end of placement, the foster care youths committed substantially fewer crimes than the youths in customary group care. The authors conclude that "the lynchpin in the [foster care] placement is not a therapist or social skills trainer but the foster parent" (p. 631). Thus, the replication of high-quality social institutions goes further than clinical interventions by themselves to reduce crime. Yet the findings are only suggestive since the conditions of traditional community care may have been quite abusive as 64% of their youths were referred to detention or ran away during residence and only 36% completed their programs (compared with 31 and 73%, respectively, in the foster care program). Second, quality foster parents are very rare and a sufficient number of "lynchpins" may not be available to keep the axles of diversion programs on track. In any event, the costs of high-quality foster care are enormous while the costs of the structural changes to achieve greater social equality are an order of magnitude greater.

Both Kirigin et al. (1982) and Chamberlain and Reid (1998) hint at the same reinterpretation of their conclusions, the dose effect of decency: Long-term provision of safe and supportive environments of care reduce recidivism and are probably necessary for the successful socialization and resocialization of people. Thus, the basic assumption of clinical treatment that attitude change precedes behavioral may be inaccurate. Attitudes may be accommodations to new situations that induce behavior change. Thus, situational changes may need to be created first if behavioral changes—reduced recidivism—is to ensue. However, residential programs promising new situations may be funded inadequately to create the conditions necessary to change behavior and those that seem adequate may not be provided for an adequate period of time. The problem remains one of a willingness to fund and a willingness to find out what is effective, neither of which exists.

Conclusion

Community psychological practice and rehabilitation in corrections have failed to achieve their goals for two principal reasons. The wrong interventions are pursued and the American public is unwilling to allocate appropriate resources. Community psychological practice and rehabilitation in corrections are pursuing notions of inexpensive cure, that effective outcomes can be achieved cheaply and without disrupting current social arrangements. They define their distinctive problems as individual deviations largely amenable to limited professional interventions—in one case pills and superficial programs such as skills training and in the other as largely psychotherapy of one sort or another. Both are stolidly blind to the proposition that long-term changes in living conditions are necessary to resocialize and protect needy people—in particular, basic comparability of living conditions, starting with housing, and the provision of credible surrogates for the absent social supports of family and community. However, basic comparability is very expensive and popular values are neither humane nor attentive to arguments for distributive fairness. The issue in a wealthy industrial society with pretensions to fairness becomes one of ethics more than clinical outcomes—greater equality rather than cure.

Evidence for the service wisdom of basic comparability—the pursuit of greater equality rather than quick cure—can be teased out of the literature. Training in community living, the clubhouses, and a variety of small-scale correctional programs are valuable as occasional demonstrations of successful programs, but only that. Even the best of the outcome literature fails to provide a warrant of successful replication or fails to adequately evaluate the programs. It is a curiosity in the literature of outcome studies that success might often be attributable to the absence of a barbaric "treatment as usual" such as prison or the streets than to the inherent value of the experimental intervention itself. Simply sending a young offender home rather than to prison might lower recidivism. Indeed, the manifest deviations of the research from standard scientific standards suggest professional complicity in creating the soothing fictions of practice—myths of concern, dreams of order, forms of denial that are coincidental with the tyrannies and indecencies of social neglect, all the more pernicious for the sincerity of professionals. More is not needed, current arrangements suffice; if all is not well, it is still pretty good.

The deficit in knowing and the weak evaluative literature are created by a committed professional community antagonistic to true neutrality in research. Here and throughout the clinical literature, there is hardly any researcher without a stake in the effectiveness of the interventions that are being evaluated. Community psychological practice and rehabilitation are social franchises of professional practice. There is no written charter that insists on obedience to social priorities; it is implicit in the socialization of professionals. Professional practice largely begins with the hope of discovery and usually through the rare, informed, specialized, and presumably rational scholarship of medicine and the social sciences. The goal is to find a cure, a bullet, a pill, a thin intervention like mentoring that efficiently and compatibly achieves socially desirable goals. The genius of discovery confers great prestige and more material rewards. Insurrections are not well funded.

There have always been mavericks but they do not lead the herd.

References

Alexander, J. F., & Parsons, B. V. (1973). Short-Term Behavioral Intervention with Delinquent Families: Impact on Family Process and Recidivism. *Journal of Abnormal Psychology, 81,* 219–225. https://doi.org/10.1037/h0034537.

Andersen, S. N., & Skardhamar, T. (2017). Pick a Number: Mapping Recidivism Measures and Their Consequences. *Crime & Delinquency, 63,* 613–635. https://doi.org/10.1177/0011128715570629.

Andrews, D. A., Zinger, I., Hoge, R. D., Bonta, J., Gendreau, P., & Cullen, F. T. (1990). Does Correctional Treatment Work? A Clinically Relevant and Psychologically Informed Meta-Analysis. *Criminology, 28,* 369–404. https://doi.org/10.1111/j.1745-9125.1990.tb01330.x.

Angell, M. (2011a, July 14). The Illusions of Psychiatry. *The New York Review of Books, 58,* 20.

Angell, M. (2011b, June 23). The Epidemic of Mental Illness: Why? *The New York Review of Books, 58,* 2–3.

Barton, R. (1999). Psychosocial Rehabilitation Services in Community Support Systems: A Review of Outcomes and Policy Recommendations. *Psychiatric Services, 50,* 525–534. https://doi.org/10.1176/ps.50.4.525.

Battin, C., Bouvet, C., & Hatala, C. (2016). A Systematic Review of the Effectiveness of the Clubhouse Model. *Psychiatric Rehabilitation Journal, 39,* 305–312.

Beard, J. H., Propst, R. N., & Malamud, T. J. (1982). The Fountain House Model of Psychiatric Rehabilitation. *Psychosocial Rehabilitation Journal, 5,* 47–53.

Becker, R. E. (2015). Policies and Consequences: How America and Psychiatry Took the Detour to Erewhon. *Psychiatric Services, 66,* 1097–1100. https://doi.org/10.1176/appi.ps.201400485.

Becker, R. E., & Greig, N. H. (2010, December 8). Lost in Translation: Neuropsychiatric Drug Development. *Science Translational Medicine, 2*(61), 1–7. http://dx.doi.org/10.1126/scitranslmed.3000446.

Benston, E. A. (2015). Housing Programs for Homeless Individuals with Mental Illness: Effects on Housing and Mental Health Outcomes. *Psychiatric Services, 66*(8), 806–816.

Bryan, A. E., & Arkowitz, H. (2015). Meta-Analysis of the Effects of Peer-Administered Psychosocial Interventions on Symptoms of Depression. *American Journal of Community Psychology, 55,* 455–471. https://doi.org/10.1007/s10464-015-9718-y.

Chamberlain, P., & Reid, J. B. (1998). Comparison of Two Community Alternatives to Incarceration for Chronic Juvenile Offenders. *Journal of Consulting and Clinical Psychology, 66,* 624–633. https://doi.org/10.1037/0022-006X.66.4.624.

Cook, T. D., & Shadish, W. R., Jr. (1982). Meta-Evaluation: An Evaluation of the CMCH Congressionally-Mandated Evaluation System. In G. J. Stahler & W. R. Tash (Eds.), *Innovative Approaches to Mental Health Evaluation* (1st ed., pp. 221–253). New York, NY: Academic Press.

Cullen, F. T., Pratt, T. C., Turanovic, J. J., & Butler, L. (2018). When Bad News Arrives: Project HOPE in a Post-Factual World. *Journal of Contemporary Criminal Justice, 34,* 13–34. https://doi.org/10.1177/1043986217750424.

Dalton, J. H., Elias, M. J., & Wandersman, A. (2001). *Community Psychology: Linking Individuals and Communities.* Belmont, CA: Wadsworth Thomson Learning.

Eckman, T. A., et al. (1992). Technology for Training Schizophrenic Patients in Illness Self-Management: A Controlled Trial. *American Journal of Psychiatry, 149,* 1549–1555.

Elliott, D. S., & Voss, H. L. (1968). Records Matching in Delinquency Research. *Social Problems, 16*(1), 120–123.

Epstein, W. M. (2013). *Empowerment as Ceremony*. New Brunswick, NJ: Transaction Publishers.

Evans, M. E., Boothroyd, R. A., & Armstrong, M. I. (1997). Development and Implementation of an Experimental Study of the Effectiveness of Intensive In-Home Crisis Services for Children and Their Families. *Journal of Emotional and Behavioral Disorders, 5,* 93–105. https://doi.org/10.1177/106342669700500204.

Evans, M. E., Boothroyd, R. A., Armstrong, M. I., Greenbaum, P. E., Brown, E. C., & Kuppinger, A. D. (2003). An Experimental Study of the Effectiveness of Intensive In-Home Crisis Services for Children and Their Families: Program Outcomes. *Journal of Emotional and Behavioral Disorders, 11,* 92–102. https://doi.org/10.1177/106342660301100203.

Fairweather, G. W. (1980). *The Fairweather Lodge: A Twenty-Year Retrospective.* San Francisco, CA: Jossey-Bass.

Gendreau, P. (1980). Recidivism Measure Reconsidered. *Canadian Journal of Criminology, 22.* Retrieved from www.heinonline.com.

Gendreau, P., & Leipciger, M. (1978). Development of a Redivism Measure and Its Application in Ontario. *Canadian Journal of Criminology, 20*(1), 3–17.

Gillig, P. M., & McQuistion, H. I. (2006). *Clinical Guide to the Treatment of the Mentally Ill Homeless*. Washington, DC: American Psychiatric Association.

Gomory, T. (unpublished). *Tautology and Coercion*. Unpublished manuscript on the Wisconsin Assertive Community Treatment Model.

Greenberg, G. A., & Rosenheck, R. A. (2010). Correlates of Past Homelessness in the National Epidemiological Survey on Alcohol and Related Conditions. *Administration and Policy in Mental Health and Mental Health Services Research, 37*(4), 357–366.

Grietens, H., Rink, J., & Hellinckx, W. (2003). Nonbehavioral Correlates of Juvenile Delinquency: Communications of Detained and Nondetained Young People About Social Limits. *Journal of Adolescent Research, 18*(1), 68–89.

Griswold, D. B. (1978). A Comparison of Recidivism Measures. *Journal of Criminal Justice, 6,* 247–252. https://doi.org/10.1016/0047-2352(78)90006-5.

Grossman, J. B., & Tierney, J. P. (1998). Does Mentoring Work? An Impact Study of the Big Brothers Big Sisters Program. *Evaluation Review, 22,* 403–426. https://doi.org/10.1177/0193841X9802200304.

Hartmann, W. E., St. Arnault, D. M., & Gone, J. P. (2018). A Return to the Clinic for Community Psychology: Lessons from a Clinical Ethnography in Urban American Indian Behavioral Health. *American Journal of Community Psychology, 61,* 62–75. http://dx.doi.org/10.1002/ajcp.12212.

Heller, K., Thompson, M. G., Trueba, P. E., Hogg, J. R., & Vlachos-Weber, I. (1991). Peer Support Telephone Dyads for Elderly Women: Was This the Wrong Intervention? *American Journal of Community Psychology, 19,* 53–74. https://doi.org/10.1007/BF00942253.

Jackson, R. L. (2001). *The Clubhouse Model: Empowering Applications of Theory to Generalist Practice.* Belmont, CA: Wadsworth/Thomson Learning.

Kagan, C., Burton, M., Duckett, P., Lawthom, R., & Siddiquee, A. (2011). *Critical Community Psychology.* West Sussex, UK: BPS Blackwell.

Kennedy, L., & Xyrichis, A. (2017). Cognitive Behavioral Therapy Compared with Non-specialized Therapy for Alleviating the Effect of Auditory Hallucinations in People with Reoccurring Schizophrenia: A Systematic Review and Meta-Analysis. *Community Mental Health Journal, 53,* 127–133. https://doi.org/10.1007/s10597-016-0030-6.

Kirigin, K. A., Braukmann, C. J., Atwater, J. D., & Wolf, M. M. (1982). An Evaluation of Teaching-Family (Achievement Place) Group Homes for Juvenile Offenders. *Journal of Applied Behavior Analysis, 15*(1), 1–16. https://doi.org/10.1901/jaba.1982.15-1.

Kirk, S. A., Gomory, T., & Cohen, D. (2013). *Mad Science.* New Brunswick, NJ: Transaction Publishers.

Knight, C. A., & Alarie, R. M. (2017). Improving Mental Health in the Community: Outcome Evaluation of a Geriatric Mental Health Day Treatment Service. *Clinical Gerontologist, 40,* 77–87. https://doi.org/10.1080/07317115.2016.1263709.

La Bonta, J., & Andrews, D. A. (2015). *The Psychology of Criminal Conduct.* New York: Routledge.

Lab, S. P., & Whitehead, J. T. (1990). From 'Nothing Works' to 'The Appropriate Works': The Last Stop on the Search for the Secular Grail. *Criminology, 28*(3), 405–418.

Larose, S., Boisclair-Chateauvert, G., De Wit, D. J., DuBois, D., Erdem, G., & Lipman, E. L. (2018). How Mentor Support Interacts with Mother and Teacher Support in Predicting Youth Academic Adjustment: An Investigation Among Youth Exposed to Big Brothers Big Sisters of Canada Programs. *The Journal of Primary Prevention, 39,* 205–228. https://doi.org/10.1007/s10935-018-0509-8.

Lerman, P. (1975). *Community Treatment and Social Control: A Critical Analysis of Juvenile Correctional Policy*. Chicago, IL: University of Chicago Press.

Lerman, P. (1984). Child Welfare, the Private Sector and Community Based Corrections. *Crime and Delinquency, 30*, 5–38.

Levine, M., & Perkins, D. V. (1997). *Principles of Community Psychology: Perspectives and Applications* (2nd ed.). New York, NY: Oxford University Press.

Lieber, J. A. (2006). Comparative Effectiveness of Antipsychotic Drugs: A Commentary on Cost Utility of the Latest Antipsychotic Drugs in Schizophrenia Study (CUtLASS 1) and Clinical Antipsychotic Trials of Intervention Effectiveness (CATIE). *Archives of General Psychiatry, 63*(10), 1069–1072.

Lipman, E. L., DeWit, D., DuBois, D. L., Larose, S., & Erdem, G. (2018). Youth with Chronic Health Problems: How Do They Fare in Main-Stream Mentoring Programs. *Journal of Emotional and Behavioral Disorders, 11*, 92–102. https://doi.org/10.1177/106342660301100203.

Lipsey, M. W., & Cullen, F. T. (2007). The Effectiveness of Correctional Rehabilitation: A Review of Systematic Reviews. *The Annual Review of Law and Social Sciences, 3*, 297–320. https://doi.org/10.1146/annurev.lawsocsci.3.081806.1128.

Marder, S. R., et al. (1996). Two-Year Outcome of Social Skills Training and Group Psychotherapy for Outpatients with Schizophrenia. *American Journal of Psychiatry, 153*, 1585–1592.

McKay, C., Nugent, K. L., Johnsen, M., Eaton, W. W., & Lidz, C. W. (2018). A Systematic Review of Evidence for the Clubhouse Model of Psychosocial Rehabilitation. *Administration and Policy in Mental Health and Mental Health Services Research, 45*, 28–47. https://doi.org/10.1007/s10488-016-0760-3.

Moller, M. D., & Murphy, M. F. (1997). The Three R's Rehabilitation Program: A Prevention Approach for the Management of Relapse Symptoms Associated with Psychiatric Diagnosis. *Psychiatric Rehabilitation Journal, 20*, 42–48. https://doi.org/10.1037/h0095365.

Morgan, R. D., et al. (2012). Treating Offenders With Mental Illness: A Research Synthesis. *Law and Human Behavior, 36*(1), 37–50.

Nelson, G., Kloos, B., & Ornelas, J. (2014). *Community Psychology and Community Mental Health*. New York, NY: Oxford University Press.

Painter, K. (2012). Evidence-Based Practices in Community Mental Health: Outcome Evaluation. *Journal of Behavioral Health Services & Research, 39*, 434–444. https://doi.org/10.1007/s11414-012-9284-0.

Palmer, T. (1974). The Youth Authority's Community Treatment Program. *Federal Probation, 38,* 3–14.

Pistrang, N., Barker, C., & Humphreys, K. (2008). Mutual Help Groups for Mental Health Problems: A Review of Effectiveness Studies. *American Journal of Community Psychology, 42,* 110–121. https://doi.org/10.1007/s10464-008-9181-0.

Repper, J., & Carter, T. (2011). A Review of the Literature on Peer Support in Mental Health Services. *Journal of Mental Health, 20,* 392–411. https://doi.org/10.3109/09638237.2011.583947.

Rickel, A. U. (1987). The 1965 Swampscott Conference and Future Topics for Community Psychology. *American Journal of Community Psychology, 15*(5), 511–513.

Rush, A. J., Trivedi, M. H., Wisniewski, S. R., Stewart, J. W., Nierenberg, A. A., Thase, M. E., et al. (2006). Bupropion-SR, Sertraline, or Venlafaxine-XR After Failure of SSRIs for Depression. *The New England Journal of Medicine, 354,* 1231–1242. https://doi.org/10.1056/NEJMoa052963.

Shepperd, S., Doll, H., Gowers, S., James, A., Fazel, M., Fitzpatrick, R., & Pollock, J. (2009). Alternatives to Inpatient Mental Health Care for Children and Young People (Review). *Cochrane Database of Systematic Reviews,* 1–58. http://dx.doi.org/10.1002/14651858.CD006410.pub2.

Smith, T. E., et al. (1996). Training Hospitalized Patients with Schizophrenia in Community Reintegration Skills. *Psychiatric Services, 47,* 1099–1103.

Staudt, M., & Drake, B. (2002). Intensive Family Preservation Services: Where's the Crisis? *Children and Youth Services Review, 24,* 777–795. https://doi.org/10.1016/S0190-7409(02)00228-1.

Stein, L. I., & Test, M. A. (1980). Alternative to Mental Hospital Treatment. I. Conceptual Model, Treatment Program, and Clinical Evaluation. *Archives of General Psychiatry, 37,* 409–412.

Stewart, L. A., et al. (2017). The Impact of a Community Mental Health Initiative on Outcomes for Offenders with a Serious Mental Disorder. *Criminal Behaviorand Mental Health, 27*(4), 371–384.

Tao, K. W., Owen, J., Pace, B. T., & Imel, Z. E. (2015). A Meta-Analysis of Multicultural Competencies and Psychotherapy Process and Outcome. *Journal of Counseling Psychology, 62,* 337–350. https://doi.org/10.1037/cou0000086.

Tebes, J. K. (2016). Reflections on the Future of Community Psychology from the Generations After Swampscott: A Commentary and Introduction to the Special Issue. *American Journal of Community Psychology,* 229–238. http://dx.doi.org/10.1002/ajcp.12110.

Timpe, Z. C., & Lunkenheimer, E. (2015). The Long-Term Economic Benefits of Natural Mentoring Relationships for Youth. *American Journal of Community Psychology, 56*(1–2), 2–24.

Turner, D. T., et al. (2018). A Meta-Analysis of Social Skills Training and Related Interventions for Psychosis. *Schizophrenia Belletin, 44*(3), 475–491.

Weisbrod, B. A., Test, M. A., & Stein, L. I. (1980). Alternative to Mental Hospital Treatment: II. Economic Benefit-Cost Analysis. *Archives of General Psychiatry*, 400–405. http://dx.doi.org/10.1001/archpsyc.1980.01780170042004.

Weisburd, D., et al. (2017). What Works in Crime Prevention and Rehabilitation. *Ciminology and Public Policy, 16*(2), 415–449.

Whitehead, J. T., & Lab, S. P. (1989). A Meta-Analysis of Juvenile Correctional Treatment. *Journal of Research in Crime and Delinquency, 26*, 276–295. https://doi.org/10.1177/0022427889026003005.

Wilson, H. A. (2014). Can Antisocial Personality Disorder Be Treated? A Meta-Analysis Examining the Effectiveness of Treatment in Reducing Recidivism for Individuals Diagnosed with ASPD. *International Journal of Forensic Mental Health, 13*, 36–46. https://doi.org/10.1080/14999013.2014.890682.

Yau, E. F., Chan, C. C., Chan, A. S., & Chui, B. K. (2005). Changes in Psychosocial and Work-Related Characteristics Among Clubhouse Members: A Preliminary Report. *Work, 25*, 287–296. Retrieved from http://content.iospress.com/articles/work/wor00466.

10

Mind and Spirit on the Fringes of the Social Clinic

The mind and spirit interventions of the social clinic—psychotherapy or other verbal interventions—are a type of alternative, fringe, complementary, integrative, folk, adjunctive, unconventional, unorthodox, nonmainstream, or irregular procedure that promises to treat mental, emotional, or physical ailments. What isolates them from the mainstream is not their strangeness but rather their use of alternative science to validate their outcomes. Yet many marginal interventions are traveling the same track on which psychoanalysis, psychotherapy, and social work moved from the odd to the commonplace and all without compelling scientific evidence of effectiveness. The achievement of clinical acceptance is a social phenomenon more often than a rational one—validation by the acceptance of use and often in the absence or defiance of clinical evidence.

Within a community of practitioners dedicated to the cannons of science, a new intervention moves from weak evidence suggesting effectiveness to a series of dispositive trials. The quintessential test of any clinical intervention must contain a randomized placebo control and a nontreatment control along with the customary protections of coherent experimentation. A persistent reliance on testimonials, practitioner

© The Author(s) 2019
W. M. Epstein, *Psychotherapy and the Social Clinic in the United States*,
https://doi.org/10.1007/978-3-030-32750-7_10

reports (e.g., evidence from the couch), research conducted by those with obvious stakes in the outcomes, subjective reports of outcomes, high attrition, convenience samples, and the other characteristics of pseudoscience begins to question the motives of practitioners and indicts the value of their practice. It is precisely the absence of scientifically valid evidence and the resistance to neutral evaluation that places an intervention at the margins of practice.

Yet the margins of practice in the social clinic—mind and spirit interventions defiant of credible science—and mainline practice are distinguished more by style than substance. That is, science is violated by both although in different ways. The professions of mainline practice have distorted science, undermining neutrality, and independence in creating exaggerated estimates of effectiveness. In contrast, the margins of practice are mockeries of science, theaters of treatment that take advantage of mysticism, intuition, ignorance, immaturity, desperation, and manipulated short-term placebo effects. In this regard, persistently untested "alternative and complementary" interventions are often the inventions of charlatans, quacks, frauds, and predators on the sufferings of humanity. Snake oil and crackpot empiricism predate science and modern medical practice by millennia and persist with undiminished force. Martin Gardner would likely agree that despite the growth of the sciences, the twentieth century was more superstitious than the nineteenth or any previous one for that matter.

Alternative and unconventional medical practice is big business (Eisenberg et al. 1998). The use of at least one of 16 unconventional and alternative medical therapies in the United States increased from 39 to 42% of the population between 1990 and 1997. Eisenberg et al. (1998) estimated that total 1997 out-of-pocket expenditures for alternative medical practices in the United States totaled $27 billion about the same as out-of-pocket expenditures for physician services. The use of alternative and unconventional interventions beyond those that Eisenberg et al. polled—including the fringe interventions of the social clinic—apparently also enjoy extensive use by the American public and earn many billions more in out-of-pocket expenditures. Holden and Barker (2017) provide some sense of their range, but there is no national survey of their use comparable to the Eisenberg et al. surveys.

Spiritual Interventions

The inclusion of spiritual elements into the social clinic has become common within counseling, pastoral and educational counseling, social work, and the psychotherapeutic community generally. Psychotherapy engages in many aspects of life, and it seems reasonable that faith and religion would be touched on. "The integration of clients' religion/spirituality in mental and behavior health treatment has the potential to improve outcomes" (Oxhandler and Pargament 2018, p. 120). The question is whether it does so, especially since the spirit—the unseen but ever present—would seem to generate antagonism toward the seen—objectivity and evaluation.

While not explicitly God-based, spiritual practice includes much of the language and assumptions of religion and faith: soul, higher powers, mystical experience, "the creative spirit or God," transformation, spiritual momentum, and others (Derezotes 2006). It makes the same claims as psychotherapy—contentment, adjustment, and life satisfaction—but adds "transpersonal" and "transrational" goals of peace with the Eternal and the Universal. It is decidedly clinic-based rather than a free-floating attempt at spontaneous self-help through the effusions of gurus.

Spiritual work is viewed as a *radical* approach to practice because the roots of human consciousness, suffering and transformation are dealt with directly. Spiritual work is a *transformational* practice method, focused on creating fundamental changes in the way individual and communities view and live in their world.... *Spiritual Practice* happens as a person takes response-ability for the development of her own consciousness in a way that is balanced between over- and under-responsibility to self and others. Spiritual practices leads to...interconnection with everything else. The terms social worker and practitioner refer to the professional helpers who serve the client. (emphasis in original Derezotes, ibid., p. 11)

Spiritually oriented practice can be conducted with all ages, in mental and physical health settings, within the criminal justice system, among the social services and school systems, and with families and groups. Advanced spiritually oriented practice reputedly achieves individual and collective transformation. Following Derezotes (2006), the methods of spiritual practice build on the "four forces of psychology: psychodynamic, cognitive behavioral, experiential humanistic, and transpersonal" but add elements of the transrational—mind, spirit, and so forth—to achieve transformation. Little appears to be defined in operational terms. The "methods" are invocations to be attentive rather than actual processes of treatment. Appeals to spirit or soul would seem to be impossible without an ability to identify spirit or soul.

Spiritual work is the same as religion, faith healing, and other elements of the common culture until announcing that its goals are both measurable and achievable as clinical practice. As clinical practice—a series of interventions with measurable effects—it is amenable to objective evaluation in the manner of cognitive behavioral therapy, eye movement desensitization, and clubhouses. However, Derezotes (2006) provides no evaluations or references to evaluations of the effectiveness of spiritual clinical practice. As one example, the assertion that "prayer and other practices of supplication can be helpful to the client" is not followed by citations or evidence that sustains the effectiveness of prayer or of any clinical intervention that incorporates prayer.

In a similar and prominent textbook on the spiritual in clinical social work published by Oxford University Press, Lee et al. (2009) attempt to bring "together insights from Eastern thought (especially Buddhism, Daoism, and Traditional Chinese Medicine), Western holistic and systemic theories, complementary and alternative therapies, and social work trends in cultural competence, spiritual sensitivity, and the strengths perspective" (Canda in Lee et al., p. vii). Yet the virtues of those insights for clinical practice are only asserted; they are not systematically tested.

Lee and many of her coauthors are either Hong Kong Chinese, western residents there or Hong Kong immigrants to the United States. Their brief and often heroicized history of American social work is not paired with a thoughtful treatment of the value of the spiritual in the East. It ignores the possibility that the spiritual East has suffered terribly at the hands of its own ancient insights. The East was not edenic before Marco Polo and is not today. Indeed, progress in the East against poverty and the occasional progress against predatory authoritarianism seem to be associated with the rejection of traditional Eastern spiritualism in favor of secularism. Unfortunately, Eastern secularism often morphs into a religion of state power as in North Korea and Maoist China.

"Body-mind-spirit connection" or "holistic health is the result of a balanced and integrated body, mind, and spirit" (Lee et al., p. 162). The holistic therapy "focuses on the process rather than the outcome," which seems an excuse to avoid outcomes (ibid., p. 164). Nonetheless, the chapter provides the cases of Kyle, Bella, Penny, Suzi, and others to demonstrate important changes including relaxation, improved socialization, and even "embodied transcendence." "In all cases, sensing through the body, thinking through the mind, and feeling through the heart open the ground for spiritual transformation" (p. 169). Rather than evaluations of clinical effects—after all only the process counts— the author invokes "research studies in the fields of psychoneuroimmunology and psychoendocrinology [that] have revealed the connection of the nervous system, immune system, and endocrine system" (ibid., p. 170). Thus, spiritual processes improve clinical outcomes even without the obligation to provide direct evidence of the relationship between spirituality and positive effects. The other chapters that discuss the elements of practice follow suit with numerous spiritual interventions to treat the range of social and individual problems.

The crucial question about spiritualism and other untested, unconventional alternatives to mainline practice should concern the benefits for clinical practice. Yet, Lee et al. in the manner of Derezotes and the spiritual literature itself offer little evidence that spiritualism leads to effective clinical practice. In fact, there is a tendency to suggest that spiritual and other subjective forms of evaluation are adequate substitutes for rational evaluation. The book is full of very short case examples provided by the different authors as testimony to the effectiveness of different treatments and the theories behind them but only five attempts in a separate section to provide standard evidence.

The five studies, reported in separate chapters, largely concerned the physical and mental benefits of spiritual interventions to patients with serious physical problems—breast cancer and colorectal cancer—depression, adjustment, and trauma. The research was consistently undercut by a variety of serious shortcomings while the interpretation of findings was often exaggerated. Insignificant findings—both statistically and clinically—were given important meaning. Many important outcomes were not statistically significant while many were subjective and elicited by the committed researchers themselves. Attrition was not reported. Blinding was often not incorporated. Only one of the five studies employed a randomized design; the "experimental" evaluation of meditation incorporated a comparison group that varied greatly from the meditation group. All of the data are suspect of bias; little of it was objective; the reliability of instruments is questionable. None provided substantial follow-up measures. Weak designs produced weak evidence whose importance was exaggerated by committed researchers. The "body-mind-spirit connection" resurrects the primitive dualism of mind and body that steps back into superstition rather than a step forward into modern clinical practice. Lee et al. is evidence of the affectation of multicultural and the charm of orientalism rather than clinical proof. It is an instance of tribalism in social clinical practice and a warning against the perils of sentimentality.

Oxhandler and Pargament (2018) reviewed the extensive literature of spiritual competence in providing counseling but only detail the presumed process qualifications of practitioners; they provide no research that measures the actual effects of pastoral counseling. There do not appear to be evaluations of spiritual social work, pastoral counseling, or spiritual clinical work. There is some vague evidence that access to a chaplain as a minor element of comprehensive medical and social supports in intensive care units may be beneficial for seriously ill patients (Penrod et al. 2011); the "spiritual" component hardly constitutes a spiritual clinical intervention.

Spiritual clinical work continues Jung's mission to restore the spiritual to modern life. It has the same weaknesses of denying objectivity and the same tendency to equate the metaphysical with the world of things, often invoking some form of a shared human consciousness that contains archetypes of knowledge. It offers transrational wisdom of the good and the authentic that is genetically endowed but without a material existence. Spiritualism in the social clinic takes heart from its companionship with the sublime to tread beyond the boundaries of science to ignore coherent evaluation. Spiritualism in any form is a language without meaning. It is perpetuated out of a strange sort of multiculturalism in the United States insisting that respect for the individual entails acceptance of the immigrant's culture, a point of thoughtless fantasy that leads to a society segregated by ethnicity and race, the plagues of American social history. It is surely better to respect the choices of other cultures within themselves while enacting a tolerant, civic culture of decency in the United States that accepts immigrants and the nation's traditional others into the communion of American society.

Spiritualism in the practice of the social clinic is an absurdity of superstition that invokes self-help manuals, the strengths perspective, the extreme individualism of the American ethos, and thus American minimalism. It reinforces the search inward rather greater social and economic equality as solutions to personal and social problems. The road to peace, contentment, hope, a good life, adjustment, and sanity, all possibilities within the individual, are unwound by the meditative will usually guided by adepts trained in the ancient, hidden wisdom of the Orient. Thus, everyone is responsible for their destiny. American stratification is just.

Mysticism, spiritualism, and the insights of ancients continue the legacy of Madam Blavatsky, her séances to speak with the dearly departed, her religion of Theosophy, and her many other hustles to make a living. A Russian emigre, she was immensely popular during her day. Yet evidence of effective spiritualism is about as credible as Dr. Duncan MacDoughall's research finding that the human soul weighs on average 21 grams (https://www.historicmysteries.com/the-21-gram-soul-theory/, July 6, 2018) or perhaps 1/3000th of an ounce (http://www.noeticscience.co.uk/weighting-the-human-soul/, July 7, 2018). Then again, the soul being immaterial cannot have weight just like spiritualism itself.

Mindfulness and Meditation

You better think (think) think about what you're trying to do to me

Yeah, think (think, think) let your mind go, let yourself be free
Oh freedom (freedom), freedom (freedom), freedom, yeah freedom
Freedom (freedom), freedom (freedom), freedom, ooh freedom
Think about it, think about it[1]

As a form of psychological practice, mindfulness and meditation promise personal transformation and specific benefits for those who suffer from a variety of emotional problems. Guided meditation is the principal technique of mindfulness. To the extent that the effectiveness of mindfulness and meditation is not credibly tested, they remain unconventional interventions sanctioned by faith and social custom rather than by scientific evidence of their value.

Mindfulness and meditation as clinical interventions do not simply enjoin patients to think about things. The clinical task lies in teaching

The skills and practices of mindfulness, self-awareness and self-compassion... Perhaps somewhat surprisingly, simply learning to keep one's attention focused in the present moment has profound positive consequences for our physical and mental health.... A growing body of medical and scientific evidence now exists, testifying to the value of practicing mindfulness for a wide variety of health and psychological conditions and purposes. (Rogers and Maytan 2012, pp. ix, x).

Often in deference to Buddhism, the mindfulness literature approximates a form of self-help. In fact, many of the mindfulness texts adopt the rhetoric and form of the self-help genre, advertising their virtues through the academic and professional reputations of their practitioners and the testimonials of both high status and presumably representative patients and glorifying the patient's achievements as self-invention. After the clinical period of instruction, mindfulness practitioners are capable of charting their own destiny with occasional touch-up and refresher sessions.

Whether devout Buddhists are more serene and functional than nominal Buddhists or the nonreligious would seem to be difficult to

---

[1] *Think* sung by Aretha Franklin in the 1980 *Blues Brothers* movie.

attribute to the practices of mindfulness. Nevertheless, it is possible to test the effectiveness of a course of mindfulness through rigorous clinical trials. Yet the best of the scientific literature does not sustain the clinical claims of mindfulness.

Rogers and Maytan (2012) provide a multitude of case examples and bits of wisdom about teaching—"Stories, not lectures, keep them engaged." However, "the research behind our teaching," despite their claims, remains weak, biased, insubstantial, and misleading (p. 39). According to Rogers and Maytan, the "classic" study by Davidson et al. (2003) "demonstrates the positive effect of meditation on our emotional state and on our immune system" (Rogers and Maytan, op. cit., p. 48). In fact, Davidson et al. (2003) only document changes in brain activity but not changes in behavior. In fact, they report that there was no significant difference between the meditation group and a waitlist control on the self-reported Positive and Negative Affect Scale; similar changes over time took place with both groups. Anxiety improvements did not persist for the meditators. Changes in brain activity were not consistent nor realized in eased emotions. Moreover, "there were no significant associations between the measures of practice and many of the biological or self-report measures" (ibid., p. 568). Further, without a placebo control it is impossible to attribute the positive immunological response to meditation or to other factors of the research situation, in particular, demand characteristics created by researchers with obvious stakes in positive outcomes. Aside from the dubious reliance on self-reported data, the samples were not representative of a troubled or needy population, and there was no extended follow-up. Travis and Arenander (2004) identify other unanswered problems with Davidson et al. (2003): misleading data analyses and questionable interpretations of brain activity. There may also well be a persistent issue with publication bias, in particular, the existence of negative findings that the many researchers committed to mindfulness interventions and their journals may refuse to publish.

Many serious pitfalls in the other mindfulness studies cited by Rogers and Maytan undercut claims of clinical effectiveness. Kabat-Zinn et al. (1998) concluded that meditation improves outcomes in treating psoriasis. However, no placebo was employed and the likelihood of demand characteristics explaining outcomes is high despite their statement that "nothing was said to create expectations of a therapeutic effect from the use of the [mindfulness] tapes" (ibid., p. 626); nothing needed to be said since the expectation of improvement is implicit in the use of the experimental intervention. Moreover, samples were small—between eight and 10 at the start—and attrition reached 39%. In addition, 30 (48%) of 67 eligible patients in the initial pool refused to participate. Many data were self-reported. The evaluators had deep stakes in demonstrating effectiveness. Still, the outcomes were not consistently positive. The value of audio-taped meditation sessions to improve treatment for psoriasis is not demonstrated.

Similar deficiencies undercut the other research Rogers and Maytan put forward as evidence of successful mindfulness and meditation interventions. The small positive effects of meditation in reducing the recurrence of depression and in tapering the use of antidepressant medications reported by Kuyken et al. (2008) may be due to a confound: Meditation patients were also pointedly encouraged to taper their medications. In addition, lower rates of relapse may have been due to less of a susceptibility to relapse among the experimental patients—i.e., a greater amount of time since the last depressive episode among meditation patients compared to the group on maintenance medication. In addition, no placebo was employed; much of the outcome data were self-reported. Differences between the mindfulness group and the medication control were neither large nor consistent. Similar problems invalidate Manzoni et al. (2008), Roberts and Danoff-Burg (2010), Rosenzweig et al. (2003), and Shapiro et al. (1998): small samples, unreliable self-reports, lack of protection against researcher expectancies, episodic problems with attrition, unrepresentative samples, mixed outcomes, and researchers who were neither independent nor neutral. The research that Rogers and Maytan cite in support of mindfulness and meditation is only a tribute to the self-promotion of the mindfulness industry. The value of meditation and mindfulness in handling psoriasis, depression, drug dependence, stress, surgery, and others is not credibly demonstrated.

Rogers and Maytan (2012) serve an advertisement for the Center for Mind-Body Medicine. The book is not a serious examination of clinical practice by members of a neutral and independent community of scholars. The mindfulness and meditation researchers often seem to have a professional and financial stake—as practitioner, researcher, apologist, or both—in particular clinical organizations.

Intuitively, "mindful" people may be less prone to depression and stress. However, it remains an open question whether the techniques of mindfulness are teachable through clinical training. Banks et al. (2015) systematically reviewed evaluations of mindfulness approaches to treat post-traumatic stress disorder. Only 12 studies conformed to their minimal inclusion criteria—standard measures of post-traumatic stress disorder, published in English, adult sample, and the employment of a mindfulness intervention. Of these 12, only four studies employed randomized designs. However, none of the four studies blinded raters and participants to group assignments; none of their samples were representative; all outcomes were self-reported.

Kearney et al. (2012), the best of the 12 and the only study that the authors rated as achieving good methodological quality, hardly provides a credible test of mindfulness. Patients were randomized to mindfulness-based stress reduction or to a standard treatment control group. Samples were small and probably not representative of those with post-traumatic stress disorder. Most important, blinding was not maintained. The mindfulness intervention was provided for eight weeks that contained one 2.5-hour session and a single 7-hour session between weeks six and seven. During the sessions, participants "received instructions on mindfulness meditation, discussed homework assignments, and had the opportunity to ask questions" (ibid., p. 18). The mindfulness intervention was apparently not successful. "Intention-to-treat analysis found no reliable effects of mindfulness based stress reduction on post-traumatic stress disorder or depression" (ibid., p. 14). The gains in quality of life and other outcomes did not persist at four-month follow-up. The study concludes with a recommendation for future research that employs better methods, i.e., blinding and large samples. They could have also listed object tests of outcomes and neutral evaluators. Authors without an obvious commitment to mindfulness might have concluded that other interventions are more promising. If anything, the growing body of evidence that Rogers and Maytan (2012) refer to is hard-pressed to come up with any credible evidence that mindfulness has clinical value.

The most recent and comprehensive meta-analyses of mindfulness interventions for mental and emotional problems consistently report small to moderate effects (and sometimes not even this) but employ low-quality research: as examples, "low quality evidence for clinically relevant effects of yoga on posttraumatic stress disorder" (Cramer et al. 2018, p. 2); "no statistically effects were found in follow-up" for mindfulness treatment of depression (Chi et al. 2018, p. 1); accounting for publication bias (unpublished studies with negative findings) wipes out any benefit for mindfulness treatment of negative affectivity (Schumer et al. 2018, p. 576) The research is typically impaired by small unrepresentative samples, self-reported outcomes, attrition, committed researchers, demonstration situations, lack of blinding, short follow-up periods, lack of appropriate controls (i.e., placebos), lack of replication, publication bias, and others.

It is extremely rare that any test of the social clinical employs a placebo control. Wolf and Abell (2003) did employ a placebo control as well as a nontreatment control in testing the effects of meditation on psychosocial functioning. They reported that maha mantra (the Hari Krishna chant) was somewhat effective compared to a nonsense chant and a no-treatment control. However, they acknowledged a number of serious problems with the research: a lack of blinding of the researchers who seemed to be partisans of the intervention, weak reliability of the instruments, self-reported outcome data, 34% attrition, no intention to treat analysis, and members of the placebo control group who were aware of the bogus chant. In the event, the reported outcomes were relatively small and episodic and usually did not persist at follow-up.

Yet a mountain of personal testimony swears to the value of prayer and religion and the different disciplineships of mindfulness and meditation but hardly any credible proof that sustains mindfulness and meditation as clinical interventions. There are no definitive tests of mindfulness and the pitfalls in the research may well account for even the modest reported findings. Mindfulness remains a modified form of spiritual psychological practice but better structured around some form of traditional religious practice, a perception of the sacred, a higher power or reference to God, and the many substitutes for the Divine.

The mindfulness and meditation literature is inattentive to the downside of the practice of ecstatic transformation, notably its use by cults. Moonies, Scientologists, Jews for Jesus, Nazis and NeoNazis, Primitive Baptists, Jim Jones (the Disciple of Christ and the purveyor of the Jonestown Massacre), Fundamentalist Latter-Day Saints, the International Society for Krishna Consciousness, and many others that incorporate some form of guided mindfulness and meditation. They are often paths to the pleasures of fanaticism—group identify, comradeship, and certainty. True belief replaces the ambiguities and terrors of existence with comforting, isolating mantras, prayers, focused thought, mental numbness, and, often, the livery of the anointed and blessed. Rather than the "clear" of Scientology or an epiphany of God's favor, romantic transformation provides fantasy and narcissism.

> Everything dissolves into feeling; everything becomes mere mood; everything becomes subjective; "thinking is only a dream of feeling." Feeling is considered valid as such; it represents the value of life which the enthusiastic disposition wants to affirm. The romantic becomes enraptured and ecstatic for the sake of ecstasy and rapture; this state becomes for him an end in itself and has its meaning within itself…. The desire to yield to illusion, justifiable in art, here characterizes the entire relation to the world. (Baeck 1958, pp. 190–191)

Mindfulness and meditation within a clinical context are not simply techniques of relaxation but subtle promises of Nirvana, pleasure, insight, peace, oneness with nature, and acceptance. Quite naturally, those lured into mind cures may also be susceptible to similar highs through illicit drugs, alcohol, and the practice of chemical psychiatry. The common pursuit of ecstatic release seems coincidental with a society that insists on heroic levels of individualism and personal responsibility but that fails to provision many of its citizens with the tools and resources for a productive life—work, family and community security, education, recreation, income, opportunities for creativity, and contribution to the civic culture. For all their deceptions, incapacities, and clinical flaws, mindfulness and meditation remain demotic soothing fictions that express and affirm the American ethos of extreme individualism, chosenness, and intuitive truth. Paul Moloney, a skeptical British psychotherapist, has it just so.

> The rise of mindfulness in the Western World as both therapy and instrument of personal development in recent decades has little to do with its superior merits – which fade under critical analysis. This situation is close to that which obtains for the more established talking therapies, from which theorists and teachers of mindfulness seek to borrow much of their authority. Rather than "science," the mindfulness movement owes its popularity (and its apparent successes) to the imperatives of fashion, to the promotional energies of the psychological therapies industry, and to its status as an officially endorsed palliative for overworked lives and troubled times. Detached from traditional Buddhist teachings and presented as a new technology of personal change, mindfulness is the latest phase in the privatization of the self that has been underway from the middle of the 20th Century, and in which the applied psychology professions have been instrumental. For governments, it presents a cheap alternative to the substantive social and economic policies needed to tackle widespread malaise. (Moloney 2016)

Centers for Positive Living

The Internet hosts many "Centers for Positive Living" including "spiritual" centers for positive living. It is difficult to discern whether they are unique organizations that found benefit in the same title or are franchises of a single enterprise. Some are religious, some secular. However, their content is similar, typically featuring exotic, unorthodox, and marginal interventions. They typically rely on faith, hyperbolic claims, unproven assumptions, and untested assertions about the ability to achieve announced goals. Many promise cure, transformation, transcendence, serenity, and even salvation. And what may seem contradictory, they wrap their marginality and strangeness in culturally conforming terms. That is, they invariably attempt to normalize themselves with academic or academically sounding degrees, an emotionally charged style appealing to superstition, faith, and at times bogus research and other references to shared values and common language. They often replicate the language and metaphors of pietistic religious revival. Many offer some form of clinical treatment, usually an unorthodox, untested intervention.

Located in Portland, Oregon, The Center for Positive Living is one of the more sophisticated centers offering "an advanced, experiential method of mind-body-spirit therapy" to achieve "extraordinary healing, life transformations, [and] profound" experiences (http://www.laurie-day.com/, Home Page, July 13, 2018). Among others, the Center promises to treat depression, anxiety, stress, and trauma, bringing into each patient's life empowerment, inner peace, inner strength, clarity, ease, tranquility, joy, and "LOVE" (emphasis in original, ibid.).

Laurie Day, a licensed clinical social worker, is the founder of the Center. More than two decades ago, she

> Experienced a spiritual awakening, an initiation, during which her heart opened and she felt Total Love, Total Trust. I was immersed in this ecstatic feeling. From a place deep inside of me I heard the words, "THIS IS THERAPY!" This life-changing event catalyzed the remarkable healing work that Laurie does now. (emphasis in original, ibid.)
>
> Her gentle energy balancing techniques allow people to release their anxiety and depression very quickly and effectively. Her abilities have evolved through years of studying many alternative healing methods, such as, Past Life therapy, MarieEl Healing, Reiki Healing, Light and Sound Therapy and Gestalt Psychotherapy….
>
> What makes Laurie's healing work so profound Is that not only does it provide a way to gently let go of the past from the core level of cell memory, it also reconnects the person with who they really are in their pure heart and soul. (ibid.)

The Center offers testimonials to Laurie Day's curative touch but no references to or systematic evidence that her interventions—past life therapy, MariEl healing, and the others—are effective. Indeed, there is no credible evidence of their effectiveness, and thus, they remain unorthodox, marginal, and eerie beyond quaintness. They fall into the category of bogus cures and quackery that have for millennia taken advantage of human ignorance, stupidity, and anguish.

On its part, MariEl Reiki healing draws on "the Healing Energy of the Mother Mary." According to the Spirit Journey Academy of the Spirits of NativeLIGHT (sic),

> MariEl is a heart-centered hands-on healing technique introduced in 1983 by its creator, Ethel Lombardi, an international healer/teacher and Reiki master taught by Mrs. Hawayo Takata of the Usui Reiki tradition. MariEL is the essence of the Feminine and was brought into existence in an effort to balance the patriarchal energy dominating Mother Earth and her people. The energy of MariEL probes to the core of the soul and facilitates the release, at a cellular level, of old blockages, patterns, memories, traumas and pain. (http://www.spiritsofnativelight.org/mari_el.asp, July 13, 2018)

The Academy markets remote and personalized sessions with Reverend Wendi, apparently the Academy's principal Reiki master, and markets her printed works and courses that teach consciousness channeling, DNA activation, shamanism, angelic empowerments, Infinite Usui Reiki among many others. Reverend Wendi's sessions include Abundance Flush Empowerment, certification in Lightarian Angel Links, and training in the 13 Crystal Skulls that are "among the most powerful objects of symbolism in human history" (ibid., n.p.). For those wishing to enroll in the 13 Crystal Skulls course, it is "highly suggested that one has significant vibrational energy work experience" (ibid.). There is an abundance of courses, reference books for sale, specials, and even the opportunity to subscribe to the Academy's newsletter. The Academy provides no reference to coherent evidence of its clinical prowess.

Light and sound therapy add sensory luster to the fringes of clinical practice. According to HealthPRO Heritage: Therapy Management and Consulting Services,

> Light and sound therapy are an increasingly popular types of Vibrational Medicine or Energy Medicine. Einstein taught us that every living thing

produces an electromagnetic field with a vibrational frequency and that energy and matter are interchangeable and transferable. Based on the principle that all mater vibrates to a precise frequency and that imbalances have frequencies that be rebalanced, light and sound therapy use resonant vibration to restore health to the body and electromagnetic field. (http://learn.healthpro.com/light-therapy-sound-therapy/, August 30, 2018, n.p.)

The tools of light and sound therapy include tuning forks, quartz crystal bowls, music, changing, Tibetan bowls, and Rife machine technologies. "Using light and sound wave frequencies which correspond to acupuncture meridians or the charka system, light and sound therapies use the 12 colors of the visible light spectrum and the 12 sound intervals of the musical scale to release blockages, correct emotional, physical, psychological and spiritual imbalances, and restore a state of harmony" (ibid.). Light and sound therapy promise success with the common problems facing the social clinic—stress, anxiety, depression, sleep disorders, low libido, creativity, pain management, self-esteem, and others along with additional goals of chakra balancing, spiritual connectedness, and the realization of higher purpose (ibid.). Apparently, spiritual awareness is its own proof but HealthPRO, among others, provides no additional evidence.

Past Life Regression Therapy

Past life regression therapy, often simply referred to as past life therapy, is a blend of Eastern religion that espouses reincarnation and modern spiritualism. The regression to earlier developmental stages in order to resolve persistent conflicts that inhibit successful emotional development characterizes both Freudian psychotherapy and psychodynamic psychotherapy generally although neither put much faith in the immortality and transmigration of souls. However, past life regression therapy asserts that human souls carry forward the failures or karma of previous, problematic incarnations that need to be addressed in any successful therapeutic intervention. Of course, the excuse can always be made that the therapist profitably begins with patients as presented and thus accepts their abiding illusions. Hypnosis is the common tool of past life regression. That mainline social clinical practice treats past life regression therapy as superstition does not seem to affect its popularity.

Brian L. Weiss, MD, the author of *Miracles Happen*, offers four signs of a past life: déjà vu, superreal dreams, unexplained talents and abilities, and the sense of a soul mate. "Through past life regression, Dr. Brian Weiss says it is possible to heal – and grow – your mind, body and soul, as well as strengthen your present-day relationships" (http://www.oprah.com/inspiration/dr-brian-weiss-past-life-regression-therapy-common-signs). As proof of earnestness and effectiveness, Dr. Weiss offers only anecdotes and an appearance on Oprah.

For $200 per session of past life regression therapy, Danielle Garcia provides "guided meditation into a trance like state where past life memories can be accessed. Danielle has the ability to see, sense and fell the client's view during this time, and leads the client through recall that can assist them in their current personal and professional life" (http://www.enchantedforestreiki.com/shop/Past-Life-Regression-Therapy-Session-Las-Vegas-Nevada). Danielle also sells shamanic tools, spiritual candles, crystal prisms, and wind ornaments, pendulums, jewelry, spiritual mists, essences, and oils, stones, dream catchers, wands, and other equipment for soul travel. Danielle practices along with 29 other therapists at the Enchanted Forest Reiki Center in Las Vegas: the Center offers no coherent data documenting outcomes, only testimonials.

It seems that social clinics providing past life regression therapy are about as ubiquitous as psychotherapy, present in just about every state and every sizable city with many outposts in suburban towns and villages. Their Web sites are similar enough to raise issues of plagiary: description of hypnosis-based therapy, claims of successful treatment for the range of emotional problems, relationship between the spiritual and the theory of soul migration, dreamlike truths, and the dangers of going through past life regression with therapists untrained in the specialty. The social clinics of past life regression therapy also offer additional spiritual services. They are often attached to gift shops.

Don Marquis' (1927) *The Lives and Times of Archy & Mehitabel* presents a more convincing testimonial for the reality of the transmigration of souls than anything the past life regression therapists have put forward. You see, Mehitabel the alley cat was once Cleopatra. Her present state is certainly many steps down from her lavish circumstances in ancient Egypt, but she has few regrets, including the absence of past life regression therapy.

> i have had my ups and downs
> but wotthehell wotthehell
> yesterday sceptres and crowns
> fried oysters and velvet gowns
> and today i herd with bums
> but wotthehell wotthehell…
> cage me and i d go frantic
> my life is so romantic
> capricious and corybantic
> and i m toujours gai toujours gai… (no punctuation in original, p. 24)

"Beam Me Up, Scotty"

The fringe of the fringe deserves attention but only because it appears to be popular and to draw considerable clinical attention at least on the Internet. Many clinics have an online presence that offers sessions by email, phone, and Skype. An enormous literature attempts to substantiate the reality of the paranormal including ghosts, poltergeists, unidentified flying objects, and notably extraterrestrials and alien abduction. Alan Boyle, a science editor at NBC News, reports that "surveys consistently indicate that about a third of all adult Americans believe extraterrestrials have visited Earth" (http://www.nbcnews.com/id/3077224/ ns/technology_and_science-science/t/alien-memories-leave-real-scars/#. W47aebgnaUk, September 4, 2018).

> In the classic alien abduction scenario, women are taken from their home, or vehicle by aliens, generally the Grays, to a UFO. Invasive procedures

performed on them that often have to do with removing ova or sperm. A short time later, the women miss their period and report unexplained pregnancies that seem to terminate after 3 months of gestation. Many of these women did not have sex at the time of conception. Physical examination will show that the women were actually pregnant, the pregnancy terminated without explanation or fetal tissue.

A child conceived under these conditions is called a hybrid-human. Later, many of these women report being taken aboard a UFO, being shown a child, told that it was theirs and is part of an experiment to create a more highly evolved race of humans. There may be a need for the child to make an emotional connection with the physical mother if the child is to survive or understand. Some women report returning later and meeting the hybrid child at an older age. These children seem to age rapidly. (http://www.crystalinks.com/removing_fetuses.html, July 16, 2018)

Alien abduction, that is, kidnapping by extraterrestrials, apparently has other unfortunate effects. Post-abduction syndrome (PAS) is similar to post-traumatic stress syndrome (PTSD) but is more difficult to treat. Symptoms of PAS include flashbacks, denial, phobic avoidance, fear, anxiety (http://aliensandchildren.org/, September 4, 2018), as well as many symptoms of trauma—"Insomnia, night sweats, trembling, muscle aches and soreness, muscle twitches, clammy hands, dry mouth, palpitations, dizziness, headaches and migraine, hyperventilation or difficulty breathing, abdominal pain, diarrhea, hypertension, gynecological problems, positive pregnancy tests with unexplainable missing fetuses, unexplainable appearance of strange lesions, scars, bruises, or burns, abdominal tenderness, loss of ovaries, joint or back pain without memory of physical injury" (https://www.mayahypnosis.com/, July 17, 2018) and even unexplained pregnancies (http://exopoliticsjournal. com/vol-3/vol-3-3-Foster.htm, September 4, 2018).

PAS differs from PTSD in that as the abductions may have occurred since early childhood it is difficult to determine precisely when the trauma began as in PTSD where there is a discrete and identifiable traumatic event (http://aliensandchildren.org/post_abduction_syn.htm, September 4, 2018).

Post-abduction syndrome is often treated as a special form of false memory syndrome or post-traumatic stress disorder. Etheric Liberation a Web site originating in the United States is a marketing hub for a multitude of apparently independent therapists including Maya Hypnosis. Unlike Maya Hypnosis, few social clinics in the United States specialize in the treatment of PAS. However, many clinics are open to handling the problem and in addition to post-abduction therapy also offer a variety of New Age and unorthodox therapies including advanced pranic energy healing, pranic crystal healing, practical psychic self-defense, soul retrieval, long-distance vibrational healing, past and future lifetime clearing and healing, psychic surgery, and others (http://ethericliberation.com/, September 4, 2018). After-death communication is also featured as a live possibility (http://www.after-death.com/Pages/About/ADC.aspx) and as a clinical tool (https://thesearchforlifeafterdeath.com/, September 4, 2018).

In addition to post-abduction therapy, Maya Hypnosis also offers hypnotherapy and numerous forms of transpersonal therapy including inner child therapy, progression, Ayurveda ("the science and wisdom of life"), and neuro-linguistic programming. Maya Hypnosis treats post-abduction syndrome as a literal event and not simply a fantasy of delusional patients. "For too many, stories of aliens and abductions are instantly dismissed as hearsay, lies or make believe, but opinion is fast changing" (https://www.mayahypnosis.com/, July 17, 2018).

Citing eminent scientists such as Stephen Hawking, Maya Hypnosis presses the argument that the vastness of the universe compels belief that there exist other intelligent life forms and probably many with technological prowess capable of visiting Earth and experimenting with humans. After all, the absence of any documented visit by an extraterrestrial is not by itself evidence of absence. Indeed, "the Roper Survey (conducted in 1991), suggests that hundreds of thousands, if not millions, of American men, women and children may have experienced abduction or abduction-related phenomena" (ibid.).

The Maya Hypnosis "treatment plan for post-abduction syndrome" lacks specific interventions and duration, containing only promises for relief of symptoms and the achievement of wisdom. Nonetheless, treatment presumably entails hypnosis and the application of one or more forms of transpersonal psychology. No systematic evidence is offered in earnest of effectiveness. Moreover, tests of the clinical value of hypnosis are dubious, often undercut by the demand characteristics of the researchers and the research situation (Orne 1962a, b). All treatments for PAS have failed to demonstrate clinical effectiveness with credible research. Nonetheless, Maya Hypnosis courageously points out that

> Individuals with frequent and intense abduction activity may approach normality, however when activity is intense symptoms of PAS may increase. We will have to determine how often you are abducted to provide you with suitable coping skills (this needs time, discipline, and patience but the out-come will be rewarding and will determine your strengths) (https://www.mayahypnosis.com/, July 17, 2018).

At first blush, the baseless absurdity of these ideas, notably alien abduction and after-death communication, is cause for ridicule. However, the intensity of belief in the paranormal and its popularity testify to the characteristic prevalence of the subjective and surreal in the American civic culture—the ascendancy of emotion over reason. Charlatans have ever taken advantage of American gullibility. However, the predators are less worrisome than the receptivity of the American population to predatory beliefs.

Certain human quirks are merely eccentricities and charming tributes to freedom of expression. Quite possibly, a patient's sincere insistence on having been abducted by space aliens is only a benign form of schizophrenia even when accompanied by unexplained pregnancy. The astute clinician might wisely prescribe play therapy with a consenting adult or refer the patient to an obstetrician.

Ho'oponopono

The search through various cultures for practices that may be clinically valuable for psychological treatment is as legitimate as the search through biodiversity for effective medicines. However, clinical practice imposes an obligation for rigor and objectivity in evaluating the effectiveness of any intervention. Social acceptance does not necessarily impose the same standard unless the intervention comes along with an explicit promise of cure, treatment, or rehabilitation through an institution such as the social clinic that claims scientific evidence of its value. The clinical standard should not be necessary and is not appropriate for cultural practices that entail important ceremonies—not treatments—for purposes of socialization, the setting of normative standards, rites of passage, and the like. The visit to a shaman, divine, minister, self-help guru, tarot card reader, or carnival gazer into the infinitude of a crystal ball is by its social role different than visiting the social clinic for depression, post-traumatic stress disorder, anorexia, or narcissism. The social clinic does not sell itself as ritual but as evidence-tested and proven treatment.

Many cultures have developed folk healing processes of body and mind—"Naikon therapy in Japan, ho'oponopono among native Hawaiians, curanderismo among Latino people, and many of the specific practices within the world's major religions (e.g., meditation, prayer, recognizing blessings, practicing compassion, and helping others)" (Hays 2014, p. 17). However, ho'oponopono—a process of "setting to rights"—is touted for clinical social work practice on grounds that cross-cultural "methods, such as ho'oponopono, *have been successfully used* with clients from other cultures" (emphasis added, Hurdle 2002, p. 183). Ho'oponopono involves four steps to resolve a psychological or personal problem: repentance, forgiveness, gratitude, and love.

Ho'oponopono distills these principles of clearing oneself into a simple, effective practice. You only have control of yourself and it's the leverage point for all change. There really is no "out there" out there. Reality is a subjective experience and our interpersonal interactions are the intermingling of unique worlds. (https://www.feelingoodfeelingreat.com/2016/09/08/how-to-practice-hoopono/, July 9, 2018, n.p.)

Have you heard of the Hawaiian therapist who cured an entire ward of criminally insane patients, without ever meeting any of them or spending a moment in the same room. It's not a joke. The therapist was Dr. Ihaleakala Hew Len. He reviewed each of the patients' files, and then he healed them by healing himself. The amazing results seem like a miracle. But the miracles do happen when you use ho'oponopono, or Dr. Len's up-dated version called Self I-Dentity Through Ho'oponopono....Do you need a miracle? (http://www.laughteronlineuniversity.com/practice-hooponopono-four-simple-steps/, July 9, 2018, n.p.)

Hawaiians are beset with more problems than other citizens of the United States: lower life expectancies, more physical disease, greater poverty and lower incomes, and more psychological and social issues. In 1988, the federal government appropriated funds for Hawaiians to receive "culturally based health care and health education and promotion" that "incorporate traditional Hawaiian values and healing practices" including ho'oponopono (Hurdle, op. cit., p. 187).

Yet Hurdle backs away from claims of effectiveness. "Although no studies have yet identified the precise nature of the effectiveness of the ho'oponopono technique, one can speculate that its basis in the culture and values of Native Hawaiians may enable families to engage in the process in a comfortable manner" (ibid., p. 189). In fact, she does not identify any credible evidence of general effectiveness, let alone the "precise" manner in which it is achieved—no changes in health status, income, life expectancy, and others that are even associated with the practice of ho'oponopono. "In addition, the spiritual component of this process is reflective of the integration of spirituality with healing in many indigenous cultures" (ibid., p. 189). Yes, indeed, and also in the nonindigenous dominant cultures but with similar absence of credible evidence that spirituality is a useful clinical intervention.

Kretzer et al. (2007) tested the ability of a one-half day session of ho'oponopono to lower blood pressure among a group of 23 Asian, Hawaiian, and other Pacific Islanders in Hawaii. Outcomes were small but positive. However, the study did not employ any control but simply took measures before and after the intervention. Thus, there was no ability to discount alternative explanations of the outcome: blood pressure artificially raised by the new procedure; blood pressures naturally declining during the day; group processes that were pleasant and lowered blood pressure; and the expectation of lower blood pressures (the demand characteristics of the research) succeeding. There were no reported follow-up measures.

The fascination with cultural competence in the professions of the social clinic often becomes patronizing. Rather than respect for different ways of doing things, it tends to justify the application of two different standards and perhaps even two different levels of treatment for similar needs. Yet, Chinese folk medicine in the East and the botanica in Latin America make claims of medical cure and not simply social participation; they coexist with modern medical practice as culturally orthodox but medically marginal—unproven and untested through rational means. It is notable that ho'oponopono has many elements of traditional Christian practice and elements of Eastern religion; it is just as notable that religion has not been a consistent broker of peace over the ages but rather a frequent justification of the very atrocities it purports to oppose. Multiculturalism seems often less a plea for tolerance and understanding than mindless enchantment with the strange and the foreign, the psychological counterpart of Orientalism, an acceptance that cheapens human difference. Many who emigrate from savage experiences have become the predatory painted birds of their failed societies, a comment that includes many native-born Americans.

Multicultural practice in the social clinic has spawned the fiction that short-term training in another culture—a course, a brief internship, and a few words in a foreign language—is sufficient to achieve cultural competence. However, true cultural competence implies approximating biculturalism and entails years of acculturation including proficiency in another language. The short course with accompanying text is a walk through stereotypes. Moreover, multicultural sensitivity is probably misplaced on immigrants whose major task should be adaptation not differentiation and preservation of their native mores. Respect for the choices that other people in their native nations make about customs and governance implies the realization that many of those choices are not appropriate for the United States or even in their own societies. Indeed, multiculturalism in the United States often masks unspoken social desires to segregate alien and marginal peoples. In a retreat to cartoon sentimentality, cultural preservation may even be more destructive.

There is an appropriate but also profoundly limited adaptation of multiculturalism to the social clinic. Patients need to be understood both linguistically and contextually in their reference to psychological and social events. These two limited goals are not easily achieved through professional training. They are not soothing fictions but seemingly rare if not unattainable goals. Adaptation can be eased or frustrated by the dominant culture.

Aspiration and Reality

Lilienfeld et al. (2015) insist on separating psychotherapies into two categories—the truly scientific and the pseudoscientific. The intent is to separate effective treatments from "the growing proliferation of questionable and unsupported techniques in clinical psychology"—"to distinguish scientifically unsupported from scientifically supported" practices (p. xxi). Their analyses of fringe interventions are right on the mark: The clinical value of many treatments such as eye movement desensitization and reprocessing, herbal remedies, recovered memory therapies, the host of New Age therapies including thought field therapy, alien abduction therapy, and many others are not sustained by credible science. The problem remains that neither are the so-called supported therapies, notably cognitive behavioral therapy, prolonged exposure, cognitive processing therapy, and others. There are no definitive tests of the effectiveness of psychotherapy. While some therapies are more "evidence-based" than others, all the tests of effectiveness have been undercut by numerous pitfalls. Problems of sample representativeness, measurement bias, blinding, follow-up, attrition, inappropriate controls, the absence of placebo controls, and others bedevil the research. However, the lack of neutrality and independence among the researchers erects the most serious barriers to credible research.

Moreover, Dawes' (1994) contention that psychotherapy is effective but only when practiced by appropriately trained practitioners with doctorates is often contradicted. The Vanderbilt studies and others demonstrate that the level of education of the therapist has little if any effect on patient outcomes (Strupp and Hadley 1979; Smith et al. 1980). At best, psychotherapists are shamans, characters in the drama of society rather than medical or psychic engineers (Frank and Frank 1991). They are the professional beneficiaries of the placebo effects of their patients. The placebo effect is in fact a biological event, yet it may be more reliably generated on grandma's lap than by an expensive practitioner.

It is quite understandable for the desperate and those in psychic and physical pain to seek relief from any source. It is quite another thing for a wealthy, scientifically sophisticated nation to ignore suffering and tolerate if not actually endorse unproven and potentially harmful practices. Yet despite manifest deficiencies, the social clinic and its many forms—mainstream and fringe—grew into prominence in response to popular demands and are sanctioned by widespread use. They comprise an institution of society, a reflection of the beliefs and values of the American public that express the nation's rejection of object coherence and indifference to many pervasive needs of its citizens for more material and effective support. The fringe elements of the social clinic are hardly fads. They have been as persistent as other elements of unconventional practice, often recast with deceptive appreciation as alternative and complementary medical practice.

The exotic, marginal, strange, unorthodox, unconventional, beyond-belief, untested, unproven, unlikely, and surreal are commonly employed in the social clinic. The assumption that professional licensure and public regulation protect citizens from ineffective treatments let alone the potential harms of crackpot cures is patently inaccurate. Many social workers, psychologists, family therapists, and the variety of counselors who practice in social clinics have earned standard academic degrees in programs accredited by recognized agencies. However, many social clinics offer unorthodox interventions that are provided by practitioners both with and without standard degrees. Nonetheless, the differences in pedigree and practice are not matched by differences in therapeutic outcomes or reliance on superstition and bogus science.

There is little difference between the practices of the mainstream social clinic and the fringe social clinic: bogus science vs anti-science, high church vs low church; and liturgical faith vs pietism. Therapeutic practice in both relies on magic, superstition, and other delusions in the history of human thought. Spiritualism, mindfulness, meditation, their offshoots, and other interventions on the fringes and at the center of the social clinical may make patients feel good for a bit but they won't make them well.[2] Rather than clinical, their meaning is mythic—the reconciliation of aspiration with reality. The social clinic in all of its incarnations propagates the soothing fiction that the genesis of individual problems and their solutions lie within the capacities of the individual rather than the circumstances in which people live. Successful treatment requires a compliant act of will. Destiny is a personal responsibility.

References

Baeck, L. (1958). *Judaism and Christianity*. Philadelphia, PA: Jewish Publication Society of America.

Banks, K., Newman, E., & Saleem, J. (2015). An Overview of the Research on Mindfulness-Based Interventions for Treating Symptoms of Posttraumatic Stress Disorder: A Systematic Review. *Journal of Clinical Psychology, 71,* 935–963. https://doi.org/10.1002/jclp.22200tyPress.

Chi, X., Bo, A., Liu, T., Zhang, P., & Chi, I. (2018). Effects of Mindfulness-Based Stress Reduction on Depression in Adolescents and Young Adults: A Systematic Review and Meta-Analysis. *Frontiers in Psychology, 9,* 1–10. https://doi.org/10.3389/fpsyg.2018.01034.

Cramer, H., Anheyer, D., Saha, F. J., & Dobos, G. (2018). Yoga for Posttraumatic Stress Disorder? A Systematic Review and Meta-Analysis. *BMC Psychiatry, 18.* http://dx.doi.org/10.1186/s12888-018-1650-x.

Davidson, R. J., Kabat-Zinn, J., Schumacher, J., Rosenkranz, M., Muller, D., Santorelli, S. F., et al. (2003). Alterations in Brain and Immune Function Produced by Mindfulness Meditation. *Psychosomatic Medicine, 65,* 564–570. https://doi.org/10.1097/01.PSY.0000077505.67574.E3.

Dawes, R. M. (1994). *House of Cards: Psychology and Psychotherapy Built on Myth*. New York, NY: Macmillan.

Derezotes, D. S. (2006). *Spiritually Oriented Social Work Practice*. Boston, MA: Pearson.

Eisenberg, D. M., et al. (1998). Trends in Alternative Medicine Use in the United States, 1990–1997: Results of a Follow-Up National Survey. *JAMA: Journal of the American Medical Association, 280*(18), 1569–1575.

---

[2]This paraphrases a comment in Science News regarding a rigorous evaluation of aromatherapy by Kiecolt-Glaser et al. (2008) (https://www.sciencedaily.com/releases/2008/03/080303093553.htm, July 4, 2018).

Frank, J. D., & Frank, J. B. (1991). *Persuasion and Healing: A Comparative Stuey of Psychotherapy*. Baltimore, MD: Johns Hopkins University Press.

Hays, P. (2014). An International Perspective on the Adaptation of CBT Across Cultures. *Australian Psychologist, 49*, 17–18.

Holden, G., & Barker, K. (2017). Should Social Workers Be Engaged in These Practices? *Journal of Evidence Informed Social Work, 15*(1), 1–13.

Hurdle, D. E. (2002). Native Hawaiian Traditional Healing: Culturally Based Interventions for Social Work Practice. *Social Work, 47*, 183–192.

Kabat-Zinn, J., Wheeler, E., Light, T., Skillings, A., Scharf, M. J., Cropley, T. G., et al. (1998). Influence of a Mindfulness Meditation-Based Stress Reduction Intervention on Rates of Skin Clearing in Patients with Moderate to Severe Psoriasis Undergoing Photo Therapy (UVB) and Photochemotherapy (PUVA). *Psychosomatic Medicine, 60*, 625–632.

Kearney, D. J., et al. (2012). Association of Participation in a Mindfulness Program with Measures of PTSD, Depression and Quality of Life in a Veteran Sample. *Journal of Clinical Psychology, 68*(1), 101–116.

Kiecolt-Glaser, J. K., et al. (2008). Olfactory Influences on Mood and Autonomic, Endocrine, and Immune Function. *Psychoneuroendocrinology, 33*(3), 328–339.

Kretzer, K., et al. (2007). Self Identity Through Ho'oponopono as Adjunctive Therapy for Hypertension Management. *Ethnicity and Disease, 17*(4), 624–628.

Kuyken, W., Taylor, R. S., Barrett, B., Evans, A., Byford, S., Watkins, E., et al. (2008). Mindfulness-Based Cognitive Therapy to Prevent Relapse in Recurrent Depression. *Journal of Consulting and Clinical Psychology, 76*, 966–978. https://doi.org/10.1037/a0013786.

Lee, M. Y., Ng, S., Leung, P. P., & Chan, C. L. (2009). *Integrative Body-Mind-Spirit Social Work: An Empirically Based Approach to Assessment and Treatment*. New York: Oxford University Press.

Lilienfeld, S. O., Lynn, S. J., & Lohr, J. M. (2015). *Science and Pseudoscience in Clinical Psychology*. New York: Guilford Press.

Marquis, D. (1927). *The Lives and Times of Archy & Mehitabel*. Garden City, NY: Doubleday.

Manzoni, G., Pagnini, F., Castelnuovo, G., & Molinari, E. (2008). Relaxation Training for Anxiety: A Ten-Years Systematic Review with Meta-Analysis. *BMC Psychiatry, 8*, 41. https://doi.org/10.1186/1471-244X-8-41.

Moloney, P. (2016). Mindfulness: The Bottled Water of the Therapy Industry. In R. E. Purser, D. Forbes, & A. Burke (Eds.), *Handbook of Mindfulness Culture, Context, and Social Engagement* (pp. 269–292). Cham: Springer.

Orne, M. T. (1962a). Implications for Psychotherapy Derived from Current Research on the Nature of Hypnosis. *The American Journal of Psychiatry, 118,* 1097–1103.

Orne, M. T. (1962b). On the Social Psychology of the Psychological Experiment: With Particular Reference to Demand Characteristics and Their Implications. *American Psychologist, 17,* 776–783. http://dx.doi.org/10.1037/h0043424.

Oxhandler, H. K., & Pargament, K. I. (2018). Measuring Religious and Spiritual Competence Across Helping Professions: Previous Efforts and Future Directions. *Spirituality in Clinical Practice, 5,* 120–132. https://doi.org/10.1037/scp0000149.

Penrod, J. D., Luhrs, C. A., Livote, E. E., Cortez, T. B., & Kwak, J. (2011). Implementation and Evaluation of a Network-Based Pilot Program to Improve Palliative Care in the Intensive Care Unit. *Journal of Pain and Symptom Management, 42,* 668–671. https://doi.org/10.1016/j.jpainsymman.2011.06.012.

Roberts, K. C., & Danoff-Burg, S. (2010). Mindfulness and Health Behaviors: Is Paying Attention Good for You. *Journal of American College Health, 59,* 165–173. https://doi.org/10.1080/07448481.2010.484452.

Rogers, H., & Maytan, M. (2012). *Mindfulness for the Next Generation.* Oxford, NY: Oxford University Press.

Rosenzweig, S., Reibel, D. K., Greeson, J. M., Brainard, G. C., & Hojat, M. (2003). Mindfulness-Based Stress Reduction Lowers Psychological Distress in Medical Students. *Teaching and Learning in Medicine, 15,* 88–92. https://doi.org/10.1207/S15328015TLM1502_03.

Schumer, M. C., Lindsay, E. K., & Creswell, J. D. (2018). Brief Mindfulness Training for Negative Affectivity: A Systematic Review and Meta-Analysis. *Journal of Consulting and Clinical Psychology, 86,* 569–583. https://doi.org/10.1037/ccp0000324.

Shapiro, S. L., Schwartz, G. E., & Bonner, G. (1998). Effects of Mindfulness-Based Stress Reduction on Medical and Premedical Students. *Journal of Behavioral Medicine, 21,* 581–599. https://doi.org/10.1023/A:1018700829825.

Smith, M. L., Glass, G. V., & Miller, T. I. (1980). *The Benefits of Psychotherapy.* Baltimore, MD: Johns Hopkins University Press.

Strupp, H. H., & Hadley, S. W. (1979). Specific vs. Nonspecific Factors in Psychotherapy: A Controlled Study of Outcome. *Archives of General Psychiatry, 36,* 1125–1136. http://dx.doi.org/10.1001/archpsyc.1979.01780100095009.

Travis, F., & Arenander, A. (2004). EEG Asymmetry and Mindfulness Meditation. *Psychosomatic Medicine, 66,* 147–152.

Wolf, D. B., & Abell, N. (2003). Examining the Effects of Meditation Techniques on Psychosocial Functioning. *Research on Social Work Practice, 13,* 27–42. https://doi.org/10.1177/104973102237471.

Part IV

Clinic and Society

11

Soothing Fictions

…The only means of fighting a plague is *common decency.* —Camus, *The Plague*

The social clinic fails to achieve its goals of treatment—cure, prevention or rehabilitation—for mental, emotional and attitudinal problems, or behavioral change. The social clinic and its community of scholars are less scientific and practical than hypocritical—obedient, intuitive, and mystical, avowing commitment to scientific truth but avoiding its obligations. The debased scholarship of the social clinic, lacking definitive tests of practice, suggests a guild mentality of loyalty to practice rather than to credible objectivity, that is, science.

The vast landscape of the social clinic is strewn with dead trees: psychotherapy, in particular, treatments for depression, trauma, addiction, and others; clinical social work's efforts at child welfare including foster care and family reunification as well as its historic failures of institutional care, home visiting, differential diagnosis, casework, charity societies, settlement houses and many others; community psychological treatments for chronic mental conditions; criminal rehabilitation; and clinical interventions at the fringes of propriety and credulity to handle emotional and social problems with MarieEl therapy, past life therapy, post-abduction syndrome therapy, Reiki, and others.

© The Author(s) 2019
W. M. Epstein, *Psychotherapy and the Social Clinic in the United States,*
https://doi.org/10.1007/978-3-030-32750-7_11

The distortions of clinical practice stem from crucial misrepresentations and spectral proofs of its vast literature that mask the ineffectiveness of the interventions—a consistent absence of independent and neutral researchers, reliance on subjective measures of outcomes, and inadequate funding and oversight of outcome tests. In fact, the field persists in the curious situation of studying phenomena that it cannot accurately measure—as though a physicist was studying heat without a thermometer. Put differently, the social clinic is market driven in the same way as the breakfast cereal industry, by consumer satisfaction rather objective value—the antithesis of the values of a modern profession. The social clinic defines an introverted commercial sector that contributes little to the civic culture. Yet it reflects in its narrow self-interest the mores of the society that have protected the sloganeering of free market individualism.

The social clinic exists as a form of social denial in two senses. In one sense, it denies the gravity of social problems by insisting that they emerge from individual moral failure—bad choices—for which the individual bears primary responsibility. In the second sense, the social clinic exists to deny access to sufficient resources to repair the consequences of society's systemic inequalities. After all, if individual responsibility is at the root of social problems, then providing resources to miscreants would simply encourage their behavior. In this spirit, the social clinic acts as an inexpensive but inadequate substitute for basic social supports, a choice that the culture has made.

In contrast with the social clinic, the universal provision of basic services—childcare, education, retirement income, health care but also personal social services of caring and support—and unconditioned by income tests sidesteps stigma and class judgments by broadening the rights of citizenship. Adequate incomes to assure that people can purchase sufficient food, clothing, and housing avoid isolating recipients from the shared culture. With each use, services intended for the poor such as Meals on Wheels, food shelters, public welfare, or even the secondhand merchandise of Goodwill Industries reinforce blame, shame, and personal failure while endorsing inequality. It is quite to the point that recipients of Supplemental Security Income, a discretionary welfare program, often prefer to speak of receiving social security insurance, a nondiscretionary program.

The social clinic has long persisted without true clinical utility. It offers other benefits, notably promotion of the American ethos of extreme individualism and personal responsibility that displace social responsibility and the sense of shared destiny. The social clinic is the material realization of the falsehood that the consequences of long-standing institutional deprivations are easily repaired through the brief, episodic enchantments of talk therapy.

Enduring and prevalent soothing fictions are not usually the deliberate lies and propaganda of a manipulative leadership acting to thwart the popular will nor are they innocent and meaningless meanders of social taste. Most often, they express a society's priority values. In this light, the soothing fictions of the American social clinic are the result of broad consent—knowing and popular expression of embedded cultural values. They are frequently promulgated by accommodating professionals in defiance of their obligations for truth. Soothing fictions that mask, soften, and justify harsh, even predatory, social choices are hardly new.

Western imperialism and colonialism in the third world were packaged in noble ideals. Lugard (1922) describes the beneficence of colonialism well.

The condition of Africa when Europe entered the continent…was deplorable…. It was the task of civilization to put an end to slavery, to establish Courts of Law, to inculcate in the natives a sense of individual responsibility, of liberty, and of justice, and to teach their rulers how to apply these principles; above all, to see to it that the system of education should be such as to produce happiness and progress. I am confident that the verdict of history will award high praise to the efforts and the achievements of Great Britain in the discharge of these great responsibilities. For, in my belief, under no other rule – be it of his own uncontrolled potentates, or of aliens – does the African enjoy such a measure of freedom and of impartial justice, or a more sympathetic treatment, and for that reason I am a profound believer in the British Empire and its mission in Africa. (Lugard 1922, p. 5)

Lugard then quotes Article 22 of the Covenant of the League of Nations in support of the "task of civilization."

> The best method of giving practical effect to this principle is that the tutelage of such peoples should be entrusted to advanced nations who, by reason their resources, their experience, or their geographical position, can best undertake this responsibility and who are willing to accept it... (Lugard 1922, p. 65)
>
> It has been well said that a nation, like an individual, must have some task higher than the pursuit of material gain, it is to escape the benumbing influence of parochialism and to fulfil its higher destiny. If high standards are maintained, the control of subject races must have an effect on national character which is not measurable in terms of material profit and loss. (ibid., p. 58)
>
> The merchant, the miner, and the manufacturer do not enter the tropics on sufferance, or employ their technical skill, their energy, and their capital as "interlopers," or as "greedy capitalists," but in fulfilment of the Mandate of civilization. America, since she became a world Power, has adopted the same standards in the Philippines. (ibid., p. 61)

The justification for the "control of subject races" and the "mandate of civilization" apparently lies in the presumed deficiencies of subject races.

> [Africans] vary in their mental and physical characteristics according to the amount of negro blood in their veins, which has shown itself extremely potent in assimilating alien strains to its own type. Perhaps the most distinctive external characteristic – much more reliable than that of colour – by which the degree of negro blood may be gauged, is the hair growth on the head and face... (ibid., p. 670)
>
> In character and temperament, the typical African of this race-type is a happy, thriftless, excitable person, lacking in self-control, discipline, and foresight, naturally courageous, and naturally courteous and polite, full of personal vanity, with little sense of veracity, fond of music, and "loving weapons as an oriental loves jewelry." His thoughts are concentrated on the events and feelings of the moment, and he suffers little from apprehension for the future, or grief for the past. "His mind,' says Sir C. Eliot, "is far nearer to the animal world than that of the European or Asiatic,

and exhibits something of the animal's placidity and want of desire to rise beyond the state he has reached," – in proof of which he cites the lack of decency in the disposal of the dead, the state of complete nudity common to one or other, or to both sexes among so many tribes, and the general (though not universal) absence of any feeling for art (other than music), and the nomadic habits of so large a section of the races. (ibid., p. 69)

In brief, the virtues and the defects of this race-type are those of attractive children, whose confidence when once it has been won is given ungrudgingly as to an older and wiser superior, without question and without envy.... But speaking generally, the characteristics of the predominantly negro races, as I have described them...extends...to the West Indies and the Southern States of America. (ibid., p. 70)

They gave a fascination of their own, for we are dealing with the child races of the world and learning at first hand the habits and customs of primitive man; not of some derelict and decadent remnant such as the aborigines of Australia, the Todas of Indiak or the Ainus of the Japanese islands, but of a virile and expanding race whose men are often models of symmetry and strength....

These demulsifiers seem harsh and raucous to modern ears but weren't then. Rather they stated the pervasive assumptions of Europe toward preindustrial peoples that moralized the obligations of wealthy nations to promote civilization to the presumably *willfully* uncivilized. They also obscured the economic exploitation of imperialism and the often harsh rule of colonialism.

Lugard rarely refers to the economic gains of the imperial European states from their control over colonies. He avoids any mention of political repression and the repeated atrocities perpetrated by the colonists to sustain their control. Yet many former colonies have freely chosen to maintain ties of culture.

Conrad's *The Heart of Darkness*, sometimes interpreted as a fierce criticism of colonialism, actually voices the author's racist and ethnocentric beliefs and Europe's exculpatory notions of imperialism that Lugard systematizes in his administrative manifesto. Conrad lamented that the ideals of the imperial mission to spread western civilization to primitives and heathens were perverted by Kurtz. Conrad's genius lay in the ability to write a dense, often opaque novel that has been interpreted in diametrically opposite fashions yet rises to the level of a literary classic (Kimbrough 1988).

The US adventures in third world empire building were also paired with the ideals of a noble mission. They continue into the present with episodic foreign policy goals of nation building that often degenerate into free market imperialism, anti-communist hysteria, and realpolitik military support of tyranny more often than peaceful economic and social development for third world citizens.

The irony of third world liberation lies in the fact that much of post-colonial nationalism in developing nations, their own soothing fiction, has often been as bad if not worse than the years of cruel paternalism under a European thumb. As examples, surely the British were not responsible for the butchery of the partition between India and Pakistan that began in 1947 during which as many as two million were slaughtered. No nation except perhaps Holland in the Congo ruled with the bloodlust of Idi Amin. Spain never presided over a civil conflict in South America that killed perhaps 500,000 in Columbia or ruled with the ruthlessness of various tyrannies in Argentina, Chile, or Central America. The former colonies all justified their wars of liberation in terms of self-determination but then went on to implement regimes of slaughter that made many of the former imperial rulers seem beneficent by comparison. The tribalism of much of the world competes at barbarity with the greed of industrial nations.

Kapuscinski's (1992) comment about newly liberated Algeria was also intended for the rest of postcolonial Africa.

Each [new leader and new regime] wants to do something good and begins to do it and then sees, after a month, after a year, after three years, that it just isn't happening, that it is slipping away, that it is bogged down in the sand. Everything is in the way: the centuries of backwardness, the primitive economy, the illiteracy, the religious fanaticism, the tribal blindness, the chronic hunger, the colonial past with its practice of debasing dulling the conquered, the blackmail by the imperialists, the greed of the corrupt, the unemployment, the red ink. Progress comes with great difficulty along such a road. The politician begins to push too hard. He looks for a way out through dictatorship. The dictatorship then fathers an opposition. The opposition organizes a coup. And the cycle begins anew. (ibid., p. 106)

The domestic record of the United States is similarly darkened by recurrent departures from humane policies: centuries of slavery without the apology of a sincere Reconstruction followed by yet another century of de jure apartheid; continuing racism, sexism, and ethnocentricity that seems to encourage widespread sectarianism at the price of progressive democracy; the slaughter, displacement, and victimization of Native Americans; the Devil in Massachusetts pursued with the bloodthirsty zeal of religious purity; lynching, false imprisonment, convict leasing; vigilantism; popular demagoguery conspicuously including Andrew Jackson, Huey Long, Father Coughlin, senators Bilbo, Long, McCarran, Stennis, and many of their colleagues; eugenics and forced lobotomies; the internment of Japanese Americans during World War II (but not German Americans or Italian Americans)—all building in some fashion to the enormous unaddressed inequality of contemporary society and the renewal of racial, ethnic, and economic segregation—the rough beast reborn.

Yet these barbarities and others have been successfully masked, excused, and propagated by popular demulsifiers drawn over time from the prevailing national ethos: white superiority, eugenics, states' rights, salvation, volunteerism, charity, social growth, progress, manifest destiny, diversity, multiculturalism, affirmative action, entrepreneurship, free markets, self-determination, self-reliance, self-help, self-invention, self-actualization, individual responsibility, and an ethos of individualism that implies heroic action, moral hazards, helping, social treatment, voluntary good works, and, repeatedly, some form of America First. And still, belief in genetic dominance over behavior persists in academia and popular belief. Demulsifies such as white superiority and heroic individualism are patently false. Others have a factual plausibility but exert an influence, or better said, represent a social preference far beyond their narrow applicability to limited situations. They are all slogans—soothing fictions—that ratify current arrangements and their implicit values.

Jefferson Davis (1881), the President of the Confederate States of America, justified slavery and racial inequality on grounds of inherent inferiority, states' rights as "sovereign communities" protected by the US Constitution, and the benefits of localism. He even minimized the culpability for slavery in the United States since "the importation of slaves into the United States continued to be carried on by northern merchants and Northern ships, without interference in the traffic from any quarter, until it was prohibited by the spontaneous action of the Southern States themselves" (p. 9)—as though the South had acted on humanitarian motives. At a minimum, Davis simply acknowledges the national consistency of racial prejudice.

Davis' "lost cause" has persisted into the present with broad support often exercising decisive influence. Madison Grant's 1916 (2017) justification of white superiority, Rushton's pseudoscience of race, the eugenics movement notably supported by Nobel Laureate William Shockley (Shurkin 2006), Kennedy and Kennedy's (2014) *The South Was Right*, Herrnstein and Murray's *The Bell Curve*, and many others tirelessly sustain the American class and caste system and the resurgent populism of white privilege. These perennially common publications voice the soothing fictions of a savage civic fundamentalism embedded in American politics and society.

In modern, wealthy America and continuous for many decades into the present, economic growth itself remains the noble national endeavor that justifies the sacrifices, and deprivations of poorer and working-class populations—the deferment of redistributive policies in order to preserve investment in an often unrealized economic bounty, a perpetually invoked just-savings principle that mocks John Rawls' (1999) intent. Ever greater economic growth with an implied dividend to be shared democratically has long been widely accepted as the solution to social malaise and economic inequalities not just poverty itself. Yet since the 1970s and during numerous previous decades, economic growth has been accumulated largely by the wealthiest while future economic growth seems unlikely to occur at levels to produce any sort of shared bounty (Gordon 2017). Nonetheless, the nation still maintains a near hermetic attachment to economic growth that denies the reality of limited resources. After all, the acceptance of a future of low growth would imply government action to repair inequalities and other social problems through greater public welfare strategies. Those strategies entail greatly increased public redistributions of income and wealth to supplement lower incomes, to invest in the marketable skills of citizens through intense education and work preparation of one sort or another and to provide the ancillary social supports that are required for successful participation in work.

The United States like other economically advanced nations is so wealthy that greater economic growth by itself is unlikely to solve many problems. Indeed, more intense industrialization and thus more environmental degradation and climate change are likely to create serious challenges to cultural survival and human health. Even worse, the demulsifier of economic growth, monotonously tied to entrepreneurship in the United States, masks the more primitive and rebarbative social motives that have contributed greatly to increased inequalities as well as to stagnant social and economic mobility. As a soothing fiction, economic growth perpetuates the class rigidities and unspoken bigotries that have poisoned American social history.

In turn, the social clinic, especially because of its often undue emphasis on work participation and self-help for its patients, has purveyed many of these soothing fallacies and with obvious popular consent. The insistence on work participation is pressed as though drudgery and inadequate pay were somehow liberating from sin and capable of ending social isolation while securing full participation in the culture. These are not hypocrisies of the society but rather core values—the romantic beliefs that defy logic in the progress toward a coherent society. They are soothing fictions of American stratification that supply the mythic endorsements of the nation's refusal to adopt an ethos of shared destiny.

Contemporary American society has softened and refashioned Lugard's prose and largely rejected racial, ethnic, and gender slights at least in public discourse. Yet its assumptions about those in need worked out through the soothing fictions of contemporary belief simply update Lugard's rhetoric. Nonetheless, the soothing fictions still powerfully affirm contemporary beliefs in the moral deficiencies of poorer and marginal citizens and thus sustain inadequate social welfare provisions including the social clinic as well as popular belief in the correctness of the nation's social and economic inequalities. Yet attributing the denigration of those in need as normal primitives—self-indulgent, cunning, lazy, inattentive, foolish, undisciplined, and unproductive—to an ascendant conservative ideology misses the broader popularity of romantic thought that has also captured the heart of even American liberals (Swigert and Farrell 1977; Epstein 2017). Kurtz was a Peace Corps volunteer gone rogue. The mission was okay; the personnel unfortunate.

Diversity and multiculturalism are soothing fictions of sectarianism, philanthropy, and tolerance that sanitize the "volksgemeinshaft" of the American people. "Volksgemeinshaft," literally "people's community," justified the Nazi reign of terror. They engineered political solidarity by promoting an ecstatic certitude in the biological, intellectual, and cultural superiority of the German people. They invented then slaughtered enemies of the nation and threats to the racial purity of the German "volk"—in particular Jews but also the Roma, the intellectually, physically, and mentally impaired, gays, and others often including political dissidents. More broadly "volksgemeinshaft" entails an emotional fundamentalism—an ecstatic seeking of oblivious communion, a mindless pursuit of transcendent oneness that arouses nationalism, tribalism, ethnocentricity, and other fanatical fantasies of social, genetic, religious, and economic superiority. The raptures of "volksgemeinshaft" provoked some of the worst collective savageries of human history that were intensified and militarized with stunning depravity during the twentieth century. As the exculpating virtue of mythic specialness, "Volksgemeinshaft" constitutes the core of multiculturalism and diversity in contemporary America encouraging each group to enjoy the pleasures of bigotry and exceptionalism. Extreme individualism perversely merges into group identity nurturing self-invention but only within the narrow tolerances of promoting tribal solidarity.

The social choice of loyalties within a politics of sectarian competition among race, ethnicity, region, gender, and sex obstructs the broader vision of a just and humane society to address needs across different and fluid communities and identities. The premise of the just society holds that no group is safe unless all are safe. An open civic culture lures people away from tribalism into an open, tolerant civic culture that protects the actual protean, fluid, and multiple roles that people perform;

unitary, dominating identities become rare and strange. However, if "sectarianism is utterly incompatible with social democracy" (Margalit 2017), then the beacon of civilization has dimmed in the United States.

Unlike the high drama of imperialism and efforts at colonizing weaker peoples, the role of the social clinic in the United States is at best marginally concerned with control since its programs and interventions are near-universally ineffective. Rather the social clinic performs deep ceremonies of citizenship that affirm the nation's romantic ideals. The domestic stability it reinforces—defining the obligations and rewards of citizenship—goes far to explain the broad satisfaction with the nation's economic and social stratification. The social clinic implements in its minimalism of service the nation's embrace of an extreme form of individual responsibility.

Rather than providing material support, the social clinic customarily offers encouragement to achieve independence through a variety of treatments. Its basic tenet holds that independence results from inner strength rather than as a result of social investment. Superior people who are able to summon up the internal magic of self-reliance succeed; inferior people without the will to overcome fail. It is not the performance that is rated but the performer who receives a summary moral judgment that implicates them in their own problems. Through the romantic logic of self-invention, failure justifies want and relieves social policy of obligations for relief. The successful are chosen by God and Darwin to the extent of their success. However, heroic individualism and its assumption of independence from society are themselves profound fallacies—soothing fictions.

> As the mantra goes, every hardworking soul can prove his or her worth in America. Everyone can climb out of the underclass and pass on that good fortune to his or her happy heirs. The flip side of the oft-told tale of mobility, what ennobling biography and autobiography cover up and Americans are loath to admit, is the fact that it is a mythic promise, a lure, a lie. For every Franklinesque tale, there are millions of Americans who can't get their feet as high as the second rung of the social ladder, which is broken for most outside of a highly unrepresentative minority – the educated elite. (Isenberg 2018, p. 16)

The absence of a credible clinical record of achievement is sufficient evidence that the propagation of myth is the essential role of the social clinic. At best, the social clinic acts as one of society's scolds along with organized religion and the self-help industry. At worst, it sanctions obedience to social norms within the sterile confines of American stratification. It is less a social welfare program than a church of the civic religion, less causative of the social order than a materialization of American belief. Certainly, from one point of view this role is a wonder of Americanism. From a different perspective, it travels the Congo River into the nation's heart of darkness—the society's inhumanity, the normalized primitiveness of its own citizens.

The gifts of genius and brilliance that drive innovation exist at all levels of society; American stratification is only economic and social; it fails to represent a meritocracy of effort, capacity, or achievement. The promise of many remains unrealized without nurturing and support. The United States has overinvested in already indulged populations. The cost of their productivity is excessive; they have not achieved enough nor contributed enough to justify their wealth. Yet the majority of Americans have been deprived of appropriate investment in their capacities with unfortunate consequences for the United States.

> Lack of support can stunt prospects for potential geniuses; they never get the chance to be productive… People born into poverty or oppression don't get a shot at working toward anything other than staying alive. (Kalb 2017, pp. 48–49)

Yet genius and brilliance are rare and inadequate by themselves to cultivate a humane society. The goal of a just and amiable society is frustrated by denying all citizens adequate resources to develop their abilities and amplify their contributions to society. Steps to a more humane society might begin by replacing the romantic demulsifier of self-invention with recognition that social support—education, wages, family and community assistance, nutrition and health care, and surrogates for other failed social institutions—determines individual outcomes. The exaggerated respect for private wealth in the United States has frustrated public purposes.

The Dream and the Promise

The American dream depends on the American promise of a decent civic culture: free speech, equal application of the law, and most important the constant responsibility seated in government to monitor and reduce great social and economic inequalities. In a democracy that cherishes merit, the government's permanent role in redistribution is necessary to protect against the tyranny of the successful. Democratic meritocracy is far more desirable than democratic populism with its constant threat of mob rule and its tendency to violate human rights.

The American promise of opportunity requires more than the absence of a predatory, coercive negation of liberty. It also requires Isaiah Berlin's (1969) positive liberty, the tools to take advantage of an open society. A full life enriched by contributions to family, community, and the civic culture takes an enormous amount of individual preparation that is often supplied naturally by families and communities but still requires the support of near universal services such as public education. Surrogates for these institutions are necessary to address their frequent failures and absence. However, the expense of provisions for failed families and communities can be enormous, and the American public has largely refused to foot the bill for supportive and surrogate care to prevent individual problems or to handle them when they emerge. American society has typically preferred the social clinic to well-funded schools, adequate foster care, full employment, universal health and mental health care, universal day care for children, and comprehensive institutions for those who cannot take care of themselves in less restrictive community settings. The social clinic, that should provide or administer social care, does not. Rather it enacts a rationale for neglect.

The value of social care as an alternative to the social clinic is repeatedly suggested in the social service literature but rarely directly addressed. Indeed, the caring function is often the unacknowledged but necessary condition of the rare instances of successful treatment. The effectiveness of "training in community living" in Wisconsin (Stein and Test 1980a, b) depended on the enormous voluntary efforts of families to provide supportive day-to-day care in addition to the services of highly trained and motivated professionals. Without willing families, it is unlikely this demonstration in the deinstitutionalization of schizophrenics would have succeeded.

The Harlem Children's Zone, a New York City charter school that enrolled poor minority students, provided exceptional schooling and was able to close the black/white educational achievement gap. It created an extraordinarily enriched learning environment with gifted, dedicated teachers and administrators that cost nearly twice as much as the average for New York City students. Yet its lottery system for enrollment assured that the children came from families that were sufficiently motivated to seek out superior schooling; they were apparently more willing than many to assure that the efforts of teachers and the learning environment of the school were carried over into the home. The costs of compensating for negligent parents would greatly increase the already large costs of the Harlem Children's Zone. It is also not clear that a sufficient number of similarly skilled and motivated teachers exist to staff out sufficient replications of the program (Yeh 2013).

Van der Kolk's (2015) argument that recovery from post-traumatic stress requires extended care within a safe and supportive community requires much greater costs than the customary short-term and ineffective psychotherapeutic treatments. Quite unusual, Van der Kolk, a psychiatrist, pressed the need for supportive care against an acknowledged backdrop of failed psychotherapeutic interventions.

Boys Town is much more expensive than the customary public foster care placement for children, but it comes much closer to fulfilling expectations to provide a decent environment for children without parents. Unfortunately, in order to qualify for public reimbursement, it seems forced to consider itself a treatment program rather than a long-term care program with the effect of returning many of its wards after a year or so to the abusive conditions that sent them to Boys Town in the first place. First published in 1908, Lucy Maud Montgomery's immensely popular novel *Ann of Green Gables* captures the social ideal of what an orphan deserves in a caring culture: loving substitute parents and a supportive community. These two conditions are provided neither by public foster care nor routinely by charitable substitutes. They are very expensive to purchase.

The clubhouse model and Fairweather Lodges that care for the seriously mentally ill apparently reach many of their goals but only for a small portion of those who would benefit from the programs (McKay et al. 2018). However, clubhouses do not have the resources to routinely offer housing for the homeless nor can they provide care for the very debilitated. Housing and a more controlled environment—two crucial elements of care and notably with an eye toward addressing homelessness—increase the cost of community mental health services substantially.

Other rare clues sustain the necessity of care. Kirigin et al. (1982) and Chamberlain and Reid (1998) suggest that the long-term provision of safe and supportive environments, rather than therapy, reduces criminal recidivism and is probably necessary for the successful socialization and resocialization of people. Palpacuer et al. (2016) hint at the possibility that a caring environment rather than psychotherapy is a defining condition of recovery from depression. Stanton and Shadish (1997) offer inklings that the degree of previous experience in a supportive family or community may predict recovery from addiction, a conclusion implicit in Hari's notion of reconnecting addicts; reconnecting addicts to the society as a feature of rehabilitation seems likely only if they had prior experience as connected.

The successful demonstrations tacitly assume, often incorrectly, that they are broadly representative of the common situations of need and service. Thus, they fail to include cost estimates to compensate for voluntary support when it must be purchased for recipients without family or substitutes for family. The necessity of long-term, high-quality special relationships among people seems also to be intuitively true. Successful socialization and its successful continuation depend on an enormous amount of time and money contributed by family and community. Indeed, more than any other factor, the caring function of deep social investments seems coincidental with middle-class economic and social achievements.

Instead, the nation substitutes the desultory interventions of the social clinic for deep social investment. The problem is exacerbated by the seeming reality that American society and its embedded economic inequalities tear at family and community, creating ever greater needs for compensatory care and notably for children.

Inspired by Smail, Feltham, and Moloney along with the critical psychology movement in England, the reformers tried but failed to define an alternative clinical practice. Becker's (1976) applied philosophy came closest but he never promised effectiveness. It was justified only as a point of civic equality that at a variety of times in life, everyone should have the opportunity of guided self-reflection to consider their role in life, society, and the cosmos. Yet the opportunity for everyone to explore their behavior at different points in life with a wise, patient, and nonjudgmental counsel, even while it has little chance of inducing large changes or perhaps even small ones in problem behavior, is at least a ceremony of great respect for the individual. Nonetheless, without the more material expressions of greater equality the practice of applied philosophy becomes simply another demulsifying detour into insensible denial.

The social clinic is a dream of order akin to nationalism, colonialism, tribalism, free markets, economic growth, autocracy, and the fallacies of social prejudice and political tyranny that are typically wrapped up in the propaganda of their unique soothing fictions. Huxley warned that the impulse to create visions of rationality and order—intellectual art that brings about "tyranny…monsters, and violence" (1948, p. 9)—also creates barbarism. The ruthless pursuit of goodness through religion, politics, the social clinic, and private behaviors generally is not good at all but rather a screen for the selfishness of a mean-spirited society.

[Gandhi] who believed only in people got himself involved in the subhuman mass-madness of nationalism, in the would-be superhuman, but actually diabolic, institutions of the nation-state. He got himself involved in these things, imagining that he could mitigate the madness and convert what was satanic in the state to something like humanity. But nationalism and the politics of power had proved too much for him. (ibid., p. 8)

In offering ineffective assistance in pursuit of the impossible goals of heroic individualism and self-invention, the social clinic commits the irremissible civic sins of willful ignorance, unconcern, blame, and scapegoating that belie the promise of the United States. The psychologically troubled, the socially marginal, and the economically needy become trapped in perpetual self-accusation. Even worse, it is done with popular consent.

The United States is wealthy enough to assure the basics and then a lot more to fulfill its promise—crucially and fundamentally, education at levels to assure an American workforce sufficient for its economic needs and adequate to create an informed, literate, and even sharing citizenry. But also and necessarily, the American promise includes a floor under income, assured housing, health and mental health care, family supports (respite care, paid parental leave, and childcare), and community services including recreation, access to the arts, and opportunities for political, social, and civic participation. If American society expects people to behave well and sustain its ideals, then it needs to treat its citizens well. Wisdom lies in seeding fertile, unplowed soil—the deprived, marginalized, and needy American masses. Yet none of this is possible within the current social ethos of the United States.

References

Becker, E. (1976). *Denial of Death* (2nd ed.). New York, NY: Macmillan.

Berlin, I. (1969). Two Concepts of Liberty. In I. Berlin (Ed.), *Four, Essays on Liberty*. London: Oxford University Press.

Chamberlain, P., & Reid, J. B. (1998). Comparison of Two Community Alternatives to Incarceration for Chronic Juvenile Offenders. *Journal of Consulting and Clinical Psychology, 66,* 624–633. https://doi.org/10.1037/0022-006X.66.4.624.

Davis, J. (1881). *The Rise and Fall of the Confederate Government.* Pantianos Classics.

Epstein, W. M. (2017). *The Masses Are the Ruling Classes: Policy Romanticism, Democratic Populism, and Social Welfare.* New York, NY: Oxford University Press.

Grant, M. (2017 [1916]). *The Passing of the Great Race.* Eastford, CT: Martino Fine Books.

Gordon, R. J. (2017). *The Rise and Fall of Economic Growth: The US Standard of Living Since the Civil War*. Princeton, NJ: Princeton University Press.

Huxley, A. (1948). *Ape and Essence*. New York, NY: Harper.

Isenberg, N. (2018, June 28). Left Behind. *New York Review of Books*. https://www.pressreader.com/usa/the-new-york-review-of-books/20180628/282492889545431.

Kalb, K. (2017). Genius. *National Geographic Magazine*, pp. 48–49.

Kapuscinski, R. (1992). *The Soccer War*. New York: Vintage.

Kennedy, J. R., & Kennedy, W. D. (2014). *The South Was Right Gretna*. Louisiana: Pelican Publishing.

Kimbrough, R. (1988). *Joseph Conrad: Heart of Darkness*. New York: Norton.

Kirigin, K. A., Braukmann, C. J., Atwater, J. D., & Wolf, M. M. (1982). An Evaluation of Teaching-Family (Achievement Place) Group Homes for Juvenile Offenders. *Journal of Applied Behavior Analysis, 15*(1), 1–16. https://doi.org/10.1901/jaba.1982.15-1.

Lugard, F. (1922). *The Dual Mandate in British Tropical Africa*. London: William Blackwood and Sons.

Margalit, A. (2017). *On Betrayal*. Cambridge, MA: Harvard University Press.

McKay, C., et al. (2018). Systematic Review of Evidence for the Clubhouse Model of Psychosocial Rehabilitation. *Administration and Policy in Mental Health and Mental Health Services Administration, 45*(1), 28–47. https://doi.org/10.1007/s10488-016-0760-3.

Palpacuer, C., Gallet, L., Drapier, D., Reymann, J., Falissard, B., & Naudet, F. (2016). Specific and Non-specific Effects of Psychotherapeutic Interventions for Depression: Results from a Meta-Analysis of 84 Studies. *Journal of Psychiatric Research, 87,* 95–104. https://doi.org/10.1016/j.jpsychires.2016.12.015.

Rawls, J. (1999). *A Theory of Justice*. Cambridge, MA: Harvard University Press.

Shurkin, J. N. (2006). *Broken Genius: The Rise and Fall of William Shockley, Creator of the Electronic Age*. New York: Palgrave Macmillan.

Stanton, M., & Shadish, W. R. (1997). Outcome, Attrition, and Family-Couples Treatment for Drug Abuse: A Meta-Analysis and Review of the Controlled, Comparative Studies. *Psychological Bulletin, 122,* 170–191. https://doi.org/10.1037/0033-2909.122.2.170.

Stein, L. I., & Test, M. A. (1980a). Alternative to Mental Hospital Treatment. I. Conceptual Model, Treatment Program, and Clinical Evaluation. *Archives of General Psychiatry, 37,* 409–412.

Stein, L. I., & Test, M. A. (1980b). Alternative to Mental Hospital Treatment. III. Social Cost. *Archives of General Psychiatry, 37,* 409–412.

Swigert, V. L., & Farrell, R. A. (1977). Normal Homicides and the Law. *American Sociological Review, 42,* 16–32.

Van der Kolk, B. (2015). *The Body Keeps the Score: Brain, Mind, and Body in the Healing of Trauma.* New York, NY: Penguin Books.

Yeh, S. S. (2013). A Re-analysis of the Effects of KIPP and the Harlem Promise Academies. *Teachers College Record, 115.*

Afterword

Global warming will be calamitous; it will deplete national wealth, productive capacity, and land. It will create unimaginable competition over basic necessities. American society will be forced to adapt quickly. Along with other nations, it will face the choice of sharing or restricting protections and resources among its citizens—being broadly generous and accepting or imposing stringent standards of worth.

The democratic barbarism of contemporary American life cherishes each citizen's separate myth of creation and their long struggle for unique cultural virtue. The broad popularity of multicultural segregation deposes a nurturing, protective civic culture—the promise of America—and rekindles the flames of nationalism and bigotry with the combustible narcotic, the soothing fiction of "volksgemeinshaft" for all: the supreme righteousness and superiority of everyone over everyone else.

The social clinic in the United States is a bleak omen of civic intent. It recalls Camus' worst sense of the plague: to live through civic indifference in which each person "bears the load of his troubles alone" (p. 69). If the plague of isolating individualism and greed continues in America, then this experiment in democracy will choke on unbreathable air, drown in rising oceans, and provoke the rough beast of prejudice, strife, and slaughter.

No one is safe unless all are safe.

© The Editor(s) (if applicable) and The Author(s), under exclusive license to Springer Nature Switzerland AG 2019
W. M. Epstein, *Psychotherapy and the Social Clinic in the United States*, https://doi.org/10.1007/978-3-030-32750-7

References

Abrams, M. H. (1953). *The Mirror and the Lamp*. New York: Oxford University Press.

Addams, J. (1938). *Twenty Years at Hull-House*. New York, NY: Macmillan.

Addams, J. (1998 [1923]). *Twenty Years at Hull-House*. New York: Penguin Books.

Ahola, P., et al. (2017). Effects of Scheduled Waiting for Psychotherapy in Patients with Major Depression. *Journal of Nervous and Mental Disease, 205*(8), 611–617.

Al, C. M., Stams, G. J., Bek, M. S., Damen, E. M., Asscher, J. J., & Van der Laan, P. H. (2012). A Meta-Analysis of Intensive Family Preservation Programs: Placement Prevention and Improvement of Family Functioning. *Children and Youth Services Review, 34,* 1472–1479. https://doi.org/10.1016/j.childyouth.2012.04.002.

Alexander, J. F., & Parsons, B. V. (1973). Short-Term Behavioral Intervention with Delinquent Families: Impact on Family Process and Recidivism. *Journal of Abnormal Psychology, 81,* 219–225. https://doi.org/10.1037/h0034537.

Allen-Meares, P. (2013, May 8, 2018). School Social Work. *Encyclopedia of Social Work*. http://dx.doi.org/10.1093/acrefore/9780199975839.013.351.

Amato, L., Minozzi, S., Davoli, M., & Vecchi, S. (2004). Psychosocial Combined with Agonist Maintenance Treatments Versus Agonist Maintenance Treatments Alone for Treatment of Opioid Dependence. *Cochrane Database of Systematic Reviews*. http://dx.doi.org/10.1002/14651858.CD004147.pub4.

© The Editor(s) (if applicable) and The Author(s), under exclusive license to Springer Nature Switzerland AG 2019
W. M. Epstein, *Psychotherapy and the Social Clinic in the United States*,
https://doi.org/10.1007/978-3-030-32750-7

Amato, L., Minozzi, S., Davoli, M., & Vecchi, S. (2011). Psychosocial Combined with Agonist Maintenance Treatments Versus Agonist Maintenance Treatments Alone for Treatment of Opioid Dependence. *Cochrane Database of Systematic Reviews*, 1–93. http://dx.doi.org/10.1002/14651858.CD004147.pub4.

Amick, H. R., Gartlehner, G., Gaynes, B. N., Forneris, C., Asher, G. N., Morgan, L. C., et al. (2015). Comparative Benefits and Harms of Second Generation Antidepressants and Cognitive Behavioral Therapies in Initial Treatment of Major Depressive Disorder: Systematic Review and Meta-Analysis. *British Medical Journal, 351*, 1–10. http://dx.doi.org/10.1136/bmj.h6019.

Andersen, S. N., & Skardhamar, T. (2017). Pick a Number: Mapping Recidivism Measures and Their Consequences. *Crime & Delinquency, 63*, 613–635. https://doi.org/10.1177/0011128715570629.

Andrews, D. A., Zinger, I., Hoge, R. D., Bonta, J., Gendreau, P., & Cullen, F. T. (1990). Does Correctional Treatment Work? A Clinically Relevant and Psychologically Informed Meta-Analysis. *Criminology, 28*, 369–404. https://doi.org/10.1111/j.1745-9125.1990.tb01330.x.

Angell, M. (2011, July 14). The Illusions of Psychiatry. *The New York Review of Books, 58*, 20.

Angell, M. (2011, June 23). The Epidemic of Mental Illness: Why? *The New York Review of Books, 58*, 2–3.

Armstrong, J. S., & Green, K. C. (2017). *Guidelines for Science: Evidence and Checklists Scholarly Commons*. https://papers.ssrn.com/sol3/papers.cfm?abstract_id=3055874.

Baeck, L. (1958). *Judaism and Christianity*. Philadelphia, PA: Jewish Publication Society of America.

Banks, K., Newman, E., & Saleem, J. (2015). An Overview of the Research on Mindfulness-Based Interventions for Treating Symptoms of Posttraumatic Stress Disorder: A Systematic Review. *Journal of Clinical Psychology, 71*, 935–963. https://doi.org/10.1002/jclp.22200tyPress.

Barbuto, D. M. (1999). *American Settlement Houses and Progressive Social Reform*. Phoenix, AZ: The Oryx Press.

Barlow, D. H. (2010). Negative Effects from Psychological Treatments. *American Psychologist, 65*, 13–19. https://doi.org/10.1037/a0015643.

Barrera, T., Mott, J., Hofstein, R., & Teng, E. (2013). A Meta-Analytic Review of Exposure in Group Cognitive Behavioral Therapy for Posttraumatic Stress Disorder. *Clinical Psychology Review, 33*, 24–32. https://doi.org/10.1016/j.cpr.2012.09.005.

Barton, R. (1999). Psychosocial Rehabilitation Services in Community Support Systems: A Review of Outcomes and Policy Recommendations. *Psychiatric Services, 50,* 525–534. https://doi.org/10.1176/ps.50.4.525.

Battin, C., Bouvet, C., & Hatala, C. (2016). A Systematic Review of the Effectiveness of the Clubhouse Model. *Psychiatric Rehabilitation Journal, 39,* 305–312.

Bausell, R. B. (2007). *Snake Oil Science: The Truth About Complementary and Alternative Medicine.* New York, NY: Oxford University Press.

Beam, C. (2013). *To the End of June.* Boston, MA: Houghton Mifflin Harcourt.

Beard, J. H., Propst, R. N., & Malamud, T. J. (1982). The Fountain House Model of Psychiatric Rehabilitation. *Psychosocial Rehabilitation Journal, 5,* 47–53.

Becker, E. (1976). *Denial of Death* (2nd ed.). New York, NY: Macmillan.

Becker, R. E. (2015). Policies and Consequences: How America and Psychiatry Took the Detour to Erewhon. *Psychiatric Services, 66,* 1097–1100. https://doi.org/10.1176/appi.ps.201400485.

Becker, R. E., & Greig, N. H. (2010, December 8). Lost in Translation: Neuropsychiatric Drug Development. *Science Translational Medicine, 2*(61), 1–7. http://dx.doi.org/10.1126/scitranslmed.3000446.

Bender, K., Tripodi, S. J., Sarteschi, C., & Vaughn, M. G. (2011). A Meta-Analysis of Interventions to Reduce Adolescent Cannabis Use. *Research on Social Work Practice, 21,* 153–164. https://doi.org/10.1177/1049731510380226.

Benishek, L. A., Dugosh, K. L., Kirby, K. C., Matejkowski, J., Clements, N. T., Seymour, B. L., et al. (2014). Prize-Based Contingency Management for the Treatment of Substance Abusers: A Meta-Analysis. *Addiction, 109,* 1426–1436. https://doi.org/10.1111/add.12589.

Benston, E. A. (2015). Housing Programs for Homeless Individuals with Mental Illness: Effects on Housing and Mental Health Outcomes. *Psychiatric Services, 66*(8), 806–816.

Bergin, A. E. (1971). The Evaluation of Therapeutic Outcomes. In S. L. Garfield & A. E. Bergin (Eds.), *Handbook of Psychotherapy and Behavior Change.* New York: Wiley and Sons.

Bergin, A. E. & Lambert, M. J. (1978). The Evaluation of Therapeutic Outcomes. In S. L. Garfield & A. E. Bergin (Eds.), *Handbook of Psychotherapy and Behavior Change.* New York: Wiley and Sons.

Berlin, S. B. (2002). *Clinical Social Work Practice: A Cognitive Perspective.* New York, NY: Oxford University Press.

Berlin, I. (1969). Two Concepts of Liberty. In I. Berlin (Ed.), *Four, Essays on Liberty.* London: Oxford University Press.

Bermingham, C., Manlick, C. F., & Liu, W. M. (2015). Mental Health, Permanent Housing, and Peer Support Through Community Living in the Fairweather Lodge: Implementation Through Collaboration. *Housing, Care and Support, 18,* 26–30. https://doi.org/10.1108/HCS-0202015-0002.

Berzoff, J., & Drisko, J. (2015). Preparing PhD-Level Clinical Social Work Practitioners for the 21st Century. *Journal of Teaching in Social Work, 35,* 82–100. https://doi.org/10.1080/08841233.2014.993107.

Bisson, J. I., Shepherd, J. P., Joy, D., Probert, R., & Newcombe, R. G. (2004). Early Cognitive-Behavioural Therapy for Post-Traumatic Stress Symptoms After Physical Injury. *British Journal of Psychiatry, 184,* 63–69. https://doi.org/10.1192/bjp.184.1.63.

Blau, J. (2017). Science as a Strategy for Social Work. *Journal of Progressive Human Services, 28,* 73–90. https://doi.org/10.1080/10428232.2017.1310543.

Blazey, D., Child Trends, & DeVooght, K. (2013). *Family Foster Care Reimbursement Rates in the U.S.: A Report from a 2012 National Survey on Family Foster Care Provider Classifications and Rates.* Retrieved from https://www.childtrends.org/publications/family-foster-care-reimbursement-rates-in-the-u-s-a-report-from-a-2012-national-survey-on-family-foster-care-provider-classifications-and-rates/.

Bledsoe, S. E., & Grote, N. K. (2006). Treating Depression During Pregnancy and the Postpartum: A Preliminary Meta-Analysis. *Research on Social Work Practice, 16,* 109–120. https://doi.org/10.1177/1049731505282202.

Blumstein, A., & Larson, R. C. (1971). Problems in Modeling and Measuring Recidivism. *Journal of Research in Crime and Delinquency, 8,* 124–132. https://doi.org/10.1177/002242787100800202.

Bond, C., Woods, K., Humphrey, N., Symes, W., & Green, L. (2013). Practitioner Review: The Effectiveness of Solution Focused Brief Therapy with Children and Families: A Systematic and Critical Evaluation of the Literature from 1990–2010. *Journal of Child Psychology and Psychiatry, 54,* 707–723. https://doi.org/10.1111/jcpp.12058.

Bond, G. R. (1992). Vocational Rehabilitation. In R. Liberman (Ed.), *Handbook of Psychiatric Rehabilitation* (pp. 244–275). New York, NY: Macmillan.

Bryan, A. E., & Arkowitz, H. (2015). Meta-Analysis of the Effects of Peer-Administered Psychosocial Interventions on Symptoms of Depression. *American Journal of Community Psychology, 55,* 455–471. https://doi.org/10.1007/s10464-015-9718-y.

Bryant, R. A., Moulds, M. L., Guthrie, R. M., Dang, S. T., & Nixon, R. D. (2003). Imaginal Exposure Alone and Imaginal Exposure with Cognitive Restructuring in Treatment of Posttraumatic Stress Disorder. *Journal of*

Consulting and Clinical Psychology, 71, 706–712. Retrieved from https://doi.org/10.1037/0022-006X.71.4.706.

Bryant, R. A., Moulds, M. L., Guthrie, R. M., & Nixon, R. D. (2005). The Additive Benefits of Hypnosis and Cognitive-Behavioral Therapy in Treating Acute Stress Disorder. *American Psychological Association, 73,* 334–340. https://doi.org/10.1037/0022-006X.73.2.334.

Bryant, R. A., Moulds, M. L., Nixon, R. D., Mastrodomenico, J., Felmingham, K., & Hopwood, S. (2006). Hypnotherapy and Cognitive Behaviour Therapy of Acute Stress Disorder: A Three-Year Follow-Up. *Behaviour Research and Therapy, 44,* 1331–1335. https://doi.org/10.1016/j.brat.2005.04.007.

Bryant, R. A., Moulds, M. L., & Nixon, R. V. (2003). Cognitive Behaviour Therapy of Acute Stress Disorder: A Four-Year Follow-Up. *Behaviour Research and Therapy, 41,* 489–494. https://doi.org/10.1016/S0005-7967(02)00179-1.

Bugg, A., Turpin, G., Mason, S., & Scholes, C. (2009). A Randomised Controlled Trial of the Effectiveness of Writing as a Self-Help Intervention for Traumatic Injury Patients at Risk of Developing Post-Traumatic Stress Disorder. *Behaviour Research and Therapy, 47*(1), 6–12. https://doi.org/10.1016/j.brat.2008.10.006.

Byrne, G., & Egan, J. (2018). A Review of the Effectiveness and Mechanisms of Change for Three Psychological Interventions for Borderline Personality Disorders. *Clinical Social Work Journal,* 1–13. http://dx.doi.org/10.1007/s10615-018-0652-y.

Caplan, G. (1976). The Family as a Support System. In G. Caplan & M. Killilea (Eds.), *Support Systems and Mutual Help.* New York, NY: Grune & Stratton.

Caplan, G., & Killilea, M. (1976). *Support Systems and Mutual Help Multidisciplinary Explorations.* New York: Grune & Stratton.

Carson, M. (1990). *Settlement Folk: Social Thought and the American Settlement Movement, 1885–1930.* Chicago: The University of Chicago Press.

Chamberlain, P. (1990). Comparative Evaluation of Specialized Foster Care for Seriously Delinquent Youth: A First Step. *Community Alternatives International Journal of Family Care, 2,* 21–36.

Chamberlain, P., et al. (2008). Prevention of Behavior Problems for Children in Foster Care: Outcomes and Mediation Effects. *Prevention Science, 9*(1), 17–27.

Chamberlain, P., & Gilbert Rosicky, J. (1995). The Effectiveness of Family Therapy in the Treatment of Adolescents with Conduct Disorders and

Delinquency. *Journal of Marital & Family Therapy, 21.* http://dx.doi. org/10.1111/j.1752-0606.1995.tb00174.x.

Chamberlain, P., Price, J., Leve, L. D., Laurent, H., Landsverk, J. A., & Reid, J. B. (2007). Prevention of Behavior Problems for Children in Foster Care: Outcomes and Mediation Effects. *Prevention Science, 9,* 17–27. https://doi. org/10.1007/s11121-007-0080-7.

Chamberlain, P., & Reid, J. B. (1994). Differences in Risk Factors and Adjustment for Male and Female Delinquents in Treatment Foster Care. *Journal of Child and Family Studies, 3,* 23–39. https://doi.org/10.1007/BF02233909.

Chamberlain, P., & Reid, J. B. (1998). Comparison of Two Community Alternatives to Incarceration for Chronic Juvenile Offenders. *Journal of Consulting and Clinical Psychology, 66,* 624–633. https://doi.org/10. 1037/0022-006X.66.4.624.

Channa, M. W., et al. (2012). A Meta-Analysis of Intensive Family Preservation Programs: Placement Prevention and Improvement of Family Functioning. *Children and Youth Services Review, 34*(8), 1472–1479.

Chard, K. M. (2005). An Evaluation of Cognitive Processing Therapy for the Treatment of Posttraumatic Stress Disorder Related to Childhood Sexual Abuse. *Journal of Consulting and Clinical Psychology, 73,* 965–971.

Chi, X., Bo, A., Liu, T., Zhang, P., & Chi, I. (2018). Effects of Mindfulness-Based Stress Reduction on Depression in Adolescents and Young Adults: A Systematic Review and Meta-Analysis. *Frontiers in Psychology, 9,* 1–10. https://doi.org/10.3389/fpsyg.2018.01034.

Cloitre, M., et al. (2010). Treatment for PTSD Related to Childhood Abuse: A Randomized Controlled Trial. *American Journal of Psychiatry, 167*(8), 915–924.

Cloward, R. A., & Epstein, I. (1965). *The Adjustment of Social Welfare to Social Change.* Available from ERIC.

Cohen, N. D. (1990). *Psychiatry Takes to the Streets: Outreach and Crisis Intervention for the Mentally Ill.* New York: Guilford.

Communities and Schools of Nevada. (n.d.). https://www.cisnevada.org/.

Conrad, J. (1988). *Heart of Darkness* (3rd ed.). London: W. W. Norton.

Cook, T. D., & Shadish, W. R., Jr. (1982). Meta-Evaluation: An Evaluation of the CMCH Congressionally-Mandated Evaluation System. In G. J. Stahler & W. R. Tash (Eds.), *Innovative Approaches to Mental Health Evaluation* (1st ed., pp. 221–253). New York, NY: Academic Press.

Cooperrider, D. L., & Whitney, D. (2005). *Appreciative Inquiry: A Positive Revolution in Change.* San Francisco: Berrett-Koehler.

Coren, E., et al. (2016). Interventions for Promoting Reintegration and Reducing Harmful Behaviour and Lifestyles in Street-Connected Children and Young People. *Cochrane Database of Systematic Reviews, 1*, article number CD009823.

Cramer, H., Anheyer, D., Saha, F. J., & Dobos, G. (2018). Yoga for Posttraumatic Stress Disorder? A Systematic Review and Meta-Analysis. *BMC Psychiatry, 18*. http://dx.doi.org/10.1186/s12888-018-1650-x.

Crews, F. (1993). The Unknown Freud. *New York Review, 30*(19), 55–66.

Crews, F. (2017). *The Making of an Illusion*. New York: Metropolitan Books.

Cristea, I. A., Gentili, C., Pietrini, P., & Cuijpers, P. (2017, February 3). Is Investigator Background Related to Outcome in Head to Head Trials of Psychotherapy and Pharmacotherapy for Adult Depression? A Systematic Review and Meta-Analysis. *PLoS One, 12*, 1–18. http://dx.doi.org/10.1371/journal.pone.0171654.

Crumlish, N., & O'Rourke, K. (2010). A Systematic Review of Treatments for Post-Traumatic Stress Disorder Among Refugees and Asylum-Seekers. *The Journal of Nervous and Mental Disease, 198*, 237–251. https://doi.org/10.1097/NMD.0b013e3181d61258.

Cuijpers, P. (2017). Four Decades of Outcome Research on Psychotherapies for Adult Depression: An Overview of a Series of Meta-Analyses. *Canadian Psychology, 58*(1), 7–19.

Cuijpers, P., Cristea, I. A., Weitz, E., Gentili, C., & Berking, M. (2016). The Effects of Cognitive and Behavioural Therapies for Anxiety Disorders on Depression: A Meta-Analysis. *Psychological Medicine, 46*, 3451–3462. https://doi.org/10.1017/S0033291716002348.

Cuijpers, P., Dekker, J., Hollon, S. D., & Andersson, G. (2009). Adding Psychotherapy to Pharmacotherapy in the Treatment of Depressive Disorders in Adults: A Meta-Analysis. *Journal of Clinical Psychiatry, 70*, 1219–1229. https://doi.org/10.4088/JCP.09r05021.

Cuijpers, P., Donker, T., Weissman, M. M., Ravitz, P., & Cristea, I. A. (2016). Interpersonal Psychotherapy for Mental Health Problems: A Comprehensive Meta-Analysis. *American Journal of Psychiatry, 173*, 680–687. https://doi.org/10.1176/appi.ajp.2015.15091141.

Cuijpers, P., Geraedts, A. S., Van Oppen, P., Andersson, G., Markowitz, J. C., & Van Straten, A. (2011). Interpersonal Psychotherapy for Depression: A Meta-Analysis. *American Journal of Psychiatry, 168*, 581–592. https://doi.org/10.1176/appi.ajp.2010.10101411.

Cuijpers, P., Karyotaki, E., Weitz, E., Andersson, G., Hollon, S. D., & Van Straten, A. (2014). The Effects of Psychotherapies for Major Depression in Adults on Remission, Recovery and Improvement: A Meta-Analysis.

Journal of Affective Disorders, 159, 118–126. https://doi.org/10.1016/j. jad.2014.02.026.

Cuijpers, P., Van Straten, A., Andersson, G., & Van Oppen, P. (2008). Psychotherapy for Depression in Adults: A Meta-Analysis of Comparative Outcome Studies. *Journal of Consulting and Clinical Psychology, 76,* 909–922. https://doi.org/10.1037/a0013075.

Cuijpers, P., Van Straten, A., Bohlmeijer, E., Hollon, S. D., & Andersson, G. (2010). The Effects of Psychotherapy for Adult Depression Are Overestimated: A Meta-Analysis of Study Quality and Effect Size. *Psychological Medicine, 40,* 211–223. https://doi.org/10.1017/S0033291709006114.

Cullen, F. T., Pratt, T. C., Turanovic, J. J., & Butler, L. (2018). When Bad News Arrives: Project HOPE in a Post-Factual World. *Journal of Contemporary Criminal Justice, 34,* 13–34. https://doi. org/10.1177/1043986217750424.

Cusack, K., Jonas, D. E., Forneris, C. A., Wines, C., Sonis, J., Cook Middleton, J., et al. (2016). Psychological Treatments for Adults with Posttraumatic Stress Disorder: A Systematic Review and Meta-Analysis. *Clinical Psychology Review, 43,* 128–141. https://doi.org/10.1016/j. cpr.2015.10.003.

Dagenais, C., Begin, J., Bouchard, C., & Fortin, D. (2004). Impact of Intensive Family Support Programs: A Synthesis of Evaluation Studies. *Children and Youth Services Review, 26,* 249–263. https://doi.org/10.1016/j. childyouth.2004.01.015.

Dal-Re, R., Bobes, J., & Cuijpers, P. (2017). Why Prudence Is Needed When Interpreting Articles Reporting Clinical Trial Results in Mental Health. *TRIALS,18*(March) Article Number: 143.

Dalton, J. H., Elias, M. J., & Wandersman, A. (2001). *Community Psychology: Linking Individuals and Communities.* Belmont, CA: Wadsworth Thomson Learning.

Danto, E. A. (2005). *Freud's Free Clinics: Psychoanalysis & Social Justice, 1918–1938.* New York, NY: Columbia University Press.

Davidson, H. (1957). *Fads and Fallacies in the Name of Science.* New York: Dover Publications.

Davidson, R. J., Kabat-Zinn, J., Schumacher, J., Rosenkranz, M., Muller, D., Santorelli, S. F., et al. (2003). Alterations in Brain and Immune Function Produced by Mindfulness Meditation. *Psychosomatic Medicine, 65,* 564–570. https://doi.org/10.1097/01.PSY.0000077505.67574.E3.

Davies, G. (1996). *From Opportunity to Entitlement: The Transformation and Decline of Great Society Liberalism.* Lawrence: University Press of Kansas.

Davis, J. (1881). *The Rise and Fall of the Confederate Government*. Pantianos Classics.

Dawes, R. M. (1994). *House of Cards: Psychology and Psychotherapy Built on Myth*. New York, NY: Macmillan.

Day, P. J. (2006). *A New History of Social Welfare* (5th ed.). Boston, MA: Pearson Education.

Derezotes, D. S. (2006). *Spiritually Oriented Social Work Practice*. Boston, MA: Pearson.

DeRubeis, R. J., Hollon, S. D., Amsterdam, J. D., Shelton, R. C., Young, P. R., Salomon, R. M., et al. (2005). Cognitive Therapy vs. Medications in the Treatment of Moderate to Severe Depression. *Archives of General Psychiatry, 62*, 409–416. https://doi.org/10.1001/archpsyc.62.4.409.

Devilly, G. J., & Spence, S. H. (1999). The Relative Efficacy and Treatment Distress of EMDR and a Cognitive-Behavior Trauma Treatment Protocol in the Amelioration of Posttraumatic Stress Disorder. *Journal of Anxiety Disorders, 13*, 131–157.

DeVooght, K., Fletcher, M., & Cooper, H. (2012). *Federal, State, and Local Spending to Address Child Abuse and Neglect in SFY 2012*. The Annie E. Casey Foundation. https://www.childtrends.org/wp-content/uploads/2014/09/SFY-2012-Report-for-Posting-July2015.pdf.

Dimidjian, S., Dobson, K. S., Kohlenberg, R. J., Gallop, R., Markley, D. K., Atkins, D. C., et al. (2006). Randomized Trial of Behavioral Activation, Cognitive Therapy, and Antidepressant Medication in the Acute Treatment of Adults with Major Depression. *Journal of Consulting and Clinical Psychology, 74*, 658–670. https://doi.org/10.1037/0022-006X.74.4.658.

Dimidjian, S., & Hollon, S. D. (2010). How Would We Know If Psychotherapy Were Harmful. *American Psychologist, 65*, 21–33. https://doi.org/10.1037/a0017299.

Dineen, T. (1996). *Manufacturing Victims*. Montreal: Robert Davies Publishing.

Dinnen, S., Simiola, V., & Cook, J. M. (2015). Post-Traumatic Stress Disorder in Older Adults: A Systematic Review of the Psychotherapy Treatment Literature. *Aging & Mental Health, 19*, 144–150. https://doi.org/10.1080/13607863.2014.920299.

Dobbie, W., & Fryer, R. G. (2011). Are High-Quality Schools Enough to Increase Achievement Among the Poor? Evidence from the Harlem Children's Zone. *American Economic Journal: Applied Economics, 3*, 158–187. https://doi.org/10.1257/app.3.3.158.

Dorwick, C., Dunn, G., Ayuso-Mateos, J., Dalgard, O., Page, H., Lehtinen, V., et al. (2000). Problem Solving Treatment and Group Psychoeducation for Depression: Multicenter Randomised Controlled Trial. *British Medical Journal, 321*, 1–6. http://dx.doi.org/10.1136/bmj.321.7274.1450.

Dossa, N. I., & Hatem, M. (2012). Cognitive-Behavioral Therapy Versus Other PTSD Psychotherapies as Treatment for Women Victims of War-Related Violence: A Systematic Review. *The Scientific World Journal, 2012*, 1–19. https://doi.org/10.1100/2012/181847.

Dragioti, E., et al. (2017). Does Psychotherapy Work? An Umbrella Review of Meta-Analyses of Randomized Controlled Trials. *Acta Psychiatrica Scandinacica, 136*(3), 236–246.

Drisko, J. (2014). Research Evidence and Social Work Practice: The Place of Evidence Based Practice. *Clinical Social Work Journal, 42*(2), 123–133.

Drisko, J. W., & Grady, M. D. (2012). *Evidence-Based Practice in Clinical Social Work*. New York, NY: Springer.

Dryden, W., & Feltham, C. (1992). *Psychotherapy and Its Discontents*. Buckingham: Open University Press.

Dunn, N., Rehm, L. P., Schillaci, J., Souchek, J., Mehta, P., Ashton, C. M., et al. (2007). A Randomized Trial of Self-Management and Psychoeducational Group Therapies for Comorbid Chronic Posttraumatic Stress Disorder and Depressive Disorder. *Journal of Traumatic Stress, 20*, 221–237. https://doi.org/10.1002/jts.20214.

Dutra, L., Stathopoulou, G., Basden, S. L., Leyro, T. M., Powers, M. B., & Otto, M. W. (2008). A Meta-Analytic Review of Psychosocial Interventions for Substance Use Disorders. *American Journal of Psychiatry, 165*, 179–187. https://doi.org/10.1176/appi.ajp.2007.06111851.

Ebert, D. D., Donkin, L., Andersson, G., Andrews, G., Berger, T., Carlbring, P., et al. (2016). Does Internet-Based Guided-Self-Help for Depression Cause Harm? An Individual Participant Data Meta-Analysis on Deterioration Rates and Its Moderators in Randomized Controlled Trials. *Psychological Medicine, 46*, 2679–2693. https://doi.org/10.1017/S0033291716001562.

Echeburua, E., De Corral, P., Zubizarreta, I., & Sarasua, B. (1997). Psychological Treatment of Chronic Posttraumatic Stress Disorder in Victims of Sexual Aggression. *Behavior Modification, 21*, 433–456.

Eckman, T. A., et al. (1992). Technology for Training Schizophrenic Patients in Illness Self-Management: A Controlled Trial. *American Journal of Psychiatry, 149*, 1549–1555.

Eckman, T. A., Marder, S. R., Wirshing, W. C., Mintz, J., Mckenzie, J., Johnston, K., et al. (1996). Two-Year Outcome of Social Skills Training and Group Psychotherapy for Outpatients with Schizophrenia. *American Journal of Psychiatry, 153,* 1585–1592. https://doi.org/10.1176/ajp.153.12.1585.

Education Development Center. (2012). *Positive Behavioral Interventions and Supports: Snapshots from the Safe Schools/Healthy Students Initiative.* Retrieved from http://www.promoteprevent.org/sites/www.promoteprevent.org/files/resources/positive_behavioral_interventions_snapshots.pdf.

Ehlers, A., Bisson, J., Clark, D. M., Creamer, M., Pilling, S., Richards, D., et al. (2010). Do All Psychological Treatments Really Work the Same in Posttraumatic Stress Disorder? *Clinical Psychology Review, 30,* 269–276. https://doi.org/10.1016/j.cpr.2009.12.001.

Ehlers, A., Clark, D. M., Hackmann, A., McManus, F., Fennell, M., Herbert, C., et al. (2003). A Randomized Controlled Trial of Cognitive Therapy, a Self-Help Booklet, and Repeated Assessments as Early Interventions for Posttraumatic Stress Disorder. *Archive of General Psychiatry, 60,* 1024–1032.

Ehring, T., et al. (2014). Meta-Analysis of Psychological Treatments for Posttraumatic Stress Disorder in Adult Survivors of Childhood Abuse. *Clinical Psychology Review, 34*(8), 645–657.

Eisenberg, D. M., Davis, R. B., & Ettner, S. L., et al. (1998). Trends in Alternative Medicine Use in the United States: Results of a Follow-Up National Survey. *JAMA, 280*(18), 1569–1575.

Eisenberg, D. M., Kessler, R. C., Foster, C., Norlock F. E., Calkins D. R., & Delbanco T. L. (1993). Unconventional medicine in the United States. *NEnglJMed, 328,* 246–252.

Eisner, D. A. (2000). *The Death of Psychotherapy.* Westport, CT: Praeger.

Elkin, I., Shea, M. T., Watkins, J. T., Imber, S. D., Sotsky, S. M., Collins, J. F., et al. (1989). National Institute of Mental Health Treatment of Depression Collaborative Research Program. *Archives of General Psychiatry, 46,* 971–982. https://doi.org/10.1016/j.ctrv.2017.03.012.

Elliott, D. S., & Voss, H. L. (1968). Records Matching in Delinquency Research. *Social Problems, 16*(1), 120–123.

Elliott, D. S., & Voss, H. L. (2014). *Delinquency and Dropout.* New York, NY: Oxford University Press.

Elshtain, J. B. (2002). *Jane Addams and the Dream of American Democracy.* New York, NY: Basic Books.

Enea, V., & Dafinoiu, I. (2009). Motivational/Solution-Focused Intervention for Reducing School Truancy Among Adolescents. *Journal of Cognitive and Behavioral Psychotherapies, 9,* 185–198.

Epstein, W. M. (1993a). *The Dilemma of American Social Welfare*. New Brunswick, NJ: Transaction Publishers.

Epstein, W. M. (1993b). *The Illusion of Psychotherapy*. New Brunswick, NJ: Transaction Publishers.

Epstein, W. M. (1997). Social Science, Child Welfare, and Family Preservation: A Failure of Rationality in Public Policy. *Children and Youth Services Review, 19,* 41–60.

Epstein, W. M. (2003). The Futility of Pragmatic Reform: The Casey Foundation in New York City. *Children and Youth Services Review, 25,* 683–701. https://doi.org/10.1016/S0190-7409(03)00067-7.

Epstein, W. M. (2006). *Psychotherapy as Religion: The Civil Divine in America*. Reno, NV: University of Nevada Press.

Epstein, W. M. (2013). *Empowerment as Ceremony*. New Brunswick, NJ: Transaction Publishers.

Epstein, W. M. (2017). *The Masses Are the Ruling Classes: Policy Romanticism, Democratic Populism, and Social Welfare*. New York, NY: Oxford University Press.

Evans, M. E., Boothroyd, R. A., & Armstrong, M. I. (1997). Development and Implementation of an Experimental Study of the Effectiveness of Intensive In-Home Crisis Services for Children and Their Families. *Journal of Emotional and Behavioral Disorders, 5,* 93–105. https://doi.org/10.1177/106342669700500204.

Evans, M. E., Boothroyd, R. A., Armstrong, M. I., Greenbaum, P. E., Brown, E. C., & Kuppinger, A. D. (2003). An Experimental Study of the Effectiveness of Intensive In-Home Crisis Services for Children and Their Families: Program Outcomes. *Journal of Emotional and Behavioral Disorders, 11,* 92–102. https://doi.org/10.1177/106342660301100203.

Eysenck, H. J. (1952). The Effects of Psychotherapy: An Evaluation. *Journal of Consulting Psychology, 16,* 319.

Eysenck, H. J., & Rachman, S. (1965). *The Causes and Cures of Neuroses*. San Diego, CA: R. R. Knapp.

Fabricant, M. B., & Fisher, R. (2002). *Settlement Houses Under Siege*. New York, NY: Columbia University.

Fairweather, G. W. (1980). *The Fairweather Lodge: A Twenty-Year Retrospective*. San Francisco, CA: Jossey-Bass.

Fairweather, G. W., Sanders, D. H., Maynard, H., & Cressler, D. L. (1969). *Community Life for the Mentally Ill*. Chicago, IL: Aldine.

Fals-Stewart, W., Birchler, G. R., & O'Farrell, T. J. (1996). Behavioral Couples Therapy for Male Substance-Abusing Patients: Effects on Relationship Adjustment and Drug-Using Behavior. *Journal of Consulting and Clinical Psychology, 64,* 959–972.

Farkas, M. D., & Anthony, W. A. (1989). *Psychiatric Rehabilitation Programs: Putting Theory into Practice.* Baltimore, MD: Johns Hopkins University Press.

Feldman, L. H. (1991). Evaluating the Impact of Intensive Family Preservation Services in New Jersey. In D. Biegel (Ed.), *Family Preservation Services: Research and Evaluation.* Newbury Park, CA: Sage.

Filges, T., & Jorgensen, A. K. (2018). Cognitive-Behavioral Therapies for Young People in Outpatient Treatment for Nonopiod Drug Use. *Research on Social Work Practice, 28,* 363–385. https://doi.org/10.1177/1049731516629803.

Fischer, J. (1973). Is Casework Effective: A Review. *Social Work, 18*(1), 5–20.

Fischer, J. (1981). The Social Work Revolution. *Social Work, 26*(3), 199–207.

Flannery, K., Sugai, G., & Anderson, C. M. (2009). School-Wide Positive Behavior Support in High School. *Journal of Positive Behavior Intervention, 11,* 177–185. https://doi.org/10.1177/1098300708316257.

Flexner, A. (1915). Is Social Work a Profession? *Research on Social Work Practice, 11,* 152–165. https://doi.org/10.1177/104973150101100202.

Foa, E. B., Hembree, E. A., Cahill, S. P., Rauch, S. A., Riggs, D. S., Yadin, E., et al. (2005). Randomized Trial of Prolonged Exposure for Posttraumatic Stress Disorder With and Without Cognitive Restructuring: Outcome at Academic and Community Clinics. *Journal of Consulting and Clinical Psychology, 73,* 953–964. https://doi.org/10.1037/0022-006X.73.5.953.

Forman-Hoffman, V. L. (2003). Comparative Effectiveness of Interventions for Children Exposed to Nonrelational Traumatic Events. *Pediatrics, 131*(3), 526–539.

Forma-Stewart, L. A., Farrell-Macdonald, S., & Feeley, S. (2017). The Impact of a Community Mental Health Initiative on Outcomes for Offenders with a Serious Mental Disorder. *Criminal Behavior and Mental Health, 27,* 371–384. https://doi.org/10.1002/cbm.2005.

Forneris, C. A., Gartlehner, G., Brownley, K. A., Gaynes, B. N., Sonis, J., Coker-Schwimmer, E., et al. (2013). Interventions to Prevent Post-Traumatic Stress Disorder: A Systematic Review. *American Journal of Preventative Medicine, 44,* 635–650. https://doi.org/10.1016/j.amepre.2013.02.013.

Frank, J. D. (1961). *Persuasion and Healing: A Comparative Study of Psychotherapy*. Baltimore: Johns Hopkins Press.

Frank, J. D., & Frank, J. B. (1991). *Persuasion and Healing: A Comparative Stuey of Psychotherapy*. Baltimore, MD: Johns Hopkins University Press.

Franklin, C. (2016). *Social Work Essentials: Selections from the Encyclopedia of Social Work*. Washington, DC: NASW Press.

Franklin, C., & Belciug, C. (2015). Solution-Focused Brief Therapy in Schools. *Encyclopedia of Social Work*. https://doi.org/10.1093/acrefore/9780199975839.013.1040.

Franklin, C., Biever, J., Moore, K., Clemons, D., & Scamardo, M. (2001). The Effectiveness of Solution-Focused Therapy with Children in a School Setting. *Research on Social Work Practice, 11,* 411–434. https://doi.org/10.1177/104973150101100401.

Franklin, C., Moore, K., & Hopson, L. (2008). Effectiveness of Solution-Focused Brief Therapy in a School Setting. *National Association of Social Workers, 30,* 15–26. https://doi.org/10.1093/cs/30.1.15.

Franklin, C., Streeter, C. L., Kim, J. S., & Tripodi, S. J. (2007). The Effectiveness of a Solution-Focused Public Alternative School for Dropout Prevention and Retrieval. *Children and Schools, 29,* 133–144.

Frederico, M., Long, M., McNamara, P., McPherson, L., & Rose, R. (2016). Improving Outcomes for Children in Out-of-Home Care: The Role of Therapeutic Foster Care. *Child and Family Social Work, 22,* 1064–1074. https://doi.org/10.1111/cfs.12326.

Froeschle, J. G., Smith, R. L., & Ricard, R. (2007). The Efficacy of a Systematic Substance Abuse Program for Adolescent Females. *Professional School Counseling, 10.* http://dx.doi.org/10.1177/2156759X0701000507.

Furukawa, T. A., Weitz, E. S., Tanaka, S., Hollon, S. D., Hofmann, S. G., Andersson, G., et al. (2017). Initial Severity of Depression and Efficacy of Cognitive-Behavioural Therapy: Individual-Participant Data Meta-Analysis of Pill-Placebo-Controlled Trials. *The British Journal of Psychiatry, 210,* 190–196. https://doi.org/10.1192/bjp.bp.116.187773.

Gardner, M. (1998). *Martin Gardner's Table Magic*. Mineola, NY: Dover Publications.

Gaylin, W., Glasser, I., Marcus, S., & Rothman, D. (1978). *Doing Good: The Limits of Benevolence*. New York, NY: Pantheon Books.

Gellis, Z. D., & Kenaley, B. (2008). Problem-Solving Therapy for Depression in Adults: A Systematic Review. *Research on Social Work Practice, 18,* 117–131. https://doi.org/10.1177/1049731507301277.

Gellis, Z. D., McGinty, J., Tierney, L., Jordan, C., Burton, J., & Misener, E. (2008). Randomized Controlled Trial of Problem-Solving Therapy for Minor Depression in Home Care. *Research on Social Work Practice, 18,* 596–606. https://doi.org/10.1177/1049731507309821.

Gendreau, P. (1980). Recidivism Measure Reconsidered. *Canadian Journal of Criminology, 22.* Retrieved from www.heinonline.com.

Gendreau, P., & Leipciger, M. (1978). Development of a Redivism Measure and Its Application in Ontario. *Canadian Journal of Criminology, 20*(1), 3–17.

Gerger, H., Munder, T., & Barth, J. (2013). Specific and Nonspecific Psychological Interventions for PTSD Symptoms: A Meta-Analysis with Problem Complexity as a Moderator. *Journal of Clinical Psychology, 70*(7), 601–615.

Gergor, H., Munder, T., & Barth, J. (2014). Specific and Nonspecific Psychological Interventions for PTSD Symptoms: A Meta-Analysis with Problem Complexity as a Moderator. *Journal of Clinical Psychology, 70,* 601–615. https://doi.org/10.1002/jclp.22059.

Gibelman, M. (2004). *What Social Workers Do* (2nd ed.). Washington, DC: NASW Press.

Gillig, P. M., & McQuistion, H. I. (2006). *Clinical Guide to the Treatment of the Mentally Ill Homeless.* Washington, DC: American Psychiatric Association.

Goldhaber-Fiebert, J. D., Snowden, L. R., Wulczyn, F., Landsverk, J., & Horwitz, S. M. (2011). Economic Evaluation Research in the Context of Child Welfare Policy: A Structured Literature Review and Recommendations. *Child Abuse & Neglect: The International Journal, 35,* 722–740. https://doi.org/10.1016/j.chiabu.2011.05.012.

Gomory, T. (unpublished). *Tautology and Coercion.* Unpublished manuscript on the Wisconsin Assertive Community Treatment Model.

Gonzalez, M. J., & Gelman, C. R. (2015). Clinical Social Work Practice in the Twenty-First Century: A Changing Landscape. *Clinical Social Work Journal, 43,* 257–262. https://doi.org/10.1007/s10615-015-0550-5.

Goodman, J. D., McKay, J. R., & DePhilippis, D. (2013). Progress Monitoring in Mental Health and Addiction Treatment: A Means of Improving Care. *Professional Psychology: Research and Practice, 44,* 231–246. https://doi.org/10.1037/a0032605.

Gordon, R. J. (2016). *The Rise and Fall of American Growth: The U.S. Standard of Living Since the Civil War.* Princeton, NJ: Princeton University Press.

Gordon, R. J. (2017). *The Rise and Fall of Economic Growth: The US Standard of Living Since the Civil War*. Princeton, NJ: Princeton University Press.

Gorey, K. M. (1996). Effectiveness of Social Work Intervention Research: Internal Versus External Evaluations. *National Association of Social Workers*. https://doi.org/10.1093/swr/20.2.119.

Grant, D. (2013). Clinical Social Work. In *Encyclopedia of Social Work*. New York: Oxford University Press.

Grant, M. (2017 [1916]). *The Passing of the Great Race*. Eastford, CT: Martino Fine Books.

Green, S., Grant, A., & Rynsaardt, J. (2007, March 1). Evidence-Based Life Coaching for Senior High School Students: Building Hardiness and Hope. *International Coaching Psychology Review, 2*, 24–32.

Greenberg, G. A., & Rosenheck, R. A. (2010). Correlates of Past Homelessness in the National Epidemiological Survey on Alcohol and Related Conditions. *Administration and Policy in Mental Health and Mental Health Services Research, 37*(4), 357–366.

Greenbert, G. A., & Rosenheck, R. A. (2010). Mental Health Correlates of Past Homelessness in the National Comorbidity Study Replication. *Journal of Health Care for the Poor and Underserved, 21*(3), 1234–1249.

Grietens, H., & Hellinckx, W. (2004). Evaluating Effects of Residential Treatment for Juvenile Offenders by Statistical Meta Analysis: A Review. *Aggression and Violent Behavior, 9*, 401–415. https://doi.org/10.1016/S1359-1789(03)00043-0.

Grietens, H., Rink, J., & Hellinckx, W. (2003). Nonbehavioral Correlates of Juvenile Delinquency: Communications of Detained and Nondetained Young People About Social Limits. *Journal of Adolescent Research, 18*(1), 68–89.

Griswold, D. B. (1978). A Comparison of Recidivism Measures. *Journal of Criminal Justice, 6*, 247–252. https://doi.org/10.1016/0047-2352(78)90006-5.

Grob, G. N. (1983). *Mental Illness and American Society 1875–1940*. Princeton, NJ: Princeton University Press.

Grossman, J. B., & Tierney, J. P. (1998). Does Mentoring Work? An Impact Study of the Big Brothers Big Sisters Program. *Evaluation Review, 22*, 403–426. https://doi.org/10.1177/0193841X9802200304.

Gross, M. L. (1978). *The Psychological Society*. New York: Random House.

Grunbaum, A. (1984). *The Foundations of Psychoanalysis: A Philosophical Critique*. Berkeley, CA: University of California Press.

Gurman, A. S., & Kniskern, D. P. (1978). Behavioral Marriage Therapy: II. Empirical Perspective. *Family Process, 17,* 139–148.

Gusfield, J. R. (1972). *Symbolic Crusade: Status Politics and the American Temperance Movement* (3rd ed.). Urbana: University of Illinois.

Gustafsson, C., Ojenagen, A., Hansson, L., Sandlund, M., Nystrom, M., Glad, J., et al. (2009). Effects of Psychosocial Interventions for People with Intellectual Disabilities and Mental Health Problems. *Research on Social Work Practice, 19,* 281–290. https://doi.org/10.1177/1049731508329403.

Guttinger, F., et al. (2003). Evaluating Long-Term Effects of Heroin-Assisted Treatment: The Results of a 6-Year Follow-Up. *European Addiction Research, 9*(2), 73–79.

Hahn, R. A., Bilukha, O., Lowy, J., Crosby, A., Fullilove, M. T., Liberman, A., et al. (2005). The Effectiveness of Therapeutic Foster Care for the Prevention of Violence. *American Journal of Preventative Medicine, 28,* 72–90. https://doi.org/10.1016/j.ampre.2004.10.007.

Hale, J., Alfonso, V., Berninger, V., Bracken, B., Christo, C., Clark, E., et al. (2010). Critical Issues in Response-to-Intervention, Comprehensive Evaluation, and Specific Learning Disabilities Identification and Intervention: An Expert White Paper Consensus. *Learning Disability Quarterly, 33,* 223–236. https://doi.org/10.1177/073194871003300310.

Hari, J. (2015). *Chasing the Scream.* New York: Bloomsbury.

Hari, J. (2018). *Lost Connections: Uncovering the Real Causes of Depression—And the Unexpected Solution.* New York, NY: Bloomsbury.

Hartmann, W. E., St. Arnault, D. M., & Gone, J. P. (2018). A Return to the Clinic for Community Psychology: Lessons from a Clinical Ethnography in Urban American Indian Behavioral Health. *American Journal of Community Psychology, 61,* 62–75. http://dx.doi.org/10.1002/ajcp.12212.

Haugen, P. T., Evces, M., & Weiss, D. S. (2012). Treating Posttraumatic Stress Disorder in First Responders: A Systematic Review. *Clinical Psychology Review, 32,* 370–380. https://doi.org/10.1016/j.cpr.2012.04.001.

Hayes, S. C., Wilson, K. G., Gifford, E. V., Bissett, R., Piasecki, M., Batten, S. V., et al. (2004). A Preliminary Trial of Twelve-Step Facilitation and Acceptance and Commitment Therapy with Polysubstance-Abusing Methadone-Maintained Opiate Addicts. *Behavior Therapy, 35,* 667–688. https://doi.org/10.1016/S0005-7894(04)80014-5.

Hays, P. (2014). An International Perspective on the Adaptation of CBT Across Cultures. *Australian Psychologist, 49,* 17–18.

Heineman, M. (1981). The Obsolete Scientific Imperative in Social Work Research. *Social Service Review, 55,* 371–397. Retrieved from http://www.jstor.org.ezproxy.library.unlv.edu/stable/30011495.

Heineman, M. B. (1982). The Obsolete Scientific Imperative in Social Work. *Social Service Review, 63*(3), 175–185.

Heller, K., Thompson, M. G., Trueba, P. E., Hogg, J. R., & Vlachos-Weber, I. (1991). Peer Support Telephone Dyads for Elderly Women: Was This the Wrong Intervention? *American Journal of Community Psychology, 19,* 53–74. https://doi.org/10.1007/BF00942253.

Hernandez, J. P., & Macgowan, M. J. (2015). Psychosocial Interventions for Women with HIV/AIDS: A Critical Review. *Research on Social Work Practice, 25,* 103–116. https://doi.org/10.1177/1049731514527799.

Herrnstein, R. J., & Murray, C. (2010). *The Bell Curve: Intelligence and Class Structure in American Life.* New York: The Free Press.

Hoffman, V. L., Zolotor, A. J., McKeeman, J. L., Blanco, R., Knauer, S. R., Lloyd, S. W., et al. (2013). Comparative Effectiveness of Interventions for Children Exposed to Nonrelational Traumatic Events. *Pediatrics: Official Journal of the American Academy of Pediatrics, 131,* 526–539. http://dx.doi.org/10.1542/peds.2012-3846.

Hofmann, S. G., Curtiss, J., Carpenter, J. K., & Kind, S. (2017). Effect of Treatment for Depression on Quality of Life: A Meta-Analysis. *Cognitive Behaviour Therapy, 46,* 265–286. https://doi.org/10.1080/16506073.2017.1304445.

Holden, G., & Barker, K. (2017). Should Social Workers Be Engaged in These Practices? *Journal of Evidence Informed Social Work, 15*(1), 1–13.

Holden, G., & Barker, K. (2018). Should Social Workers Be Engaged in These Practices? *Journal of Evidence-Informed Social Work, 15*(1), 1–13. https://doi.org/10.1080/23761407.2017.1422075.

Holden, G., et al. (2017). Self-Efficacy Regarding Social Work Competencies. *Research on Social Work Practice, 27*(5), 594–606.

Holt, M. I. (1992). *The Orphan Trains: Placing Out in America.* Lincoln and London: University of Nebraska Press.

Horner, R. H., et al. (2009). A Randomized, Wait-List Controlled Effectiveness Trial Assessing School-Wide Positive Behavior Support in Elementary Schools. *Journal of Positive Behavior Interventions, 11*(3), 133–144.

Horwitz, A. V., & Wakefield, J. C. (2007). *The Loss of Sadness.* New York: Oxford University Press.

How to Practice Ho'oponopono in Four Simple Steps. (n.d.). Retrieved from https://www.laughteronlineuniversity.com/practice-hooponopono-four-simple-steps/.

Hurdle, D. E. (2002). Native Hawaiian Traditional Healing: Culturally Based Interventions for Social Work Practice. *Social Work, 47*, 183–192.

Huxley, A. (1948). *Ape and Essence*. New York, NY: Harper.

Isenberg, N. (2018, June 28). Left Behind. *New York Review of Books*. https://www.pressreader.com/usa/the-new-york-review-of-books/20180628/282492889545431.

Jackson, R. L. (2001). *The Clubhouse Model: Empowering Applications of Theory to Generalist Practice*. Belmont, CA: Wadsworth/Thomson Learning.

Jakobsen, J. C., Hansen, J. L., Simonsen, S., Simonsen, E., & Gluud, C. (2012). Effects of Cognitive Therapy Versus Interpersonal Psychotherapy in Patients with Major Depressive Disorder: A Systematic Review of Randomized Clinical Trials with Meta-Analyses and Trial Sequential Analyses. *Psychological Medicine, 42*, 1343–1357. https://doi.org/10.1017/S0033291711002236.

Jarrett, R. B., Schaffer, M., McIntire, D., Witt-Browder, A., Kraft, D., & Risser, R. C. (1999). Treatment of Atypical Depression with Cognitive Therapy or Phenelzine. *Archives of General Psychiatry, 56*, 431–437. https://doi.org/10.1001/archpsyc.56.5.431.

Joanning, H., Thomas, F., Quinn, W., & Mullen, R. (1992). Treating Adolescent Drug Abuse: A Comparison of Family Systems Therapy, Group Therapy, and Family Drug Education. *Journal of Marital and Family Therapy, 18*, 345–356. https://doi.org/10.1111/j.1752-0606.1992.tb00948.x.

Johnson, J. E., Back Price, A., Chienwen Kao, J., Fernandes, K., Stout, R., Gobin, R. L., et al. (2016). Interpersonal Psychotherapy (IPT) for Major Depression Following Perinatal Loss: A Pilot Randomized Controlled Trial. *Archives of Women's Mental Health, 19*, 845–859. https://doi.org/10.1007/s00737-016-0625-5.

Kabat-Zinn, J., Wheeler, E., Light, T., Skillings, A., Scharf, M. J., Cropley, T. G., et al. (1998). Influence of a Mindfulness Meditation-Based Stress Reduction Intervention on Rates of Skin Clearing in Patients with Moderate to Severe Psoriasis Undergoing Photo Therapy (UVB) and Photochemotherapy (PUVA). *Psychosomatic Medicine, 60*, 625–632.

Kagan, C., Burton, M., Duckett, P., Lawthom, R., & Siddiquee, A. (2011). *Critical Community Psychology*. West Sussex, UK: BPS Blackwell.

Kalb, K. (2017). Genius. *National Geographic Magazine*, pp. 48–49.

Kamenov, K., Twomey, C., Cabello, M., Prina, A. M., & Ayuso-Mateos, J. L. (2017). The Efficacy of Psychotherapy, Pharmacotherapy and Their Combination on Functioning and Quality of Life in Depression: A Meta-Analysis. *Psychological Medicine, 47,* 414–425. https://doi.org/10.1017/S0033291716002774.

Kapuscinski, R. (1992). *The Soccer War.* New York: Vintage.

Karger, H. J. (1984). *The Sentinels of Order: A Case Study of Social Control and the Minneapolis Settlement House Movement, 1897–1950.* University of Illinois at Urbana-Champaign, ProQuest Dissertations Publishing.

Karyotaki, E., Smit, Y., De Beurs, D. P., Holdt Henningsen, K., Robays, J., Huibers, M. J., et al. (2016). The Long-Term Efficacy of Acute-Phase Psychotherapy for Depression: A Meta-Analysis of Randomized Trials. *Depression and Anxiety, 33,* 370–383. https://doi.org/10.1002/da.22491.

Kaufmann, W. (1970). *Judaism and Christianity.* New York, NY: Atheneum.

Kearney, D. J., et al. (2012). Association of Participation in a Mindfulness Program with Measures of PTSD, Depression and Quality of Life in a Veteran Sample. *Journal of Clinical Psychology, 68*(1), 101–116.

Kearney, D. J., McDermott, K., Malte, C., Martinez, M., & Simpson, T. L. (2013). Effects of Participation in a Mindfulness Program for Veterans with Posttraumatic Stress Disorder: A Randomized Controlled Pilot Study. *Journal of Clinical Psychology, 69,* 14–27. https://doi.org/10.1002/jclp.21911.

Keeley, R. D., Engel, M., Nordstrom, K., Dickinson, L. M., Brody, D. S., Burke, B. L., et al. (2016). Motivational Interviewing Improves Depression Outcome in Primary Care: A Cluster Randomized Trial. *Journal of Consulting and Clinical Psychology, 84,* 993–1007. https://doi.org/10.1037/ccp0000124.

Kelly, M. S. (2014). Response to Intervention in Schools. *Encyclopedia of Social Work.* https://doi.org/10.1093/acrefore/9780199975839.013.1013.

Kelly, M. S., Frey, A. J., Alvarez, M., Cosner Berzin, S., Shaffer, G., & O'Brien, K. (2010). School Social Work Practice and Response to Intervention. *Children & Schools, 32,* 201–209. http://dx.doi.org/10.2137/145960610792912602.

Kennedy, J. R., & Kennedy, W. D. (2014). *The South Was Right Gretna.* Louisiana: Pelican Publishing.

Kennedy, L., & Xyrichis, A. (2017). Cognitive Behavioral Therapy Compared with Non-specialized Therapy for Alleviating the Effect of Auditory Hallucinations in People with Reoccurring Schizophrenia: A Systematic Review and Meta-Analysis. *Community Mental Health Journal, 53,* 127–133. https://doi.org/10.1007/s10597-016-0030-6.

Kessler, R. C., Pecora, P. J., Williams, J., Hiripi, E., O'Brien, K., English, D., et al. (2008). Effects of Enhanced Foster Care on Long-Term Physical and Mental Health of Foster Care Alumni. *Archives of General Psychiatry, 65,* 625–633. https://doi.org/10.1001/archpsyc.65.6.625.

Kiecolt-Glaser, J. K., et al. (2008). Olfactory Influences on Mood and Autonomic, Endocrine, and Immune Function. *Psychoneuroendocrinology, 33*(3), 328–339.

Kim, J. S., Brook, J., & Akin, B. A. (2018). Solution-Focused Brief Therapy with Substance-Using Individuals: A Randomized Controlled Trial Study. *Research on Social Work Practice, 28,* 452–462. https://doi.org/10.1177/1049731516650517.

Kim, J. S., & Franklin, C. (2009). Solution-Focused Brief Therapy in Schools: A Review of the Outcome Literature. *Children and Youth Services Review, 31,* 464–470. http://dx.doi.org/10.1016/j.childyouth.2008.10.002.

Kimbrough, R. (1988). *Joseph Conrad: Heart of Darkness.* New York: Norton.

Kinney, J., Haapala, D., & Booth, C. (1991). *Keeping Families Together: The Homebuilders Model.* New York: Transaction Publishers.

Kirigin, K. A., Braukmann, C. J., Atwater, J. D., & Wolf, M. M. (1982). An Evaluation of Teaching-Family (Achievement Place) Group Homes for Juvenile Offenders. *Journal of Applied Behavior Analysis, 15*(1), 1–16. https://doi.org/10.1901/jaba.1982.15-1.

Kirk, S. A., Gomory, T., & Cohen, D. (2013). *Mad Science.* New Brunswick, NJ: Transaction Publishers.

Kirk, S. A., & Kutchins, H. (1992). *The Selling of DSM: The Rhetoric of Science in Psychiatry.* New York, NY: Aldine De Gruyter.

Kitchiner, N. J., et al. (2012). Systematic Review and Meta-Analyses of Psychosocial Interventions for Veterans of the Military. *European Journal of Psychotraumatology, 3,* 1–16. http://dx.doi.org/10.3402/ejpt.v3i0.19267.

Klimas, J., Field, C. A., Cullen, W., O'Gorman, C. S., Glynn, L. G., Keenan, E., et al. (2012). Psychosocial Interventions to Reduce Alcohol Consumption in Concurrent Problem Alcohol and Illicit Drug Users. *Cochrane Database of Systematic Reviews,* 1–43. http://dx.doi.org/10.1002/14651858.CD009269.pub2.

Knight, C. A., & Alarie, R. M. (2017). Improving Mental Health in the Community: Outcome Evaluation of a Geriatric Mental Health Day Treatment Service. *Clinical Gerontologist, 40,* 77–87. https://doi.org/10.1080/07317115.2016.1263709.

Kolovos, S., Van Tulder, M. W., Cuijpers, P., Prigent, A., Chevreul, K., Riper, H., et al. (2017). The Effect of Treatment as Usual on Major Depressive Disorder: A Meta-Analysis. *Journal of Affective Disorders, 210,* 72–81. https://doi.org/10.1016/j.jad.2016.12.013.

Kraemer Tebes, J. (2016). Reflections on the Future of Community Psychology from the Generations After Swampscott: A Commentary and Introduction to the Special Issue. *American Journal of Community Psychology,* 229–238. http://dx.doi.org/10.1002/ajcp.12110.

Kretzer, K., et al. (2007). Self Identity Through Ho'oponopono as Adjunctive Therapy for Hypertension Management. *Ethnicity and Disease, 17*(4), 624–628.

Kushel, M. B., Yen, I. H., Gee, L., & Courtney, M. E. (2007). Homelessness and Health Care Access After Emancipation: Results from the Midwest Evaluation of Adult Functioning of Former Foster Youth. *Archives of Pediatrics & Adolescent Medicine, 161,* 986–993. https://doi.org/10.1001/archpedi.161.10.986.

Kutchins, H., & Kirk, S. A. (1997). *Making Us Crazy: DSM: The Psychiatric Bible and the Creation of Mental Disorders.* New York, NY: The Free Press.

Kuyken, W., Taylor, R. S., Barrett, B., Evans, A., Byford, S., Watkins, E., et al. (2008). Mindfulness-Based Cognitive Therapy to Prevent Relapse in Recurrent Depression. *Journal of Consulting and Clinical Psychology, 76,* 966–978. https://doi.org/10.1037/a0013786.

Kvarme, L. G., Helseth, S., Sorum, R., Luth-Hansen, V., Haugland, S., & Natvig, G. K. (2010). The Effect of a Solution-Focused Approach to Improve Self-Efficacy in Socially Withdrawn School Children: A Non-randomized Controlled Trial. *International Journal of Nursing Students, 47,* 1389–1396. https://doi.org/10.1016/j.ijnurstu.2010.05.001.

Lab, S. P., & Whitehead, J. T. (1990). From 'Nothing Works' to 'The Appropriate Works': The Last Stop on the Search for the Secular Grail. *Criminology, 28*(3), 405–418.

La Bonta, J., & Andrews, D. A. (2015). *The Psychology of Criminal Conduct.* New York: Routledge.

Lambert, M. F., & Bergin, A. E., (1994). The Effectiveness of Psychotherapy. In A. E. Begin & S. L. Garfield (Eds.), *Handbook of Psychotherapy and Behavior Change.* New York: Wiley and Sons.

Lambert, M. J., Christensen, E. R., & DeJulio, S. S. (1984). The Assessment of Psychotherapy Outcome. *Psychological Bulletin, 83*(1), 23–62.

Lambert, M. J., et al. (1993). Psychotherapy Versus Placebo Therapies: A Review of the Meta-Analysis Literature. Poster Presented at the Annual Meeting of the Western Psychological Association, Phoenix Arizone.

Larney, S., Gowing, L., Mattick, R. P., Farrell, M., Hall, W., & Degenhardt, L. (2014). A Systematic Review and Meta-Analysis of Naltrexone Implants for the Treatment of Opioid Dependence. *Drug and Alcohol Review, 33,* 115–128. https://doi.org/10.1111/dar.12095.

Larose, S., Boisclair-Chateauvert, G., De Wit, D. J., DuBois, D., Erdem, G., & Lipman, E. L. (2018). How Mentor Support Interacts with Mother and Teacher Support in Predicting Youth Academic Adjustment: An Investigation Among Youth Exposed to Big Brothers Big Sisters of Canada Programs. *The Journal of Primary Prevention, 39,* 205–228. https://doi.org/10.1007/s10935-018-0509-8.

Lasch-Quinn, E. (1993). *Black Neighbors: Race and the Limits of Reform in the American Settlement House Movement, 1890–1945.* Chapel Hill: University of North Carolina Press.

Lee, C., Gavriel, H., Drummond, P., Richards, J., & Greenwald, R. (2002). Treatment of PTSD: Stress Inoculation Training with Prolonged Exposure Compared to EMDR. *Journal of Clinical Psychology, 58,* 1071–1089. https://doi.org/10.1002/jclp.10039.

Lee, M. Y., Ng, S., Leung, P. P., & Chan, C. L. (2009). *Integrative Body-Mind-Spirit Social Work: An Empirically Based Approach to Assessment and Treatment.* New York: Oxford University Press.

Leiby, J. (1978). *A History of Social Welfare and Social Work in the United States.* New York: Columbia University Press.

Leichsenring, F., et al. (2017). Biases in Research: Risk Factors for Non-Replicability in Psychotherapy and Pharmacotherapy Research. *Psychological Medicine, 47*(6), 1000–1011.

Lerman, P. (1975). *Community Treatment and Social Control: A Critical Analysis of Juvenile Correctional Policy.* Chicago, IL: University of Chicago Press.

Lerman, P. (1984). Child Welfare, the Private Sector and Community Based Corrections. *Crime and Delinquency, 30,* 5–38.

Leuchtenburg, W. E. (1963). *Franklin D. Roosevelt and the New Deal: 1932–1940.* New York: Harper and Row.

Levine, M., & Perkins, D. V. (1997). *Principles of Community Psychology: Perspectives and Applications* (2nd ed.). New York, NY: Oxford University Press.

Lewis, R. E. (2005). The Effectiveness of Families First Services: An Experimental Study. *Children and Youth Services Review, 27,* 499–509. https://doi.org/10.1177/106342669700500204.

Li, L., Zhu, S., Tse, N., Tse, S., & Wong, P. (2015). Effectiveness of Motivational Interviewing to Reduce Illicit Drug Use in Adolescents: A Systematic Review and Meta-Analysis. *Addiction, 111*, 795–805. https://doi.org/10.1111/add.13285.

Lieber, J. A. (2006). Comparative Effectiveness of Antipsychotic Drugs: A Commentary on Cost Utility of the Latest Antipsychotic Drugs in Schizophrenia Study (CUtLASS 1) and Clinical Antipsychotic Trials of Intervention Effectiveness (CATIE). *Archives of General Psychiatry, 63*(10), 1069–1072.

Liberman, J. A., Stroup, S., McEvoy, J. P., Swartz, M. S., Rosenheck, R. A., Perkins, D. O., et al. (2005). Effectiveness of Antipsychotic Drugs in Patients with Chronic Schizophrenia. *The New England Journal of Medicine, 353*, 1209–1223. https://doi.org/10.1056/NEJMoa051688.

Lilienfeld, S. O., Lynn, S. J., & Lohr, J. M. (2003). *Science and Pseudoscience in Clinical Psychology*. New York, NY: The Guilford Press.

Lilienfeld, S. O., Lynn, S. J., & Lohr, J. M. (2015). *Science and Pseudoscience in Clinical Psychology*. New York: Guilford Press.

Lindstrom, M., Filges, T., & Jorgensen, A. (2016). Brief Strategic Family Therapy for Young People in Treatment for Drug Use. *Research on Social Work Practice, 25*(1), 61–80.

Lipman, E. L., DeWit, D., DuBois, D. L., Larose, S., & Erdem, G. (2018). Youth with Chronic Health Problems: How Do They Fare in Main-Stream Mentoring Programs. *Journal of Emotional and Behavioral Disorders, 11*, 92–102. https://doi.org/10.1177/106342660301100203.

Lipsey, M. W., & Cullen, F. T. (2007). The Effectiveness of Correctional Rehabilitation: A Review of Systematic Reviews. *The Annual Review of Law and Social Sciences, 3*, 297–320. https://doi.org/10.1146/annurev.lawsocsci.3.081806.1128.

Lo, H. H., Ng, S., & Chan, C. L. (2015). Evaluating Compassion-Mindfulness Therapy for Recurrent Anxiety and Depression: A Randomized Control Trial. *Research on Social Work Practice, 25*, 715–725. https://doi.org/10.1177/1049731514537686.

Lubove, R. (1965). *The Professional Altruist*. Cambridge, MA: Harvard University Press.

Lubove, R. (1967). *The Professional Altrusit*. Cambridge, MA: Harvard University Press.

Luborsky, et al. (1975). Comparative Studies of Psychotherapies: Is It True That Everyone Has Won and All Must Have Prizes? *Archives of General Psychiatry, 32*, 995–1008.

Lugard, F. (1922). *The Dual Mandate in British Tropical Africa*. London: William Blackwood and Sons.

Lugard, F. J. (2012). *The Dual Mandate in British Tropical Africa*. London, UK: William Blackwood and Sons.

Lundahl, B. W., et al. (2008). Process-Based Forgiveness Interventions: A Meta-Analytic Review. *Research on Social Work Practice, 18*(5), 465–478.

Macmillan, C. (1997). *Freud Evaluated: The Completed Arc*. Cambridge, MA: MIT Press.

Macy, J. T., Seo, D., Chassin, L., Presson, C. C., & Sherman, S. J. (2007). Prospective Predictors of Long-Term Abstinence Versus Relapse Among Smokers Who Quit as Young Adults. *The American Journal of Public Health, 97,* 1470–1475.

Madigan, S., Paton, K., & Mackett, N. (2017). The Springfield Project Service: Evaluation of a Solihull Approach Course for Foster Carers. *Adopting & Fostering, 41,* 254–267. https://doi.org/10.1177/0308575917719373.

Maegowan, M. J. (2004). Psychosocial Treatment of Youth Suicide: A Systematic Review of the Research. *Research on Social Work Practice, 14,* 147–162. https://doi.org/10.1177/1049731503257889.

Magill, M., & Ray, L. A. (2009). Cognitive-Behavioral Treatment with Adult Alcohol and Illicit Drug Users: A Meta-Analysis of Randomized Controlled Trials. *Journal of Studies on Alcohol and Drugs, 70,* 516–527. http://dx.doi.org/10.15288/jsad.2009.70.516.

Manzoni, G., Pagnini, F., Castelnuovo, G., & Molinari, E. (2008). Relaxation Training for Anxiety: A Ten-Years Systematic Review with Meta-Analysis. *BMC Psychiatry, 8,* 41. https://doi.org/10.1186/1471-244X-8-41.

Marder, S. R., et al. (1996). Two-Year Outcome of Social Skills Training and Group Psychotherapy for Outpatients with Schizophrenia. *American Journal of Psychiatry, 153,* 1585–1592.

Margalit, A. (2017). *On Betrayal*. Cambridge, MA: Harvard University Press.

Margolin, L. (1997). *Under the Cover of Kindness: The Invention of Social Work*. Charlottesville, NC: University Press of Virginia.

Markowitz, J. C., Kocsis, J. H., Fishman, B., Spielman, L. A., Jacobsberg, L. B., Frances, A. J., et al. (1998). Treatment of Depressive Symptoms in Human Immunodeficiency Virus-Positive Patients. *Archives of General Psychiatry, 55,* 452–457. https://doi.org/10.1001/archpsyc.55.5.452.

Marks, I., Lovell, K., Noshirvani, H., Livanou, M., & Thrasher, S. (1998). Treatment of Posttraumatic Stress Disorder by Exposure and/or Cognitive Restructuring. *Archive of General Psychiatry, 55,* 317–325. Retrieved from http://jamanetwork.com.

Marquis, D. (1927). *The Lives and Times of Archy & Mehitabel.* Garden City, NY: Doubleday.

Masson, J. M. (1988). *Against Therapy: Emotional Tyranny and the Myth of Psychological Healing.* New York: Atheneum.

Mayet, S., et al. (2005). Psychosocial Treatment for Opiate Abuse and Dependence. *Cochrane Database of Systematic Reviews* (1): CD004330.

Mayet, S., Farrell, M., Ferri, M., Amato, L., & Davoli, M. (2010). Psychosocial Treatment for Opiate Abuse and Dependence. *The Cochrane Collaboration,* 1–20. http://dx.doi.org/10.1002/14651858.CD004330.pub2.

McCree Bryan, M., & Davis, A. F. (1969). *100 Years at Hull-House.* Bloomington: Indiana University Press.

McDonagh, A., et al. (2005). Randomized Trial of Cognitive-Behavioral Therapy for Chronic Posttraumatic Stress Disorder in Adult Female Survivors of Childhood Sexual Abuse. *Journal of Consulting and Clinical Psychology, 73*(3), 515–524.

McKay, C., Nugent, K. L., Johnsen, M., Eaton, W. W., & Lidz, C. W. (2018). A Systematic Review of Evidence for the Clubhouse Model of Psychosocial Rehabilitation. *Administration and Policy in Mental Health and Mental Health Services Research, 45*(1), 28–47. https://doi.org/10.1007/s10488-016-0760-3.

McLellan, A. T., Arndt, I. O., Metzger, D. S., Woody, G. E., & O'Brien, C. P. (1993, April 21). The Effects of Psychological Services in Substance Abuse Treatment. *Journal of the American Medical Society, 269,* 1953–1959. http://dx.doi.org/10.1001/jama.1993.03500150065028.

McPherson, J. (2012). Does Narrative Exposure Therapy Reduce PTSD in Survivors of Mass Violence? *Research on Social Work Practice, 21,* 153–164. https://doi.org/10.1177/1049731511414147.

Meezan, W., & McCroskey, J. (1996). Improving Family Functioning Through Family Preservation Services: Results of the Los Angeles Experiment. *Journal of Family Strengths, 1*(2), 1–21. Retrieved from http://digitalcommons.library.tmc.edu/jfs.

Meezan, W., & O'Keefe, M. (1998). Evaluating the Effectiveness of Multifamily Group Therapy in Child Abuse and Neglect. *Research on Social Work Practice, 8,* 330–353. https://doi.org/10.1177/104973159800800306.

Meltzoff, J., & Kornreich, M. (1970). *Research in Psychotherapy.* New York: Atherton.

Mencher, S. (1967). *Poor Law to Poverty Program: Economic Security Policy in Britain and the United States.* Pittsburgh: University of Pittsburgh Press.

Mendes, D. D., Mello, M. F., Ventura, P., De Medeiros Passarela, C., & De Jesus Mari, J. (2008). A Systematic Review on the Effectiveness of Cognitive Behavioral Therapy for Posttraumatic Stress Disorder. *International Journal of Psychiatry in Medicine, 38,* 241–259. https://doi.org/10.2190/PM.38.3.b.

Milgrom, J., Negri, L. M., Gemmill, A. W., McNeil, M., & Martin, P. R. (2005). A Randomized Controlled Trial of Psychological Interventions for Postnatal Depression. *British Journal of Clinical Psychology, 44,* 529–542. https://doi.org/10.1348/014466505X34200.

Miranda, J., Chung, J. Y., Green, B. L., Krupnick, J., Siddique, J., Revicki, D. A., et al. (2003). Treating Depression in Predominately Low-Income Young Minority Women. *Journal of the American Medical Association, 290,* 57–65. https://doi.org/10.1001/jama.290.1.57.

Mizrahi, T., & Davis, L. E., (2005). *Encyclopedia of Social Work* (20th ed.). Washington, DC: NASW Press.

Mohr, D. C., Ho, J., Hart, T. L., Baron, K. G., Berendsen, M., Beckner, V., et al. (2014). Control Condition Design and Implementation Features in Controlled Trials: A Meta-Analysis of Trials Evaluating Psychotherapy for Depression. *Translational Behavioral Medicine Journal, 4,* 407–423. https://doi.org/10.1007/s13142-014-0262-3.

Moller, M. D., & Murphy, M. F. (1997). The Three R's Rehabilitation Program: A Prevention Approach for the Management of Relapse Symptoms Associated with Psychiatric Diagnosis. *Psychiatric Rehabilitation Journal, 20,* 42–48. https://doi.org/10.1037/h0095365.

Moloney, P. (2013). *The Therapy Industry: The Irresistible Rise of the Talking Cure, and Why It Doesn't Work.* London, UK: Pluto Press.

Moloney, P. (2016). Mindfulness: The Bottled Water of the Therapy Industry. In R. E. Purser, D. Forbes, & A. Burke (Eds.), *Handbook of Mindfulness Culture, Context, and Social Engagement* (pp. 269–292). Cham: Springer.

Montgomery, L. M. (2000). *Anne of Green Gables.* Mineola, NY: Dover Publications.

Moore, K. C. (2002). *The Effectiveness of Solution-Focused Therapy on Students with School-Related Behavioral Problems.* Doctoral Dissertation. Available from ProQuest Information and Learning Company (3110661).

Morgan, R. D., et al. (2012). Treating Offenders With Mental Illness: A Research Synthesis. *Law and Human Behavior, 36*(1), 37–50.

Morrow-Howell, N., Becker-Kemppainen, S., & Judy, L. (1998). Evaluating an Intervention for the Elderly at Increased Risk of Suicide. *Research on Social Work Practice, 8,* 28–46. https://doi.org/10.1177/104973159800800104.

Moxley, D. P., Mowbray, C. T., & Brown, K. S. (1993). Supported Education. In R. Flexer & P. Solomon (Eds.), *Psychiatric Rehabilitation in Practice* (pp. 137–153). New York, NY: Butterworth.

Mufson, L., Dorta, K. P., Wickramaratne, P., Nomura, Y., Olfson, M., & Weissman, M. M. (2004). A Randomized Effectiveness Trial of Interpersonal Psychotherapy for Depressed Adolescents. *Archives of General Psychiatry, 61,* 577–584. https://doi.org/10.1001/archpsyc.61.6.577.

Mufson, L., Weissman, M. M., Moreau, D., & Garfinkel, R. (1999). Efficacy of Interpersonal Psychotherapy for Depressed Adolescents. *Archives of General Psychiatry, 56,* 573–579. http://dx.doi.org/10-1001/pubs. ArchGenPsychiatry-ISSN-0003-990x-56-6-yoa8163.

Murray, L., Cooper, P. J., Wilson, A., & Romaniuk, H. (2003). Controlled Trial of Short- and Long-Term Effect of Psychological Treatment of Post-Partum Depression. *British Journal of Psychiatry, 182,* 420–427.

NASW Center for Workforce Studies. (2010). *2009 Compensation and Benefits Study: Summary of Key Compensation Findings.* Washington, DC: NASW.

Negt, P., Brakemeier, E., Michalak, J., Winter, L., Bleich, S., & Kahl, K. G. (2016). The Treatment of Chronic Depression with Cognitive Behavioral Analysis System of Psychotherapy: A Systematic Review and Meta-Analysis of Randomized-Controlled Clinical Trials. *Brain and Behavior, 6*(8), 1–15. https://doi.org/10.1002/brb3.486.

Neuner, F., Schauer, M., & Klaschik, C. (2004). A Comparison of Narrative Exposure Therapy, Supportive Counseling, and Psychoeducation for Treating Posttraumatic Stress Disorder in an African Refugee Settlement. *Journal of Consulting and Clinical Psychology, 72,* 579–587. https://doi.org/10.1037/0022-006X.72.4.579.

Nelson, G., Kloos, B., & Ornelas, J. (2014). *Community Psychology and Community Mental Health.* New York, NY: Oxford University Press.

Newsome, W. S. (2004). Solution-Focused Brief Therapy Groupwork with At-Risk Junior High School Students: Enhancing the Bottom Line. *Research on Social Work Practice, 14,* 336–343. https://doi.org/10.1177/1049731503262134.

Newsome, W. S. (2005). The Impact of Solution-Focused Brief Therapy with At-Risk Junior High School Students. *Children & Schools, 27,* 83–90. https://doi.org/10.1093/cs/27.2.83.

Norcross, J. C., VandenBos, G. R., & Freedheim, D. K. (Eds.). (2011). *History of Psychotherapy: Continuity and Change* (2nd ed.). Washington, DC, USA: American Psychological Association.

Nugent, W. R. (2017). Variability in the Results of Meta-Analysis as a Function of Comparing Effect Sizes Based on Scores From Noncomparable Measures: A Simulation Study. *Education and Psychological Measurement, 77*(3), 449–470.

O'Connor, A. (2001). *Poverty Knowledge: Social Science, Social Policy, and the Poor in the Twentieth-Century U.S. History.* Princeton, NJ: Princeton University Press.

O'Connor, S. (2001). *Orphan Trains: The Story of Charles Loring Brace and the Children He Saved and Failed.* Boston, MA: Houghton Mifflin.

Office of Technology Assessment (1980). The Implication sof Cost Effectiveness Analysis of Medical Technology. Background Paper #3: The Efficacy and Cost Effectiveness of Psychotherapy. Washington, DC: United States Congress.

Okuyama, T., Akechi, T., Mackenzie, L., & Furukawa, T. A. (2017). Psychotherapy for Depression Among Advanced, Incurable Cancer Patients: A Systematic Review and Meta-Analysis. *Cancer Treatment Reviews, 56,* 16–27. https://doi.org/10.1016/j.ctrv.2017.03.012.

Orford, J. (2008). *Community Psychology: Challenges, Controversies and Emerging Consensus.* West Sussex, UK: Wiley.

Orne, M. T. (1962a). Implications for Psychotherapy Derived from Current Research on the Nature of Hypnosis. *The American Journal of Psychiatry, 118,* 1097–1103.

Orne, M. T. (1962b). On the Social Psychology of the Psychological Experiment: With Particular Reference to Demand Characteristics and Their Implications. *American Psychologist, 17,* 776–783. http://dx.doi.org/10.1037/h0043424.

Oxhandler, H. K., & Pargament, K. I. (2018). Measuring Religious and Spiritual Competence Across Helping Professions: Previous Efforts and Future Directions. *Spirituality in Clinical Practice, 5,* 120–132. https://doi.org/10.1037/scp0000149.

Pacey, L. M. (1950). *Readings in the Development of Settlement Work.* Freeport, NY: Books for Libraries Press.

Painter, K. (2012). Evidence-Based Practices in Community Mental Health: Outcome Evaluation. *Journal of Behavioral Health Services & Research, 39,* 434–444. https://doi.org/10.1007/s11414-012-9284-0.

Palmer, T. (1974). The Youth Authority's Community Treatment Program. *Federal Probation, 38,* 3–14.

Palpacuer, C., Gallet, L., Drapier, D., Reymann, J., Falissard, B., & Naudet, F. (2016). Specific and Non-specific Effects of Psychotherapeutic Interventions for Depression: Results from a Meta-Analysis of 84 Studies. *Journal of Psychiatric Research, 87,* 95–104. https://doi.org/10.1016/j.jpsychires.2016.12.015.

Parker, B., & Turner, W. (2014). Psychoanalytic/Psychodynamic Psychotherapy for Sexually Abused Children and Adolescents: A Systematic Review. *Research on Social Work Practice, 24,* 389–399. https://doi.org/10.1177/1049731514525477.

Parker, I. (2007). *Revolution in Psychology: Alienation to Emancipation.* Ann Arbor, MI: Pluto Press.

Pecora, P. J., Kessler, R. C., O'Brien, K., White, C. R., Williams, J., Hiripi, E., et al. (2006). Educational and Employment Outcomes of Adults Formerly Placed in Foster Care: Results from the Northwest Foster Care Alumni Study. *Children and Youth Services Review, 28,* 1459–1481. https://doi.org/10.1177/030857590703100126.

Penrod, J. D., Luhrs, C. A., Livote, E. E., Cortez, T. B., & Kwak, J. (2011). Implementation and Evaluation of a Network-Based Pilot Program to Improve Palliative Care in the Intensive Care Unit. *Journal of Pain and Symptom Management, 42,* 668–671. https://doi.org/10.1016/j.jpainsymman.2011.06.012.

Peron, J., et al. (2013). Influence of Statistician Involvement on Reporting of Randomized Clinical Trials in Medical Oncology. *Anti-Cancer Drugs, 24*(3), 306–309.

Pistrang, N., Barker, C., & Humphreys, K. (2008). Mutual Help Groups for Mental Health Problems: A Review of Effectiveness Studies. *American Journal of Community Psychology, 42,* 110–121. https://doi.org/10.1007/s10464-008-9181-0.

Prioleau, L., Murdock, M., & Brody, N. (1983). An Analysis of Psychotherapy Versus Placebo Studies. *Behavioral and Brain Sciences, 6,* 275–310.

Pu, J., Zhou, X., Liu, L., Zhang, Y., Yang, L., Yuan, S., et al. (2017). Efficacy and Acceptability of Interpersonal Psychotherapy for Depression in Adolescents: A Meta-Analysis of Randomized Controlled Trials. *Psychiatry Research, 253,* 226–232. https://doi.org/10.1016/j.psychres.2017.03.023.

Quay, H., & Peterson, D. (1975). *Manual for the Behavior Problem Check List.* Champaign: University of Illinois.

Rachman, S. (1970). *The Effects of Psychological Treatment.* Oxford: Paragon Press.

Rapp, R. C., Van Den Noortgate, W., Broekaert, E., & Vanderplasschen, W. (2014). The Efficacy of Case Management with Persons Who Have Substance Abuse Problems: A Three-Level Meta-Analysis of Outcomes. *Journal of Consulting and Clinical Psychology, 82,* 605–618. http://dx.doi.org/10.10.7/a0036750.

Ravetz, J. (1971). *Scientific Knowledge and Its Social Problems.* Oxford: Clarendon Press.

Rawls, J. (1999). *A Theory of Justice.* Cambridge, MA: Harvard University Press.

Rehm, J., et al. (2005). Mortality in Heroin-Assisted Treatment in Switzerland 1994–2000. *Drug and Alcohol Dependence, 79*(2), 137–143.

Reid, W. J., & Hanrahan, P. (1982). Recent Evaluations of Social Work: Grounds for Optimism. *Social Work, 27*(4), 328–340.

Repper, J., & Carter, T. (2011). A Review of the Literature on Peer Support in Mental Health Services. *Journal of Mental Health, 20,* 392–411. https://doi.org/10.3109/09638237.2011.583947.

Resick, P. A., et al. (2008). A Randomized Clinical Trial to Dismantle Components of Cognitive Processing Therapy for Posttraumatic Stress Disorder in Female Victims of Interpersonal Violence. *Journal of Consulting and Clinical Psychology, 76*(2), 243–258.

Resick, P. A., Nishith, P., Weaver, T. L., Astin, M. C., & Feuer, C. A. (2002). A Comparison of Cognitive-Processing Therapy with Prolonged Exposure and a Waiting Condition for the Treatment of Chronic Posttraumatic Stress Disorder in Female Rape Victims. *Journal of Consulting and Clinical Psychology, 70,* 867–879. https://doi.org/10.1037/0022-006X.70.4.867.

Reynolds, C. R., & Shaywitz, S. E. (2009). Response to Intervention: Prevention and Remediation, Perhaps. Diagnosis, No. *Child Development Perspectives, 3,* 44–47. https://doi.org/10.1111/j.1750-8606.2008.00075.x.

Richmond, M. (1917). *Social Diagnosis.* New York: Russell Sage Foundation.

Rieff, P. (1966). *Triumph of the Therapeutic: Uses of Faith After Freud.* New York: Harper and Row.

Roberts, K. C., & Danoff-Burg, S. (2010). Mindfulness and Health Behaviors: Is Paying Attention Good for You. *Journal of American College Health, 59,* 165–173. https://doi.org/10.1080/07448481.2010.484452.

Roberts, N. P., Kitchiner, N. J., Kenardy, J., & Bisson, J. I. (2010). Multiple Session Early Psychological Interventions for the Prevention of Posttraumatic Stress Disorder (Review). *Cochrane Database of Systematic Reviews,* 1–44. http://dx.doi.org/10.1002/14651858.CD006869.pub2.

Roberts, N. P., Kitchiner, N. J., Kenardy, J., & Bisson, J. I. (2012). Early Psychological Interventions to Treat Acute Traumatic Stress Symptoms (Review). *Cochrane Database of Systematic Reviews*, 1–81. http://dx.doi.org/10.1002/14651858.CD007944.pub2.

Roberts, N. P., Roberts, P. A., Jones, N., & Bisson, J. I. (2015). Psychological Interventions for Post-Traumatic Stress Disorder and Comorbid Substance Use Disorder: A Systematic Review and Meta-Analysis. *Clinical Psychology Review, 38,* 25–38. https://doi.org/10.1016/j.cpr.2015.02.007.

Rothbaum, B. O., Astin, M. C., & Marsteller, F. (2005). Prolonged Exposure Versus Eye Movement Desensitization and Reprocessing (EMDR) for PTSD Rape Victims. *Journal of Traumatic Stress, 18,* 607–616. https://doi.org/10.1002/jts.20069.

Rickel, A. U. (1987). The 1965 Swampscott Conference and Future Topics for Community Psychology. *American Journal of Community Psychology, 15,* 511–513. https://doi.org/10.1007/BF00929903.

Rieaud, D. (2004). Long-Term Impacts of the Swiss Heroin Prescription Trials on Crime of Treated Heroin Users. *Journal of Drug Issues, 34,* 163–194. https://doi.org/10.1177/002204260403400108.

Rogers, H., & Maytan, M. (2012). *Mindfulness for the Next Generation.* Oxford, NY: Oxford University Press.

Rosen, A., Proctor, E. K., Staudt, M. M. (1999). Social Work Research and the Quest for Effective Practice. *Social Work Research, 23*(1), 4–14.

Rosenthal, R., & Rubin, D. B. (1978). Interpersonal Expectancy Effects—The First 345 Studies. *Behavioral and Brain Sciences, 1,* 377–386. https://doi.org/10.1017/S0140525X00075506.

Rosenzweig, S., Reibel, D. K., Greeson, J. M., Brainard, G. C., & Hojat, M. (2003). Mindfulness-Based Stress Reduction Lowers Psychological Distress in Medical Students. *Teaching and Learning in Medicine, 15,* 88–92. https://doi.org/10.1207/S15328015TLM1502_03.

Rothman, D. J. (1971). *The Discovery of the Asylum: Social Order and Disorder in the New Republic.* Boston and Toronto, Canada: Little, Brown.

Rubin, A., & Yu, M. (2017). Within-Group Effect-Size Benchmarks for Problem-Solving Therapy for Depression in Adults. *Research on Social Work Practice, 27,* 552–560. https://doi.org/10.1177/1049731515592477.

Rush, A. J., Trivedi, M. H., Wisniewski, S. R., Stewart, J. W., Nierenberg, A. A., Thase, M. E., et al. (2006). Bupropion-SR, Sertraline, or Venlafaxine-XR After Failure of SSRIs for Depression. *The New England Journal of Medicine, 354,* 1231–1242. https://doi.org/10.1056/NEJMoa052963.

Rushton, J. P. (1999). *Race, Evolution and Behavior*. New Brunswick, NJ: Transaction Publishers.

Saleebey, D. (1996). The Strengths Perspective in *Social Work* Practice: Extensions and Cautions. *Social Work, 41,* 296–305. http://dx.doi.org/ezproxy.library.unlv.edu/10.1093/sw/41.3.296.

Sarnoff, S. K. (2001). *Sanctified Snake Oil: The Effect of Junk Science on Public Policy*. Westport, CT: Praeger.

Scannapieco, M., Connell-Carrick, K., & Painter, K. (2007). In Their Own Words: Challenges Facing Youth Aging Out of Foster Care. *Child and Adolescent Social Work Journal, 24,* 423–435. https://doi.org/10.1007/s10560-007-0093-x.

Schuerman, J. R., Rzepnicki, T. L., & Littell, J. H. (1994). *Putting Families First: An Experiment in Family Preservation*. New York: Aldine de Gruyter.

Schumer, M. C., Lindsay, E. K., & Creswell, J. D. (2018). Brief Mindfulness Training for Negative Affectivity: A Systematic Review and Meta-Analysis. *Journal of Consulting and Clinical Psychology, 86,* 569–583. https://doi.org/10.1037/ccp0000324.

Scott, J., & Young, A. H. (2016). Psychotherapies Should Be Assessed for Both Benefit and Harm. *British Journal of Psychiatry, 208*(3), 208–209.

Segal, S. P. (1972). Research on Outcome of Social Work Therapeutic Interventions—Review of Literature. *Journal of Health and Social Behavior, 13*(1), 3–17.

Shapiro, F. (1989a). Efficacy of the Eye Movement Desensitization Procedure in the Treatment of Traumatic Memories. *Journal of Traumatic Stress, 2,* 199–223.

Shapiro, F. (1989b). Eye Movement Desensitization: A New Treatment for Post-Traumatic Stress Disorder. *Journal of Behavioral Therapy and Experimental Psychiatry, 20,* 211–217.

Shapiro, S. L., Schwartz, G. E., & Bonner, G. (1998). Effects of Mindfulness-Based Stress Reduction on Medical and Premedical Students. *Journal of Behavioral Medicine, 21,* 581–599. https://doi.org/10.1023/A:1018700829825.

Sheldon, B. (1986). Social Work Effectiveness Experiments—Review and Implications. *British Journal of Social Work, 16*(2), 223–242.

Shepperd, S., Doll, H., Gowers, S., James, A., Fazel, M., Fitzpatrick, R., & Pollock, J. (2009). Alternatives to Inpatient Mental Health Care for Children and Young People (Review). *Cochrane Database of Systematic Reviews,* 1–58. http://dx.doi.org/10.1002/14651858.CD006410.pub2.

Shin, S. (2009). Effects of a Solution-Focused Program on the Reduction of Aggressiveness and the Improvement of Social Readjustment for Korean Probationers. *Journal of Social Service Research, 35,* 274–284. https://doi.org/10.1080/01488370902901079.

Shurkin, J. N. (2006). *Broken Genius: The Rise and Fall of William Shockley, Creator of the Electronic Age.* New York: Palgrave Macmillan.

Singh, J. P., Grann, M., & Fazel, S. (2013). Authorship Bias in Violence Risk Assessment? A Systematic Review and Meta-Analysis. *PLoS One, 8.* http://dx.doi.org/10.1371/journal.pone.0072484.

Singh, S., & Ernst, E. (2008). *Trick or Treatment: The Undeniable Facts About Alternative Medicine.* New York, NY: Norton.

Sinniah, A., Oei, T., Maniam, T., & Subramaniam, P. (2017). Positive Effects of Individual Cognitive Behavioral Therapy for Patients with Unipolar Mood Disorders with Suicidal Ideation in Malaysia: A Randomised Controlled Trial. *Psychiatry Research, 254,* 179–189. https://doi.org/10.1016/j.psychres.2017.04.026.

Smail, D. (1993). *The Origins of Unhappiness: A New Understanding of Personal Distress.* London: HarperCollins.

Smail, D. (2005). *Power, Interest and Psychology.* London: PCCS Books.

Smit, A., Kluiter, H., Conradi, H. J., Van der Meer, K., Tiemens, B. G., Jenner, J. A., et al. (2006). Short-Term Effects of Enhanced Treatment for Depression in Primary Care: Results from a Randomized Controlled Trial. *Psychological Medicine, 36,* 15–26. https://doi.org/10.1017/S0033291705006318.

Smith, A. (2019 [1776]). *An Inquiry into the Nature and Causes of the Wealth of Nations.* Amazon Digital Services.

Smith, M. L., Glass, G. V., & Miller, T. I. (1980). *The Benefits of Psychotherapy.* Baltimore, MD: Johns Hopkins University Press.

Smith, T. E., Hull, J. W., MacKain, S. J., Wallace, C. J., Rattenni, L. A., Goodman, M., et al. (1996). Training Hospitalized Patients with Schizophrenia in Community Reintegration Skills. *Psychiatric Services, 47,* 1099–1103. https://doi.org/10.1176/ps.47.10.1099.

Specht, H., & Courtney, M. (1994). *Unfaithful Angels: How Social Work Has Abandoned Its Mission.* New York, NY: The Free Press.

Springer, D. W., Lynch, C., & Rubin, A. (2000). Effects of a Solution-Focused Mutual Aid Group for Hispanic Children of Incarcerated Parents. *Human Sciences Press, 17,* 431–442. https://doi.org/10.1023/A:1026479727159.

Stahler, G. J., & Tash, W. R. (1982). *Innovative Approaches to Mental Health Evaluation* (1st ed.). New York, NY: Academic Press.

Stanton, M., & Shadish, W. R. (1997). Outcome, Attrition, and Family-Couples Treatment for Drug Abuse: A Meta-Analysis and Review of the Controlled, Comparative Studies. *Psychological Bulletin, 122,* 170–191. https://doi.org/10.1037/0033-2909.122.2.170.

Staudt, M., & Drake, B. (2002). Intensive Family Preservation Services: Where's the Crisis? *Children and Youth Services Review, 24,* 777–795. https://doi.org/10.1016/S0190-7409(02)00228-1.

Stein, L. I., & Test, M. A. (1975). *Conference on Alternatives to Mental Hospital Treatment.* New York, NY: Plenum Press.

Stein, L. I., & Test, M. A. (1980a). Alternative to Mental Hospital Treatment. I. Conceptual Model, Treatment Program, and Clinical Evaluation. *Archives of General Psychiatry, 37,* 409–412.

Stein, L. I., & Test, M. A. (1980b). Alternative to Mental Hospital Treatment. III. Social Cost. *Archives of General Psychiatry, 37,* 409–412.

Stewart, L. A., et al. (2017). The Impact of a Community Mental Health Initiative on Outcomes for Offenders with a Serious Mental Disorder. *Criminal Behavior and Mental Health, 27*(4), 371–384.

Stoesz, D., Karger, H. J., & Carrilio, T. (2010). *A Dream Deferred: How Social Work Education Lost Its Way and What Can Be Done.* New Brunswick, NJ: Aldine Transaction.

Stokey Kelly, M., Cosner Berzin, S., Frey, A., Alvarez, M., Shaffer, G., & O'Brien, K. (2010). The State of School Social Work: Findings from the National School Social Work Survey. *School Mental Health, 2,* 132–141. https://doi.org/10.1007/s12310-010-9034-5.

Strupp, H. H., & Hadley, S. W. (1979). Specific vs. Nonspecific Factors in Psychotherapy: A Controlled Study of Outcome. *Archives of General Psychiatry, 36,* 1125–1136. http://dx.doi.org/10.1001/archpsyc.1979.01780100095009.

Stuart, R. B. (1973). *Trick or Treatment.* Champaign, IL: Research Press.

Subramaniam, G. A., Warden, D., Minhajuddin, A., Fishman, M. J., Stitzer, M. L., Adinoff, B., et al. (2011, November). Predictors of Abstinence: National Institute of Drug Abuse Multisite Buprenorphine/Naloxone Treatment Trial in Opioid-Dependent Youth. *Journal of the American Academy of Child and Adolescent Psychiatry, 11,* 1120–1128. Retrieved from http://www.clinicaltrials.gov.

Sugarman, M. A. (2016). Are Antidepressants and Psychotherapy Equally Effective in Treating Depression? *A Critical Commentary Journal of Mental Health, 25*(6), 475–478.

Surles, R., Blanch, A., Shern, D., & Donahue, S. (1992). Case Management Strategy for Systems Change. *Health Affairs, 11,* 151–163.

Swan, S., Keen, N., Reynolds, N., & Onwumere, J. (2017). Psychological Interventions for Post-Traumatic Stress Symptoms in Psychosis: A Systematic Review of Outcomes. *Frontiers in Psychology, 8,* 1–14.

Swenson, C. R. (1995). Clinical Social Work. In R. L. Edwards (Ed. in Chief), *Encyclopedia of Social Work* (19th ed., pp. 502–513). Washington, DC: NASW Press.

Swigert, V. L., & Farrell, R. A. (1977). Normal Homicides and the Law. *American Sociological Review, 42,* 16–32.

Szasz, T. (1974). *Myth of Mental Illness: Foundations of a Theory of Personal Conduct.* New York: Harper and Row.

Tao, K. W., Owen, J., Pace, B. T., & Imel, Z. E. (2015). A Meta-Analysis of Multicultural Competencies and Psychotherapy Process and Outcome. *Journal of Counseling Psychology, 62,* 337–350. https://doi.org/10.1037/cou0000086.

Thomas, C., & Corcoran, J. (2001). Empirically Based Marital and Family Interventions for Alcohol Abuse: A Review. *Research on Social Work Practice, 11,* 549–575. https://doi.org/10.1177/104973150101100502.

Thomlison, R. J. (1984). Something Works—Evidence from Practice Effectiveness Studies. *Social Work, 29*(1), 51–56.

Thompson, A. E., & Greeson, J. K. (2017). Prosocial Activities and Natural Mentoring Among Youth at Risk of Aging Out of Foster Care. *Journal of the Society for Social Work and Research, 8,* 421–440. https://doi.org/10.1086/693119.

Throop, E. A. (2009). *Psychotherapy, American Culture, and Social Policy: Immoral Individualism.* New York: Palgrave Macmillan.

Thyer, B. A. (2015). A Bibliography of Randomized Controlled Experiments in Social Work (1949–2013): Solvitur Ambulando. *Research on Social Work Practice, 25,* 753–793. https://doi.org/10.1177/1049731515599174.

Timpe, Z. C., & Lunkenheimer, E. (2015). The Long-Term Economic Benefits of Natural Mentoring Relationships for Youth. *American Journal of Community Psychology, 56,* 12–24. https://doi.org/10.1007/s10464-015-9735-x.

Tosone, C. (2016). Clinical Social Work Education, Mental Health, and the DSM-5. *Social Work in Mental Health, 14,* 103–111. https://doi.org/10.1080/15332985.2015.1083513.

Townley, G., Brown, M., & Sylvestre, J. (2018). Community Psychology and Community Mental Health: A Call for Reengagement. *American Journal of Community Psychology, 61,* 3–9. https://doi.org/10.1002/ajcp.12225.

Towvim, L., et al. (2012). *Positive Behavioral Interventions and Supports.* National Center for Mental Health Promotion and Youth Violence Prevention. http://www.promoteprevent.org/sites/www.promoteprevent.org/files/resources/positive_behavioral_interventions_snapshots.pdf.

Trattner, W. I. (1999). *From Poor Law to Welfare State: A History of Social Welfare in America* (6th ed.). New York, NY: The Free Press.

Travis, F., & Arenander, A. (2004). EEG Asymmetry and Mindfulness Meditation. *Psychosomatic Medicine, 66,* 147–152.

Trolander, J. A. (1975). *Settlement House and the Great Depression.* Detroit, MI: Wayne State University Press.

Turner, D. T., McGlanaghy, E., Cuijpers, P., Van der Gaag, M., Karyotaki, E., & MacBeth, A. (2018). A Meta-Analysis of Social Skills Training and Related Interventions for Psychosis. *Schizophrenia Bulletin, 44,* 475–491. https://doi.org/10.1093/schbul/sbx146.

Tusek, D. L., Church, J. M., Strong, S. A., Grass, J. A., & Fazio, V. W. (1996). A Significant Advance in the Care of Patients Undergoing Elective Colorectal Surgery. *Diseases of the Colon & Rectum, 40,* 172–178. https://doi.org/10.1007/BF02054983.

Uchtenhagen, A., Dobler-Mikola, A., Steffen, T., Gutzwiller, F., Blattler, R., & Pfeifer, S. (1999). *Prescription of Narcotics for Heroin Addicts: Main Results of the Swiss National Cohort Study.* New York, NY: Karger.

U.S. Department of Housing and Urban Development. (2017). *HUD 2017 Continuum of Care Homeless Assistance Programs Homeless Populations and Subpopulation.* Retrieved from https://www.hudexchange.info/resource/reportmanagement/published/CoC_PopSub_NatlTerrDC_2017.pdf.

Van Dam, D., Vedel, E., Ehring, T., & Emmelkamp, P. M. (2012). Psychological Treatments for Concurrent Posttraumatic Stress Disorder and Substance Use Disorder: A Systematic Review. *Clinical Psychology Review, 32,* 202–214. https://doi.org/10.1016/j.cpr.2012.01.004.

Van der Kolk, B. A. (2007). A Randomized Clinical Trial of Eye Movement Desensitization and Reprocessing (EMDR), Fluoxetine, and Pill Placebo in the Treatment of Posttraumatic Stress Disorder: Treatment Effects and Long-Term Maintenance. *Journal of Clinical Psychiatry, 68*(1), 37–46.

Van der Kolk, B. (2015). *The Body Keeps the Score: Brain, Mind, and Body in the Healing of Trauma.* New York, NY: Penguin Books.

Vandivere, S., Malm, K. E., Allen, T. J., Williams, S., & McKlindon, A. (2017). A Randomized Controlled Trial of Family Finding: A Relative Search and Engagement Intervention for Youth Lingering in Foster Care. *Evaluation Review, 41,* 542–567. https://doi.org/10.1177/0193841X17689971.

Van Emmerik, A. A., Kamphuis, J. H., & Emmelkamp, P. M. (2008). Treating Acute Stress Disorder and Posttraumatic Stress Disorder with Cognitive Behavior Therapy or Structured Writing Therapy: A Randomized Controlled Trial. *Psychotherapy and Psychosomatics, 77,* 93–100. https://doi.org/10.1159/000112886.

Verduyn, C., et al. (2003). Maternal Depression and Child Behaviour Problems: Randomised Placebo-Controlled Trial of a Cognitive-Behavioural Group Intervention. *British Journal of Psychiatry, 183,* 342–348.

Violeta, E., & Dafinoiu, I. (2009). Motivational/Solution-Focused Intervention for Reducing School Truancy Among Adolescents. *Journal of Cognitive & Behavioral Psychotherapies, 9,* 185–198.

Visser, E., et al. (2015). The Course, Prediction, and Treatment of Acute and Posttraumatic Stress in Trauma Patients: A Systematic Review. *Journal of Trauma and Acute Care Surgery, 82*(6), 1158–1183.

Visser, E., Gosens, T., Leontine Den Oudsten, B., & De Vries, J. (2017). The Course, Prediction, and Treatment of Acute and Posttraumatic Stress in Trauma Patients: A Systematic Review. *Journal of Trauma and Acute Care Surgery, 82,* 1158–1183. https://doi.org/10.1097/TA.0000000000001447.

Wakefield, J. C. (1988a, June). Psychotherapy, Distributive Justice, and Social Work. Part 1: Distributive Justice as a Conceptual Framework for Social Work. *Social Service Review, 62,* 187–210.

Wakefield, J. C. (1988b). Psychotherapy, Distributive Justice, and Social Work Part 2: Psychotherapy and the Pursuit of Justice. *Social Service Review, 62*(3), 353–382.

Waldron, H. B., & Turner, C. W. (2008). Evidence-Based Psychosocial Treatments for Adolescent Substance Abuse. *Journal of Clinical Child & Adolescent Psychology, 37,* 238–261. https://doi.org/10.1080/15374410701820133.

Wallerstein, R. S. (1995). *The Talking Cures: The Psychoanalyses and the Psychotherapies.* New Haven: Yale University Press.

Warren, A. (1996). *Orphan Train Rider: One Boy's True Story.* Boston, MA: Houghton Mifflin.

Weisbrod, B. A., Test, M. A., & Stein, L. I. (1980). Alternative to Mental Hospital Treatment: II. Economic Benefit-Cost Analysis. *Archives of General Psychiatry,* 400–405. http://dx.doi.org/10.1001/archpsyc.1980.01780170042004.

Weisburd, D., et al. (2017). What Works in Crime Prevention and Rehabilitation. *Ciminology and Public Policy, 16*(2), 415–449.

Weisz, J. R., McCarty, C. A., & Valeri, S. M. (2006). Effects of Psychotherapy for Depression in Children and Adolescents: A Meta-Analysis. *Psychological Bulletin, 132*, 132–149. https://doi.org/10.1037/0033-2909.132.1.132.

Wells, K., & Biegel, D. E. (1991). *Family Preservation Services: Research and Evaluation*. Newbury Park, CA: Sage.

Whitehead, J. T., & Lab, S. P. (1989). A Meta-Analysis of Juvenile Correctional Treatment. *Journal of Research in Crime and Delinquency, 26*, 276–295. https://doi.org/10.1177/0022427889026003005.

Wilensky, H. L., & Lebeaux, C. N. (1965). *Industry Society and Social Welfare*. New York, NY: The Free Press.

Williams, J. W., Barrett, J., Oxman, T., Frank, E., Katon, W., Sullivan, M., et al. (2000). Treatment of Dysthymia and Minor Depression in Primary Care: A Randomized Controlled Trial in Older Adults. *Journal of the American Medical Association, 27*, 1519–1526. https://doi.org/10.1001/jama.284.12.1519.

Wilson, H. A. (2014). Can Antisocial Personality Disorder Be Treated? A Meta-Analysis Examining the Effectiveness of Treatment in Reducing Recidivism for Individuals Diagnosed with ASPD. *International Journal of Forensic Mental Health, 13*, 36–46. https://doi.org/10.1080/14999013.2014.890682.

Wolf, D. B., & Abell, N. (2003). Examining the Effects of Meditation Techniques on Psychosocial Functioning. *Research on Social Work Practice, 13*, 27–42. https://doi.org/10.1177/104973102237471.

Wood, K. M. (1978). Casework Effectiveness: New Look at Research Evidence. *Social Work, 23*(6), 437–458.

Woodroofe, K. (1971 [1962]). *From Charity to Social Work in England and the United States*. Toronto: University of Toronto Press.

Woods, R. A., & Kennedy, A. J. (1990). *The Settlement Horizon*. New Brunswick, NJ: Transaction Publishers.

Wootton, B. (1959). *Social Science and Social Pathology*. London: George Allen and Unwin.

Yang, L., Zhou, X., Zhou, C., Zhang, Y., Pu, J., Liu, L., et al. (2017). Efficacy and Acceptability of Cognitive Behavioral Therapy for Depression in Children: A Systematic Review and Meta-Analysis. *Academic Pediatrics, 17*, 9–16. https://doi.org/10.1016/j.acap.2016.08.002.

Yau, E. F., Chan, C. C., Chan, A. S., & Chui, B. K. (2005). Changes in Psychosocial and Work-Related Characteristics Among Clubhouse Members: A Preliminary Report. *Work, 25*, 287–296. Retrieved from http://content.iospress.com/articles/work/wor00466.

Yeh, S. S. (2013). A Re-analysis of the Effects of KIPP and the Harlem Promise Academies. *Teachers College Record, 115.*

Yoon, S., et al. (2015). Effective Treatments of Late-Life Depression in Long-Term Care Facilities: A Systematic Review. *Research on Social Work Practice, 28*(2), 116–130.

Yoon, S., Moon, S., & Pitner, R. (2018). Effective Treatments of Late-Life Depression in Long-Term Care Facilities: A Systematic Review. *Research on Social Work Practice, 28,* 116–130. https://doi.org/10.1177/1049731515621165.

Zilbergeld, B. (1983). *The Shrinking of America: Myths of Psychological Change.* Boston: Little Brown.

Zatzick, D., Roy-Byrne, P., Russo, J., Rivara, F., Droesch, R., Wagner, A., et al. (2004). A Randomized Effectiveness Trial of Stepped Collaborative Care for Acutely Injured Trauma Survivors. *Archives of General Psychiatry, 61,* 498–506.

Index